DATE DUE

OC 27 00			
JY 26 01			
DE 19 01			
JE 2 05			

DEMCO 38-296

The Empty Cradle

The Henry E. Sigerist Series in the History of Medicine

Sponsored by the American Association for the History of Medicine and the Johns Hopkins University Press

The Development of American Physiology: Scientific Medicine in the Nineteenth Century

W. Bruce Fye

Save the Babies: American Public Health Reform and the Prevention of Infant Mortality, 1850–1929

Richard A. Meckel

Politics and Public Health in Revolutionary Russia, 1890–1918

John F. Hutchinson

Rocky Mountain Spotted Fever: History of a Twentieth-Century Disease

Victoria A. Harden

Quinine's Predecessor: Francesco Torti and the Early History of Cinchona

Saul Jarcho

The Citizen-Patient in Revolutionary and Imperial Paris

Dora B. Weiner

Subjected to Science: Human Experimentation in America before the Second World War

Susan E. Lederer

The Empty Cradle: Infertility in America from Colonial Times to the Present

Margaret Marsh and Wanda Ronner

R

THE
Empty Cradle

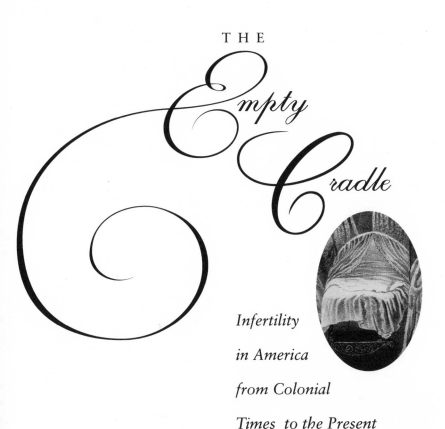

Infertility

in America

from Colonial

Times to the Present

Margaret Marsh

and

Wanda Ronner

The Johns Hopkins University Press

Baltimore & London

This book has been brought to publication with the generous assistance of the American Association for the History of Medicine.

Printed in the United States of America on acid-free paper

05 04 03 02 01 00 99 98 97 96   5 4 3 2 1

The Johns Hopkins University Press
2715 North Charles Street
Baltimore, Maryland 21218-4319
The Johns Hopkins Press Ltd., London

ISBN 0-8018-5228-5

Library of Congress Cataloging-in-Publication Data will be found at the end of this book.
A catalog record for this book is available from the British Library.

In Memory of Nana

Contents

Preface and Acknowledgments

This book is a collaboration between sisters, one of us a historian and the other a gynecologist. Close since childhood, we have always included each other in our interests, so it was natural, when we came to have careers, that we would care about what the other was doing. Margaret, the historian, has gone on hospital rounds and been present in the operating room. For the latter event Wanda, not trusting Margaret's declaration that she could stand the sight of blood, had a nurse stand by with smelling salts. Wanda, the physician, has been to history conferences and lectures. She claims not to have felt faint on those occasions, too. For several years, we talked casually about writing a book together. In the summer of 1987, more than a year after Margaret decided against undergoing in vitro fertilization for her infertility problem, which had resulted from endometriosis, and more than three years before Wanda's infertility problem would be successfully treated, we began to think seriously about tackling the history of infertility.

It was not our own situations that gave us the initial idea, however. In June of that year, at the Berkshire Conference on Women's History, Margaret was introduced to medical historian Janet Golden. When told of the interest we had in a collaborative project, Janet replied that no one had yet written a history of infertility and that, given our fields, it seemed like a perfect project for us. Margaret at that time was writing *Suburban Lives,* a book on the transformation of middle-class family life in American suburbs from the mid–nineteenth to the mid–twentieth century. Gender roles within the household and community, and the significance of children within the family, were very much on her mind. Wanda was just beginning her final year of residency in obstetrics and gynecology. Our more personal experiences undoubtedly figured in our decision, as well.

Within a few months, we had applied for and received an ACOG-ORTHO Fellowship in the History of American Obstetrics and Gynecology from the American College of Obstetricians and Gynecologists. We then set out to see if two sisters, trained intellectually in very dissimilar ways, could collaborate harmoniously. As was perhaps inevitable when collaborators come from different intellectual traditions, we did not approach the subject in the same way. Wanda stressed the importance of gathering data that could be analyzed empirically. Margaret, who as a graduate student in the 1970s was a devotee of quantitative methods, had long since lapsed into cultural history. Wanda was cautious about generalizing; Margaret constantly looked for the larger implications in documents and stories. Wanda expressed a belief in the significance of medical progress; Margaret was reluctant even to use the words together. But in spite of our very different approaches—or perhaps because of them—our initial collaboration, a paper on nineteenth-century surgical and instrumental treatments for infertility (or sterility, as it was then called), which we presented at the 1989 meeting of the American College of Obstetricians and Gynecologists, demonstrated that we could work well together. The following year we began this book.

Perhaps surprisingly, given where we started, over the course of our research Wanda became particularly interested in the experiences of the patients, and Margaret found the scientific history fascinating in its own right. As collaborators, what we have tried to do is write a book that would reflect our two perspectives and the perspectives of two disciplines while being united by our commonly held intellectual values. *The Empty Cradle* is a history both of the ways in which Americans have experienced infertility and of the ways in which medical practitioners have diagnosed and treated it. We—one of us a historian of women and the other a medical practitioner whose work is devoted to issues of women's health—have been especially concerned to understand the nature of the relationships between women, who have historically borne and continue to bear a disproportionate burden when a couple has an infertility problem, and those practitioners who attempt to alleviate the condition.

We accumulated a large number of intellectual debts during the years in which we worked on this book. We are very grateful to the institutions that supported our work financially, and to our colleagues and friends who offered advice and assistance and kept us supplied with news clippings. The book was supported by a multiyear grant (RH-20937-90) from the National Endowment for the Humanities. We would like to express our gratitude to the Endowment and especially to Elizabeth Arndt and Daniel Jones. The administrators at Stockton State College, Margaret's employer for the first year of the grant, agreed to administer the grant for the entire four-year period. We would like to thank President Vera King Farris, Vice-President Charles Tantillo, Vice-President Russell Nazzaro, and Dean Robert Regan, as well as grants administrators Anna Mae Bensel, Linda McNeil, and Beth Olsen. Temple University, where Margaret currently works, provided released time and a semester's study leave, for which we thank her former department chair, James Hilty, Dean Carolyn Adams, and Provost James England. Thanks are also due to Beverly Vaughn, with whom Wanda practices obstetrics and gynecology at Pennsylvania Hospital in Philadelphia, for acceding to Wanda's three-month absence for her initial stint of historical research, to Keith Owens for covering her practice during that time, and to Ruth Friel, Wanda's secretary, for her constant support. At the American College of Obstetricians and Gynecologists, where we spent a month as History Fellows, we are grateful to then-Executive Director Dr. Warren Pearse; Pamela Van Hine and Kathie DeGeorges of the Resource Center; and former history librarian Gay Takakoshi and her successor, Susan Rishworth. ORTHO Pharmaceutical Corporation funded the fellowship. ACOG also granted us permission to reprint material on the process of conception in the Appendix. The illustration for that Appendix is the work of Robert Colleluori and has been drawn specifically for *The Empty Cradle*.

Archivists and librarians at a number of institutions kindly and patiently assisted us with their expertise. At the Rare Books and Manuscripts Division of the Countway Library of Medicine, Harvard University, we are grateful to Richard Wolfe and his staff for their help, and to the library for permission to quote from the papers of John Rock and to reproduce photographs from the collection. At the College of Physicians of Philadelphia, Thomas Horrocks, Tracy Byrd, and Jean Carr were unfailingly helpful; and we are especially grateful to Kevin Crawford, who researched illustrations for us and arranged to have them reproduced. We would also like to thank the archivists and librarians at the History of Medicine Division of the National Library of Medicine, particularly John Parascandola; the Library of Congress, especially Jane Van Nimmen of the Prints and Photographs Division; the Bolling Medical Library at St. Luke's–Roosevelt Hospital Center, especially Nancy Panella and Joan Carvajal; the Rockefeller Archive Center, which also granted us permission to quote from the Bureau of Social Hygiene Archives; and Stanford University Library.

Without our excellent research assistants—Julie Berebitsky, Sally Dwyer-McNulty, and Susan Morse—we would still be in the archives. Julie was with us from the beginning, and we benefited not only from her finely honed research skills and her ability to ask just the right questions but also from her expertise on the history of adoption, the subject of her forthcoming dissertation. Susan tracked down articles on infertility in the popular press for us; Sally, whose own field of expertise is in Catholicism and the family, joined Margaret and Julie in researching the uncatalogued papers of John Rock and enhanced her store of medical knowledge at the Philadelphia College of Physicians. Julie and Sally also read and commented on an early draft of the manuscript as a whole.

Thanks are also due to Margaret's friends Michael and Darryl Ebner, and to former Temple University student Gail Schachter, who sent us relevant contemporary articles. Also, the family life columnist of the *Philadelphia Inquirer*, Lucia Herndon, discussed this book in her column and alerted her readers to our desire to hear from those who had experienced infertility problems from World War II through 1980. Our thanks are owed to her and especially to the women who took the time to answer our questions and tell us about their own experiences.

As newcomers to the history of medicine, we owe a special debt of gratitude to all those experienced scholars in the field who enlarged our bibiliography, offered counsel, listened to the papers that we presented at various meetings, or read parts or all of this manuscript, as did a number of Margaret's colleagues outside the history of medicine. Over the past five years we have discussed this work, separately and together, at the University of California, Health Sciences Campus, San Francisco; the College of Physicians of Philadelphia; the Hagley Institute; Lake Forest College; Rutgers University, Camden; and the University of Utah. We benefited from the comments and questions that our hearers raised. In particular, we would like to thank Barbara Kimmelman, William C. Lubenow, Colleen McDannell, James Mohr, Regina Morantz-Sanchez, Jack Pressman, Guenter Risse, and Nancy Tomes. Elaine Tyler May, engaged herself in research on the history of childlessness at the same time that we were working on this book, was a model of scholarly generosity. At the Johns Hopkins University Press, our editor, Jacqueline Wehmueller, provided us with advice and encouragement in just the right doses, and manuscript editor Carol Ehrlich made the final stages of writing this book run smoothly. Finally, there are two people who, no matter how energetically we thank them, would not be getting thanks enough. Janet Golden read and commented incisively on the penultimate draft of most of this manuscript. Howard F. Gillette put aside his own work on numerous occasions, sometimes at considerable sacrifice, to critique and provide editorial expertise for each chapter as it moved from "almost there" to final draft. If, in spite of all the good advice we received, errors remain, they are our fault.

We are also grateful for the emotional support provided by our friends, family, and loved ones. In addition to Howard Gillette, who appears above in his role as fellow scholar, we want to thank Wanda's husband, Peter Ronner, for everything he does, and our cousin Kathleen Sammartino. Margaret would also like to thank her colleagues in the Temple University Department of History, especially Allen Davis, Barbara Day, Herbert Ershkowitz, Harriet Freidenreich, Richard Immerman, Mark Haller, David Rosenberg, and Morris Vogel. Lukas Ronner was born during his mother's initiation into historical research after having spent much of his prenatal existence in the History Library at the College of Physicians of Philadelphia.

This book is dedicated to the memory of our grandmother, who was born in a small village in Italy and came to the United States as a young girl of sixteen. Nana, as we called her, had seven children and numerous grandchildren and great-grandchildren. An important presence in our lives, she passed on to us, we like to think, her perseverance and her ability to look at things from other people's points of view.

The Empty Cradle

Introduction

A quarter of a century ago, about 600,000 Americans a year visited a physician to discuss an infertility problem. By the early 1990s, that number had increased to 1.5 million, and more than a million couples a year were undergoing treatment because they had difficulty conceiving a child. One might imagine that such figures represent a dramatic rise in the incidence of infertility in the United States. Many clinicians and journalists seem to think that this country is witnessing an "epidemic" of infertility, and most contemporary analysts ascribe the upsurge in demand for treatment to a combination of an actual increase in the incidence of infertility with the development of new reproductive technologies. On the contrary, whether one counts numbers or percentages, the overall incidence of infertility has *decreased* since the mid-1960s. In 1965, when the first national fertility survey took place, some three million married women, or approximately 11 percent of married couples, claimed to have experienced an infertility problem. Some twenty years later, those figures stood at 2.5 million married women, or approximately 8 per cent of married couples. In fact, if statistics culled from a variety of sources can be believed, infertility rates have remained surprisingly consistent for more than a century, ranging from just under 10 to about 13 percent of the total number of married couples.[1]

The mistaken idea that current infertility rates reflect a fundamentally new phenomenon in American society, and the equally erroneous but commonly held belief that white middle-class couples predominate among the infertile, not only provide a distorted image of the present but also obscure the relationships between contemporary ways of coping with infertility and those of past generations. This book explores those relationships, examining the ways in which the inability to conceive a child has been experienced by individuals, perceived by society, and treated by medical practitioners since the colonial era. By putting into perspective the extraordinary interest that exists today in the problem of infertility in the United States, *The Empty Cradle* seeks to understand its historical significance as a medical and cultural phenomenon.

In the seventeenth century, when this narrative begins, very few colonists would have considered seeking medical advice; indeed, the very idea of attempting to alleviate infertility could be viewed as defiance of the will of the Lord. By the late nineteenth century, however, physicians by the score were performing surgery to restore fertility and one prominent surgeon had devised a procedure he called "ovarian transplantation," which involved transferring portions of the ovaries of fertile women into women whose own ovaries had been lost to disease. In the late twentieth century, in vitro fertilization and related reproductive technologies have both raised the hopes of many infertile couples and caused considerable controversy within the larger society over their moral and ethical implications.

Americans having difficulty conceiving a child may not have abandoned the Lord completely over the course of these three hundred years or so, but they have increasingly turned their infertility problems over to physicians. As they did so, the inability to procreate became converted from a social state into a medical condition. This process of "medicalization"—which had some roots in the late eighteenth century, began in earnest just before the Civil War, and may have reached its apogee with the arrival of technologically assisted reproduction—brought about the shift from an emphasis on coping with childlessness through social means, such as participating in the rearing of others' children, to dependence on medical intervention. This transformation, although never absolute or uncontested, dominates the history of infertility from the late nineteenth century onward.

But if infertility has become a "disease," as physicians and infertile couples alike have increasingly come to define it, like other diseases it exists neither in a medical vacuum nor in some ahistorical space but is always experienced within a social and temporal context. Embedded in the larger cultural transformations that have altered the ways in which Americans have defined the meaning of family life—in terms of expectations about appropriate family size, the proper roles of wives and husbands, the nature of the relationship between parents and children, and the connections between families and the larger community—the experience of infertility, and its treatment, have reflected changing values and social norms.

To say that infertility is culturally conditioned, however, is to deny neither its underlying physiological causes nor the importance of advances in scientific knowledge about the ways to alleviate it. New discoveries that illuminated the ways in which the human reproductive system operates— for instance, the discovery of the hormones, which led to the development of endocrinology—ultimately led to dramatic therapeutic advances for specific reproductive dysfunctions. The ability to fertilize human ova outside the human body, first reported in 1944 when Harvard physician John Rock and his assistant Miriam Menkin announced that they had fertilized four human eggs in vitro, brought to the fore the possibility of severing reproduction from sexuality. The significance of such discoveries notwithstanding, however, there appears to be little if any direct relationship between advances in reproductive science and an increase in demand for infertility services.

Changes in the culture, rather than scientific advances or greater technological expertise, have been and still are the forces most likely to bring a rush of infertile patients to clinicians' offices. Perhaps the most striking example of this phenomenon is the dramatic growth of infertility treatment that took place in the 1950s. In post–World War II America, existing infertility centers expanded and new ones multiplied, the result both of widely shared pronatalist sentiment and of a nearly unquestioning public faith in the power of science and technology. However, although advances in the field of endocrinology enriched clinicians' understanding of the reproductive processes, especially on the critical question of what went wrong when women failed to ovulate, no effective therapies for that condition existed. In fact, physicians could do little more in 1955 in terms of treatment than they could in 1940, yet their clinics and offices were jammed. Practitioners, patients, and the public all believed that the bulging clinics were a direct result of medicine's progress in treating infertility.

It is no surprise that physicians would maintain that increasing demand for infertility treatment was a natural result of new medical discoveries. Such claims have permeated the medical literature since the second half of the nineteenth century, but they should not be taken at face value. Although some physicians kept records of their successes and failures before the twentieth century, many did not. Those records that survive suggest that until the 1930s fewer than a quarter of women treated could expect to conceive; today, the figure stands at around 50 per cent overall, although some causes of infertility are more amenable to treatment than others.[2] In spite of the faith that many couples have placed in medical treatment, therefore, for most of this history more couples have had to adjust to their infertility than have been cured. That adjustment, which may have taken the form of resignation to their situation; adoption; or, beginning in the late nineteenth century or so, donor insemination if the husband were the infertile partner, also forms a part of the infertility story.

No book about reproduction—or, as in this case, the inability to reproduce—can fail to acknowledge the centrality of gender. Although men are infertile as often as women, throughout these three centuries the woman, whether or not she has been the infertile partner, has disproportionately borne the medical, social, and cultural burden of a couple's failure to conceive. From the eighteenth century, when impotence was considered to be the only cause of sterility in men, to the late twentieth century, when women undergo invasive procedures in order to maximize the fertilizing potential of a partner's barely motile sperm, women have been subject to more treatment, endured more blame, and generally felt more answerable for a couple's inability to conceive than their husbands. Infertility treatment thus provides a paradigmatic example of a medical situation in which throughout much of its history the doctors have been men, the patients women, and the focus of attention the sexual organs.

The image of a male authority figure peering into the forbidden spaces of women's bodies and wielding a knife to reconfigure those spaces, which feminist scholars have often described, is not simply a caricature. Historians of women have been rightly critical of the ways in which the medical profession has often dealt with women patients in matters of sexuality and reproduction. But such criticism does not tell the whole story. Although physicians have clearly attempted to use their medical expertise to extract compliance from their patients, the evidence shows that women can also be aggressive in seeking treatment on their own terms, rejecting what they disagree with and often demanding specific procedures. Furthermore, the doctors themselves cannot be so effortlessly fit into a single mold. The relationship between women seeking infertility treatment and their doctors thus defies easy categorization.

Also defying categorization are the women whose infertile unions cause them such pain and sorrow. It is true that throughout American history there has been, to a greater or lesser degree, a cultural expectation that all women will want to become mothers. Those who express no maternal feelings might easily find themselves accused of unwomanliness. And if a woman marries, she is *expected* to reproduce. This "motherhood mandate" can—and has—stigmatized those whose unions are involuntarily childless as well as those who choose not to have children. Historically, it has been invoked to valorize women's fertility and to castigate those with expectations for achievement beyond the confines of home and family.

Nevertheless, it is wrong to assume that those who seek to alleviate their (or their partners') infertility problems are doing so only because of a cultural imperative that restricts women's choices. Women have, as this book shows, felt subjected to the pressure to procreate, but it is undeniable that many women as well as men desire children because they want to be parents—to pass on their love, family traditions, and heritage to another generation. To suggest that women who seek medical treatment because of an intense desire to bear children are victims of a patriarchal social structure, as some critics of contemporary technology have done, is to do these women an injustice.

To tell this story—or, more precisely, these three stories—we have drawn on a wide array of historical records: from memoirs to patient records, from medical textbooks to the letters of women and men anguished over their inability to have a baby, from women's magazines to medical and scholarly journals. In recovering the voices of those who have experienced infertility, those who have sought to alleviate it, and those who have chronicled and observed its impact on the larger society, we seek both to illuminate the responses of past generations to thwarted desires for parenthood and to remind contemporary Americans that neither the anguish of childlessness nor the search for technological solutions is a new phenomenon. Once the two became intertwined toward the end of the nineteenth century, however, they began to exercise a profound reciprocal influence. History may not be able to tell us how to solve the societal dilemmas posed by assisted reproduction in contemporary America, but it does help us to understand the processes that brought us to this point.

Part I

one

Denied "a Blessing of the Lord"

Living with Barrenness in Early America

When a young couple are married, they naturally desire Children, and therefore use those means that Nature has appointed to that end. But notwithstanding their endeavors, they must know that the success of all Depend on a Blessing of the Lord; and Children are a Blessing of the Lord.

Aristotle's Master Piece Compleated, 1720

In 1728, twenty-year-old Anna Maria Boehm Miller of Philadelphia, married just two years, petitioned for divorce. Her twenty-five-year-old husband, she claimed, was unable "to have carnal copulation with me for the procreation of Children." George Miller, she told the court, was impotent. He was also, as the court conceded, "defective in the conformation of his testicles." As the four men charged with inspecting his genitals to determine the truth of his wife's allegation discovered, George had one undescended testicle, and the other seemed malformed. Cryptorchidism (the medical term for an undescended testicle) can cause sterility. But although Anna Maria's petition emphasized her husband's inability to procreate, the court cared only whether or not he could sustain an erection and produce semen. Because George was able to display both an erect penis and several drops of semen to the men called upon to examine him, Anna Maria did not get her divorce. We will never know whether George Miller was truly impotent, whether he was simply unable to have intercourse with his wife, or even whether his wife was telling the truth.[1]

To the court, Anna Maria's expressed desire for children was irrelevant. The law drew a line between George's potential ability to perform his marital duties, as indicated by his performance before the examining committee, and the success of that performance, as measured in the production of children. Proof of a husband's impotence—or a physiological incapacity to have intercourse on a wife's part, for that matter—would have constituted grounds for the dissolution of a marriage. A barren union was in a different category, since at any time the Lord could choose to bless a couple with offspring. Or so colonists reasoned from the biblical accounts of Abraham and Sarah and Hannah's conception of the prophet Samuel.

Populating the New World was, of course, a serious matter, and large families were common. However, an individual couple's childlessness in the early eighteenth century, although considered a source of personal sorrow, was not generally a compelling societal concern; neither was infertility a subject of pressing interest to most physicians. An unhappily childless colonial woman might have discussed the problem with relatives or friends, sought comfort and aid from her religious faith, and perhaps obtained assistance from a midwife. Only rarely would she have sought advice from a physician. These views underwent a gradual change over the course of the next century and a half. Infertility began to be "medicalized," that is, to be seen as a medical condition that called for a therapeutic intervention. By the middle of the nineteenth century, although a wife might also pray and consult her family, the balance would begin to tilt in medicine's favor. By then barrenness, a personal misfortune in colonial America, had become sterility, a medical condition with larger societal implications.

Running parallel with this shift toward seeking medical advice for infertility was a transformation in the nature of family life. The colonial household seemed almost infinitely expandable; it was not unusual to find a patriarchal family head presiding over a variable household that might include a wife, biological children, stepchildren, and sundry unrelated dependents, including apprentices of various kinds. While such households did not entirely disappear, by the middle of the nineteenth century they were no longer the norm. Particularly among the rising middle classes in northern and midwestern towns and cities, the family had contracted markedly, and households had lost most of their public functions.[2] The ideal family had become a married couple and their offspring, bound together at least in theory more by ties of love than of economic need, and increasingly dependent on these affectional relationships. The more the household separated from the community, the more important having one's "own" family became. The result, however, was not exactly what one might expect. The transformation of American society from one in which the community held sway to one in which Americans felt entitled to privacy changed both the medical and the social perceptions of childlessness, but with an ironic twist. As this chapter demonstrates, in an increasingly privatized society infertility became an issue that attracted growing public concern.

The ideal colonial family was large and bustling, the central unit of a household production system that served an essentially rural community. Nearly all men and women married and brought six or more children into the world. Most women's lives centered around repeated cycles of pregnancy and childbearing. Mary Vial Holyoke of Salem, Massachusetts, for example, who married physician Edward Augustus Holyoke in 1759 at the age of twenty-three, bore twelve children over a twenty-two-year period. Seven died before reaching their first birthdays, and only three reached adulthood.[3] Babies born and babies wrested from life formed the leitmotif of the lives of most colonial women as they moved through the tasks of colonial housewifery—cooking, cleaning, quilting, gardening, and sewing, punctuated by the occasional gala and more frequent visits to family and friends. Few mothers, no matter what their social status, escaped the sorrow of the death of a child. High fertility and high infant mortality continued to the end of the eighteenth century. As late as 1800 the average white woman bore seven living children, which usually meant that she had more than seven pregnancies, since many ended in miscarriage or stillbirth.[4]

Children, the more the better, served several functions in colonial society, enhancing the family economy as well as providing company and comfort. Boys worked on the farm, in the family sawmill, or at their father's trade. Girls wove and spun and sometimes took over enough of the housekeeping to allow their mothers to engage in other kinds of labor. Midwife Martha Ballard, for example, who enjoyed a large practice in late-eighteenth-century Maine, would have had a difficult time engaging in her vocation had not her daughters and nieces been at home to help with the household chores, including spinning and weaving for the family and community as well as producing food for a large household.[5]

In a society in which the large family was the rule, couples without biological children were clearly atypical, although exactly how uncommon they were remains unclear. There are no definitive statistics on the number of childless marriages in the seventeenth or eighteenth century. Neither the genealogical studies of the late nineteenth and early twentieth centuries, which asserted that colonial Americans experienced an extraordinarily low rate of infertility—2 percent—nor most of the more recent community studies, which rarely mention its existence, are very helpful. Some data do exist, however, from which historians have estimated that about 8 percent of the marriages in colonial New England were childless. The figure may have been larger for other colonies, where higher rates of mortality and morbidity prevailed. The Dutch families in New Amsterdam at the time of the English conquest were, perhaps because of particularly stressful circumstances, especially unfruitful; nearly 23 percent of marriages apparently were childless.[6]

Although childless couples were never so rare in colonial America as to be considered curiosities, neither did they conform to the colonial familial ideal. Especially in Puritan New England, it was commonly thought that childlessness signified either the Lord's disfavor or His desire to test the faith of the couple. In both cases, the best comfort would come from prayer and reflection. Or so the ministers said. Benjamin Wadsworth's famous sermon on the duties of husbands and wives is representative of clerical advice to barren women. Retelling the familiar biblical account of Hannah, eventually to be the mother of the prophet Samuel, he recounted her misery in the face of her childlessness. Her husband hoped that his love would console her for her inability to conceive—"Am I not more to you than ten sons?" he asked—but it did not. (The fact that her husband had children by another wife, a detail omitted by Wadsworth in his retelling, did not make Hannah feel any better.) Only the Lord could bring her relief. After praying and fasting, she conceived. The lesson could not have been lost on Wadsworth's hearers.[7]

Understanding "Barrenness"

Submission to the will of the Lord may have helped couples to accept their inability to conceive, even if Providence did not see fit to change Its mind. But prayer was not the only option for the childless. Various kinds of advice, both popular and learned, was offered on how to bring about a desired pregnancy, although it is impossible to know how many childless women and men availed themselves of it. From the late seventeenth century on, colonists had relied on imported English publications, but by the middle of the eighteenth century, American publishers began to produce their own editions of both popular and learned medical and sexual advice. Erudite Americans consulted the English translation from the Latin of the work of Michael Etmuller, professor of physic (medicine) at the University of Leipzig, which was available as *Etmullerus Abridg'd* after 1699; or the English edition of François Mauriceau's *Diseases of Women with Child and in Child-Bed,* translated by Hugh Chamberlen the Elder, who belonged to a prominent family of "man-midwives," famous for their pioneering use of forceps, in seventeenth-century England.[8]

The less learned, in contrast, might have had access to the pseudonymous works of "Aristotle," who was actually a number of authors, one of whom may have been Nicholas Culpeper, whose other writings included a widely used book on midwifery.[9] The most popular of these works was *Aristotle's Master Piece,* which appeared in England sometime in the late seventeenth century, went through numerous printings, both in England and America, and has been called "the best example of the popular works on sexuality" of the late seventeenth century. Although the book remained in print after the American Revolution, in the early nineteenth century its sales fell off, and the last edition published came out in 1831.[10]

Superficially very different in the audiences they sought as well as in the styles in which they expressed themselves, both learned physicians and popular writers at least until the early eighteenth century were nevertheless generally in accord about how conception occurred and what problems underlay a failure to conceive. Complete unanimity of opinion did not reign, of course, but the fault lines did not always lie between the "expert" and the popularizer. The most prevalent view of conception among the public was the so-called semence theory, which held that men and women both emitted "seed" during intercourse, and that pregnancy resulted from the mixing of the seeds. The production of seed required an orgasm in each partner. Until the late seventeenth century, many medical authorities also held to the semence theory. It was, after all, the classical view handed down from Hippocrates through Galen, although Aristotle—the real Aristotle and not the spurious one of the *Master Piece*—had dissented.[11]

Before the turn of the eighteenth century, however, scientists began to question the idea that women emitted seed; instead, they spent their time arguing over where the new being resided. In some ways, this was a re-hashing of old preformationist questions—that is, did the new being already exist, and if so, where? In the semen or the ovary? Aristotle had insisted on the former and argued that women simply provided gestational space for the new being, which was created by the man. In Aristotle's view, "the male parent supplies the seed and the female the soil, and . . . by the co-operation of these diverse elements the foetus is produced." The semence theory had long prevailed over the Aristotelian position, but the latter gained new life when microscopic views of sperm disclosed what appeared to be tiny "animalcules" in semen. In 1677, Anton van Leeuwenhoek found spermatozoa when he viewed semen under a microscope; continued observation of both human and animal semen convinced him and others that they had indeed discovered the microscopic beings in which human life originated.[12]

This discovery, however, did not immediately convert those who held to what was called the "ovist" interpretation of reproductive theory. Just a decade before Leeuwenhoek's sightings of spermatozoa, Renier de Graaf, experimenting on rabbits, found what came to be called in his honor the Graafian follicles, which contain the mammalian ova. Even though the ova themselves were not seen until 1827, the discovery of the follicles added considerable weight to the ovist argument, of which William Harvey had been the most notable early proponent. De Graaf's discovery, according to one historian of science, put the ovist position "on a scientific footing, and was responsible for its general acceptance." De Graaf did not accept Leeuwenhoek's view of the significance of the sperm; he considered semen simply a "volatile salt" that "affected the egg by contact." Other ovists agreed, insisting that semen was "mere manure for the ovum," and that "the foetus was only excited into life by the 'seminal worms.' " The animalculists countered by arguing that Leeuwenhoek's discovery showed that even if the egg existed (and not all of them were convinced on that point), its only purpose was to nourish the life already present in the animalcules.[13]

Both the ovist and the animalculist theories ran counter to the idea that each partner produced seed, although neither idea immediately undermined scientific belief in the importance for conception of the female orgasm. With the exception of Harvey, popular and medical opinion alike held until at least the early nineteenth century that female pleasure was almost always essential for pregnancy to occur.[14] According to Etmuller, for example, the "languishing" of a woman's "venereal appetite" often caused barrenness. Mauriceau went so far as to cite "the insensibility of some Women, who take no pleasure in the venereal act," as the "most frequent reason why this orifice opens not in this act to receive the Man's Seed." Unless both partners, insisted another authority, "act with befitting Ardency," conception would not take place. "The womb," declared John Marten in 1708, "must be in a state of delight," or the coupling would be fruitless.[15]

Wives and husbands desiring children, therefore, were advised to seek mutual sexual satisfaction; for those whom "the state of delight" eluded, advice was available, concerning both techniques of sexual arousal and the use of various aphrodisiacs. *Aristotle's Master Piece* advised men that the exercise of both consideration and restraint would be most likely to bring the desired result. "Women," it reminded them, "rather choose to have a thing done well, than have it often. And in this Case, to do it well and often too is inconsistent." Moderation, according to the *Master Piece,* enhanced pleasure and promoted fertility; after all, "common Whores have none, or very rarely any children; for the Grass seldom grows in a Path that is commonly trodden in."[16]

Although Mauriceau had cited women's "insensibility" as the chief cause of infertility, other authorities believed that an imbalance in a wife's bodily "humors" was at least as great a culprit. The theory that health resulted from maintaining the body in a state of equilibrium—in fluid intake and outgo, in eating and elimination—had served as the foundation of Western medical practice since classical times. Humoral medicine had decreed since Galen the necessity for a proper balance of the four bodily fluids: blood, phlegm, choler (yellow bile), and melancholy (black bile). And even when scientists no longer took the idea of humoral theory literally, the concept of "balance" was central to therapeutic practice until the nineteenth century. Belief in the importance of bodily equilibrium to good health was widely shared within the culture. As a result, practitioners of all sorts, and their patients, could recognize both the outward signs of ill health and the converse signs of a cure by understanding this system.[17]

Some imbalances affected both sexes, such as fevers, skin eruptions, various changes in bladder or bowel habits, and hemorrhaging. In addition, women had their particular disequilibria, including leucorrhea (vaginal discharges that could result from a number of causes) and menstrual disorders. Practitioners ranging from the learned European professor of physic to the village midwife agreed that these imbalances might easily lead to sterility. For retention or suppression of the menses—what physicians now call primary or secondary amenorrhea—women took em-menogogues (botanical or mineral remedies prescribed to promote the menstrual flow) and might have called in a medical practitioner for vene-section (bloodletting). For leucorrhea, prescriptions included other botan-ical and mineral remedies, which might be taken as tonics, applied to the external pelvic region, inserted into the vagina, or even given as "injec-tions" into the uterus itself.[18]

Women, as these remedies make clear, generally bore the onus of a bar-ren marriage. Only impotence or deformity, it was believed, rendered a man sterile, and treatments for both existed. Impotence, of course, called for the use of aphrodisiacs. Deformities raised more complicated issues, but at the end of the eighteenth century the English surgeon John Hunter used artificial insemination to overcome one patient's hypospadias (an anomaly in which the opening of the urethra is on the undersurface of the penis). Impotence and deformities were considered rare conditions, how-ever, and medical authorities held that as long as a man could accomplish "connection," then he could father children.[19]

Barrenness, therefore, was clearly a woman's problem, and self-treat-ment was the usual means employed to alleviate it. American women, like their counterparts in England, kept medicinal recipe books, which often contained specific preparations to treat various menstrual irregularities that were believed to cause barrenness and that could also be used for the prevention of miscarriage. Or they or their husbands could consult the popular or learned literature, depending on their access to such material. In addition, women of means could visit several mineral springs just as their counterparts in Europe took the waters at German and English spas in the hope of becoming fertile. If self-treatment failed, a woman might consult a midwife, who would have prescribed various botanical prepa-rations. Some colonial authorities, however, looked on the treatment of barrenness by midwives with suspicion. After all, the Lord was not the only supernatural being reputed to be able to cause barrenness. So could the devil. When infertility resulted from diabolical intervention, a popu-lar midwifery manual recommended that the afflicted woman should carry on her person a "loadstone" or some "St. Johns Wort." But some midwives, it was feared, might be willing to bargain more directly with the devil for a cure. John Winthrop suspected one midwife who "prac-ticed physic" of witchcraft because of the nature of the botanical medi-cines she dispensed to women desirous of conceiving.[20]

The idea of medical treatment for barrenness, especially in the eyes of pious Christians, may have seemed questionable in the seventeenth century; gradually, however, it became less suspect, although it is unclear exactly when the transition took place. By the Revolutionary era medical treatment had become more acceptable. Nevertheless, no matter what medical advice a couple took, they would have always been reminded that in the end, children were a gift from God, Who might simply choose to withhold that blessing. As the authors of *Aristotle's Master Piece* declared at the end of a full list of prescriptions for barrenness, there was no guarantee of success: "When a young Couple are married, they naturally desire Children, and therefore use those means that Nature has appointed to that end. But notwithstanding their endeavors, they must know that the success of all depends on a Blessing of the Lord; and Children are a Blessing of the Lord."[21]

Children for the Childless

Even if a couple in colonial America failed to conceive, that did not necessarily mean that they faced either a childless existence or a sense of being somehow excluded from the life of their community. Those women who never bore children nevertheless could participate in communal rituals—from the birth of a neighbor's child to the "sitting up" visits that surrounded the entrance of a child into the world. And wife and husband together had a number of means of bringing children into their families. It is true that most couples wanted to have children of their own. As Gordon Wood has noted, landowning farmers "particularly wanted . . . sons to whom they could pass on their land and who would continue the family name." But because the household, and not so much the conjugal unit, constituted the colonial family, it does not appear to have been terribly difficult for couples to accept children who came their way by various means other than conceiving them themselves. Akin to modern adoption (although no adoption laws existed in the colonies), such practices were nevertheless sufficiently different to require some explanation. First, as far as it is possible to tell, most couples took in the children of family members. Second, a childless couple might "adopt" the child of a living family member in order to provide themselves with an heir, without the biological parent having to relinquish the child completely. The concept of a couple having an absolute "right" to a child they brought up would emerge much later, in the nineteenth century, as a part of a more general transformation taking place in ideas about the family.[22]

Childless couples may have even been *expected* to rear the children of deceased siblings or cousins. From Puritan New England through the Chesapeake and southward, maternal deaths left many half-orphans. When a wife died leaving young children, a father who did not remarry quickly was likely to send the youngsters to relatives to be reared. If half-orphanhood was the rule, in some parts of the colonies full orphanhood was also common. In one Chesapeake county, for example, almost 20 percent of the children were orphaned before the age of thirteen and more than 30 percent by the age of eighteen.[23]

When a parent died, nearly everyone agreed that the bonds of blood provided the best guarantee of an orphaned child's welfare. The child's relatives, courts, and other colonial authorities viewed stepparents, in particular, with suspicion. As historian Joyce Goodfriend has noted, Dutch settlers in New York were careful in their wills to provide that relatives take charge of the upbringing and the property of orphaned children.[24] Childless couples welcomed orphaned nieces, nephews, and cousins into their homes and hearts. In Massachusetts, when Thomas and Bethiah Lothrop adopted a cousin's orphaned daughter in the 1670s, Thomas expressed thankfulness "for the providence of God in disposing of the child from one place to another till it must be brought into his house that he might be a father to it." In New York, a childless silversmith sent to Holland for his nephew, brought him into his home and business, and provided for him in his will. In Massachusetts the very rich but childless Thomas Hancock brought his nephew John, the future signer of the Declaration of Independence, into his house when the boy was eight. Thomas and Lydia Hancock had been married for thirteen years without having children. John's widowed mother, living with her children in the household of her late husband's father, kept her two daughters with her but sent John to Boston, where he became the virtual son of Thomas and Lydia, and their heir.[25]

These intimate dramas of orphanhood and adoption, of estates and guardianship, were played out against the backdrop of a distinctive kind of familial and communal life. As historian Helena Wall reminds us, colonists from New England through the Middle Atlantic states and into the South "conceived of the family almost entirely within the context of community." Families and households in the seventeenth and eighteenth centuries were often quite elastic, and most of them included the sons and daughters of kin as well as unrelated youngsters "put out" (in the parlance of the day), often when very young, to learn husbandry, housewifery, or a trade, or simply because the parents had too many younger mouths to feed.[26] A widespread practice, "putting out" was not limited to families in crisis but was a way for couples to relieve themselves of the care of a superfluity of offspring. This practice was not the same as adopting a young relative, but it too provided a means for the childless to enjoy some of the benefits of having children, ideally including both ties of affection and the more tangible attributes of extra hands on the farm or in the kitchen.[27]

Throughout the seventeenth and eighteenth centuries, adoptive practices, guardianship, and being on the receiving end of the putting-out system served the community by creating households and providing for children and childless couples by enabling them to enjoy some of the benefits of parenthood. Such solutions were possible in a society in which the boundaries between family and community were highly permeable. But as Americans in the post-Revolutionary era began to cut deeper lines of separation between the two, children took on a new significance. In the seventeenth and early eighteenth centuries, the principal value of children lay in the benefits they could bring to the family and the community. Historians have noted changes in patterns of family formation as well as cultural shifts in the meaning of family life beginning in the late eighteenth century, although they disagree on the reasons for the changes. What for some historians was a manifestation of Revolutionary democracy appears to others to have constituted evidence of the development of an individualism derived at least in part from eighteenth-century evangelistic religion. It has also been argued that the turn from communalism and hierarchy toward privacy and greater if not absolute equality, which marked the end of the dominance of the household family form and its replacement by the conjugal unit, had its origins in the rise of capitalism.[28]

However historians choose to explain them, the changes in the family—both real and ideal—had profound implications for the ways in which Americans dealt with infertility. In a communal society composed of households, it might matter somewhat less (to the society, if not to the individual couple) how the children came into those households. But in a society where the fundamental unit was the married couple and their offspring, having one's "own" children became increasingly important.[29] One consequence of such shifts in cultural attitudes toward the relationship between the family and the larger society was a change in perceptions of infertility. Elusive but unmistakable signs of such a change emerged in the closing decades of the eighteenth century and became clearly manifest in the early years of the nineteenth, making their way into the medical literature. Although it would take another half-century to accomplish, by the end of the eighteenth century barrenness was on the way to becoming sterility.

From Barrenness to Sterility

One way to highlight this transformation, as well as to emphasize the means by which new ideas built on the past, is to look at how two men, emblems of the old and the new ways of defining and treating infertility, conceptualized the condition. James Graham (1745–1794) was a flamboyant Scotsman who once practiced in the colonies just before the American Revolution, a maverick whose therapies might best be identified with those of midwives and herb doctors. James Walker, a young man at the close of the eighteenth century and the author of the first English language volume devoted entirely to infertility (which he pointedly called sterility and not barrenness), clearly thought of himself as a young doctor in the vanguard.

James Graham built a fortune by his ingenious linkage of sexual pleasure with electrotherapy in order to cure sterility in women and impotence in men. Earlier in his career Graham had traveled from his native Scotland to the American colonies; he settled in Philadelphia in the early 1770s, where he claimed to have a thriving practice in the treatment of barrenness. He then moved to England, where he reportedly cured the Duchess of Devonshire of sterility in 1779. Grateful, she rewarded him handsomely. Practicing in Bath and Bristol after returning to Great Britain, he had been relying principally on his "magnetic throne" and "electrical bath" to make men potent and women fertile. With his newfound wealth made possible by the Duchess, he moved to London and built the "Temple of Health." Here, in the "Great Apollo Apartment," an audience of men seated in chairs that provided mild electrical shocks listened to Graham lecture on potency. Women who came to the temple heard lectures on fertility given by a member of their own sex.[30]

Those not able to visit the Temple of Health could purchase a copy of Graham's *Lecture on Love; or, Private Advice to Married Ladies and Gentlemen,* in which he provided women with this "never-failing prescription" for fertility:

Take one handful of red virgin sage leaves; steep them in a bottle of old red port; then drink a glassful every morning; repeat it in two or three months; . . . with regular hours and moderate exercise, . . . with plain and simple drink; bathing is also necessary . . . ; in case of great weakness, relaxation, or debility, the sea, Bristol, or the German Spa water is preferable.[31]

Those whom the "never failing" prescription failed, if they still had faith in the prescriber, had the opportunity to purchase Dr. Graham's "aetherial or divine balsam," the recipe for which he kept to himself. It was, he claimed, "a preparation of rich gum, with . . . ether, electricity, air, or magnetism!"[32]

If the aetherial balsam did not bring about the desired result, all but the most affluent were now out of luck. The well-to-do, however, had a further option—Graham's vibrating "celestial bed." The "superior ecstasy which the parties enjoy in the Celestial Bed," promised Graham, was "really astonishing . . . ; the barren certainly must become fruitful when they are so powerfully agitated in the delights of love." Graham had good reason to enthuse. At first, he had charged 50 guineas for the use of the bed for the night, but as he (and the bed) became more well-known, he raised the price—ultimately to 500 guineas. A short comedy called *Genius of Nonsense,* in which Graham and his bed were featured, played in London for three years, bringing him both fame and fortune.[33]

In spite of Graham's well-publicized success, the bulk of his audience, no doubt, came to the Temple of Health to be titillated by the mild electrical shocks or by the lectures themselves. In fact, it was hard for his contemporaries, as it has been for generations since then, to take Graham seriously. But his actual prescriptions—regulation of diet, exercise, electricity, and balsamic preparations—were considered appropriate remedies for barrenness in his own day.[34] Besides, the simple fact that he made his fortune because at least one of his infertile patients became pregnant reminds us that such a claim of success brought him other paying clients who hoped he could repeat his accomplishment for them.

There could be no greater contrast between the flamboyant showman James Graham and the sober young medical student James Walker, who sought to recast his profession's diagnosis and treatment of infertility. If he had hopes that his work would bring him fame and fortune, he was destined for disappointment. Returning to his native Virginia after graduation, he established a small hospital and faded into obscurity. He did, however, leave a slim volume, grandly entitled *An Inquiry into the Causes of Sterility in Both Sexes; with Its Method of Cure.* Written as a dissertation at the medical school of the University of Pennsylvania in 1797, it

A N

INQUIRY

INTO THE

Causes of Sterility

I N

BOTH SEXES;

W I T H

ITS METHOD OF CURE.

By JAMES WALKER, M. P. M. S.

CITIZEN OF THE STATE OF VIRGINIA.

———— creavit Deus hominem ad imaginem suam, ad imaginem Dei creavit illum, masculum et fæminam creavit eos. Benedixitque illis Deus et ait; *crescite et multiplicamini et replete terram.* **Genesis,** *cap.* 1. *ver.* 28.

Philadelphia:

Printed by E. OSWALD, No. 179, South Second-Street.

M,DCC,XCVII.

C

Frontispiece of James Walker's *Inquiry into the Causes of Sterility*. In this slim volume, Walker attempted to recast the inability to bear a child from an unhappy personal situation to a treatable medical condition.

was an attempt both to codify "advanced" medical knowledge about sterility and to break new ground.

Walker argued forcefully that the time was ripe for regular physicians to wrest the diagnosis and treatment of infertility from the hands of midwives by defining barrenness as a condition requiring the expertise of a physician. In so doing, he was following the lead of his teachers in Philadelphia, who had already been surprisingly successful in defining childbirth in that way. Indeed, in the 1780s and 1790s the city's elite families, prodded by the medical establishment, were already turning away from midwives as their birth attendants, choosing local physicians instead. The University of Pennsylvania's medical school had taken the initiative; its students, well in advance of national trends, routinely attended obstetrical (still called midwifery) lectures. Walker's assumption that women could be encouraged to turn increasingly to physicians for advice on how to become pregnant, just as they were turning to them for their deliveries, was completely in accord with his professors' views.[35]

To "the anxiety of mind . . . universally connected with unfruitful marriages," Walker attempted to graft a new set of medical and societal dangers. Sterility, he argued, was "the cause of as much evil in the world, as any of those diseases to which we are liable." Nevertheless, he acknowledged, he had few guidelines in this attempt to define sterility as a disease—to medicalize it, as we would say in the twentieth century. Science, he believed, lagged behind in providing the knowledge required by the profession. Neither classical medical authorities nor modern scientists were able to answer definitely even the most basic question of how conception occurred. What the ancients wrote, Walker concluded, was so "unsatisfactory, that we are left nearly in the dark." And the moderns? Not one of them, he concluded, "has treated of it methodically."[36]

Walker's interpretive difficulties began, appropriately enough, with the controversy that still raged, as it would continue to do for another thirty or forty years, between the ovists and the animalculists. (In fact, as late as the 1840s, one popular medical writer would assert he could see in sperm under the microscope the rudiments of the brain and spinal column.) The locus of conception—ovaries or uterus—remained another contested issue. Walker preferred the ovarian theory, but admitted that he had no evidence on either side. No one yet argued that fertilization took place in the fallopian tubes.[37]

Walker felt on surer ground defending the need for the mutual orgasm. "When the female is not capable of gratification from debility, or against inclination," he noted, "she is scarcely ever fruitful." But Walker inter-

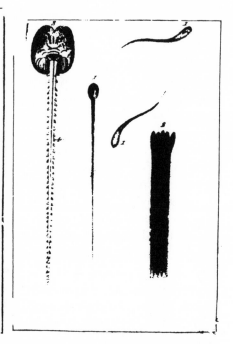

PLATE 6, p. 119.

SEMINAL ANIMALCULE.

This plate exhibits the form of the Seminal Animalcule ; and also its resemblance to that of the Brain and Spinal Marrow, to illustrate the Neuro Spermatic Theory of Generation.

No. 1–1–1.–Magnified views of the Seminal Animalculæ, enlarged many thousand times.

No. 2.—The same in bunches, as they are usually seen.

No. 3.—The Brain.

No. 4.—The Spinal Marrow proceeding from the Brain, with the nerves branching from it cut off.

The resemblance between the Brain and Spinal Marrow, and one of the Seminal Animalcules will be seen at once, by comparing them together as they are placed side by side.

As late as the 1840s, one popular medical writer argued that one could discern the rudiments of the brainstem in sperm, suggesting that the male contribution to fetal development had specifically to do with mental powers.

From Frederick Hollick, *The Origin of Life*, 1845

preted the lack of female orgasm in medical rather than sexual terms. James Graham, following traditional views, promoted fertility by suggesting ways to heighten sexual pleasure in both sexes. That was, after all, the whole point of the Celestial Bed. But Walker, although he was not above recommending the use of aphrodisiacs if necessary, believed that when a woman failed to achieve "gratification," the presence of disease was a far more likely explanation than a lack of inclination.[38]

In spite of including the words "both sexes" in his title, Walker did not challenge the idea that unless a man were impotent, sterility was a woman's problem; and the female disorder that Walker associated most closely with sterility was leucorrhea, a general term for a vaginal discharge from any cause, including gonorrhea (although at this time no one suggested that gonorrhea was a specific culprit in cases of sterility). Other causes included various "local complaints," most of which were extremely difficult to diagnose or cure. In spite of his professed optimism, Walker concluded that "we are . . . not to expect cures in all cases, and indeed but few of them comparatively speaking, according to the number which occur." He was in good company. The distinguished Edinburgh physician Alexander Hamilton also expressed doubts about how often infertility was curable. Some women, he wrote, "have original imperfections in the uterine system, which cannot be remedied by any operation of art, and which remain often concealed until after death." Such "imperfections" included various conditions affecting the reproductive organs, including blocked fallopian tubes.[39]

Hamilton had contended that only when infertility resulted from menstrual disorders, "improprieties in the manner of living," or "female weakness" (another term for leucorrhea) could it be successfully treated. Walker agreed that menstrual disorders—particularly suppression and retention of the menses—responded best to treatment. "Retention" suggested that a woman simply could not expel the menstrual blood retained within her body, while suppression implied a complete cessation of the function. The two conditions required different prescriptions. Retention warranted the use of stimulants of various kinds: tonics, exercise, "venery, when it is admissible," and electricity. "The uterus may be stimulated by shocks passed through the pelvis," he suggested. Suppression, in contrast, required bleeding "or other depleting remedies."[40] But if such remedies failed, Walker advised physicians to fall back on time-honored remedies such as dietary recommendations and to prescribe "the cold bath." Indeed, he slyly noted, doctors ought to appropriate the balsamic remedies of the midwives and other healers. After all, he said, these appeared to work when recommended by "the good women."[41]

By calling James Graham an exemplar of the "old" and James Walker the harbinger of a "new" perception of infertility, we do not mean to suggest either that Walker had better ideas or that the views he presented, especially regarding therapeutics, differed significantly from conventional wisdom. What was happening was more subtle, the earliest stages of the assertion of authority on the part of "experts." Walker's treatise, defining sterility as pathology and its cure as resting in the hands of physicians, served in short to signal the beginnings of the trend toward the medicalization of infertility in the United States. Over the course of the nineteenth century, women faced with an involuntarily childless marriage would come to rely more and more heavily on medical expertise, and to accept the definition of infertility as a disease. This process, however, would take several generations. Reliance on prayer did not die in the eighteenth century; neither did the belief in roots and herbs. Moreover, although elite physicians trained in institutions such as the University of Pennsylvania might have aspired to become authorities on infertility as early as the turn of the nineteenth century, the initial impact of medical interest in infertility in the late eighteenth and early nineteenth centuries was not so much to encourage women to seek out a physician to treat her barrenness as to give her the tools to treat it herself.

In this era, doctors could rarely exert the kind of influence that Walker conferred on them. Physicians dealt with whatever came their way in the guise of a patient, and usually only on occasions of medical crisis. As for the prospective patients themselves, as the people of the United States scattered to frontier settlements and farming communities, some had only limited access to physicians and others found the fees prohibitive. A great deal of medical advice came not in the shape of a physician but in the form of one or another of the guides to domestic medicine, beginning with the nearly ubiquitous William Buchan's *Domestic Medicine,* which became very widely used in the early nineteenth century.[42]

Buchan's popular guide, initially an English import but with numerous American "adapters," offered the traditional view of the necessity of maintaining bodily equilibrium. Many cases of barrenness, Buchan argued, resulted from the various "passions which tend to obstruct the menstrual flux," such as "grief, sudden fear, [and] anxiety." In these cases, husbands were enjoined to make their wives "as easy and cheerful as possible; all disagreeable objects are to be avoided, and every method taken to amuse and entertain the fancy."[43]

Buchan's readers would have understood this emphasis on the importance of attitudes, since it reflected their own understanding of the precariousness of bodily equilibrium and of the mental and physical disorders that might upset the body's balance and turn health into disease. Grief or anxiety could affect fertility, just as leucorrhea could, and there was no suggestion that the latter was more of a "disease" than the former. The most important indicator of the causes of a woman's inability to conceive, according to the popular guides, was irregular or painful menstruation. In addition to having their minds relieved of excessive cares, women with menstrual irregularities (generally called "obstructions") were advised to improve their overall state of health. Exercise, a diet "chiefly of milk and vegetables," cold baths, and the use of "astringent medicines" (tonics) were all recommended. Although not every domestic medical guide included a chapter on sterility, nearly all dealt with menstruation. Women attempting to conceive would not have had difficulty in finding suggestions for treatment.[44]

Purveyors of proprietary medicines gained considerable followings by promising more immediate cures. Joseph Ralph, who bottled and sold "Ralph's Domestic Medicine," promoted his product directly to "female sufferers." Claiming that women's "complaints" were "of a nature so delicate as to be far more properly treated by themselves than by any other person," he told women that by purchasing his medicine they could avoid the embarrassment of consulting personally with a (male) physician. Painful menstruation, symptomatic of inflammation, must never be left untreated, or it could result in the loss of "the capacity of having children." The solution to the problem? Self-treatment with his "domestic medicine."[45]

In the guides to domestic medicine, however, although recommendations for self-treatment such as diet and exercise dominated advice on the treatment of infertility, a number of physician-writers also discussed more invasive therapies, such as venesection for amenorrhea or uterine injections for leucorrhea. The aim of both kinds of therapies was the same. Restoration of regular menstruation and promotion of general health were considered the most promising routes to fertility. One of the many "handbooks" for medical students, for example, advised practitioners treating sterility to promote menstrual regularity, to remove local disease, and to restore "vigour" to the uterus. If self-treatment did not restore the body's natural balance, then more interventionist treatment was necessary.[46]

Medical intervention into the barren marriage in the early nineteenth century arose not only from the domestic medical guides and the increasingly popular "handbooks" for medical students and practitioners but also out of the emergent relationship between the legal and the medical professions. Medical jurisprudence originated from the growing sense that the courts required the expertise of physicians in both civil and criminal matters. To meet the need, courses in the subject became commonplace in medical schools by the middle third of the century. Physicians in practice could also consult Theodoric Romeyn Beck's *Elements of Medical Jurisprudence,* which first appeared in 1823 and which was frequently updated.[47]

Medical jurisprudence brought physicians into the courts to deal with questions of infertility as the legal system wrestled with such issues as whether sterility ought to be grounds for divorce. If so, courts eventually decided, it must be the result of absolute male impotence or female incapacity for intercourse. To allow them to judge such questions, the courts sought medical advice about the symptoms or physical manifestations that indicated the probability of sterility or impotence.

As late as 1825, New York State rejected impotence as grounds for divorce, but within a decade such grounds were allowed and an examination by a physician required to establish them. No longer would it suffice, as it had in the case of George Miller, for a committee of citizens to make a judgment about the existence of impotence; now it required expert testimony. Cases came before the courts regarding both male and female impotence. Judges everywhere demanded proof of the "absolute incapacity for sexual intercourse . . . ; mere sterility is not enough." In deciding the precedent-setting case of *Devanbaugh v. Devanbaugh*—in which the wife rather than the husband was alleged to be impotent—the court explicitly relied on the authority of T. R. Beck's *Elements*. This case established the principle that a defendant alleged to be impotent must submit to examination "by skillful and competent surgeons." Mrs. Devanbaugh, the court-appointed physician determined, did not suffer from genital malformation but only from an intact hymen, an impediment to intercourse that could easily be corrected. The judge therefore ruled, based on Beck's teachings, that she suffered from a "temporary and curable incapacity," requiring only a "slight surgical operation, without danger to the defendant, for its cure." Mrs. Devanbaugh declined to submit to the operation, but the court nevertheless refused her husband a divorce.[48]

By the 1830s, courts confronted with demands for divorce on the grounds of sexual incapacity commonly depended on medical testimony. In some states, men obtained divorces when their wives displayed no physiological impediment to intercourse but instead suffered from an "excessive sensibility" that rendered "sexual intercourse practically impossible, on account of the pain it would inflict." And if Anna Maria Boehm Miller had been seeking a divorce in New York State in the 1830s, instead of in Pennsylvania in the 1720s, she might have had more luck. In New York, "if the defendant is . . . incapable of sexual intercourse with the plaintiff, though not with other persons, if such a thing be possible, a decree of nullity may be granted."[49]

The courts relied on the expertise of physicians in such cases. Impotence could be physical or psychological, absolute or "relative," but it had to be incurable, to which a physician had to testify. Perhaps it was their experience in the divorce courts that led some physicians to conclude that in spite of the fact that no court accepted sterility alone as grounds for divorce, it would soon come to that. The most extreme warning from medical jurisprudence came from London physician Michael Ryan, writing in the 1830s. His predictions for the sterile were dire indeed: "There is no subject which distresses married persons so much as want of family, or leads to so much domestic feud and unhappiness, and finally to the nullification of marriage." Driving this theme home, he insisted that "those . . . who are not blessed with children experience daily a diminution of affection. . . . they are sad, and . . . too often violate conjugal fidelity." Couples without children, it was clear, were in grave danger.[50]

Although American courts continued to reject sterility as grounds for divorce, Ryan's words found a receptive audience among both physicians and societal observers convinced that infertility had become a grave medical problem with significant social implications. Their concern was related to what had become a national issue: the state of women's health. Perhaps it was merely coincidence that regularly trained physicians began to take on this issue just as increasing numbers of American women decided that they would rather take their health into their own hands. Perhaps not. But in the mid–nineteenth century a wave of antagonism toward regular medicine swept the middle classes and had a profound effect on women. These years marked the high point of medical democracy, and there was a broad audience for health information of all kinds. Medical self-help literature reached an enormously receptive public. Women lecturers—many of them from the increasingly popular hydropathy movement—gave health information to capacity crowds in halls throughout the East and Midwest.

Childlessness, "Debility," and the Cult of Motherhood

The public, then, as well as radical health reformers and regular practitioners, feared for the health of modern women. For most middle-class Americans, it was an article of faith that women of their generation were considerably less healthy than their grandmothers had been. Women health reformers and advice givers argued that a large cohort of women endured delicate health throughout their adult lives. Catharine Beecher's survey of two hundred American communities at midcentury convinced her, for example, that all over the country the majority of women were either "delicate or diseased," or worse, "habitual invalids." Of course, it is possible that this state of ill health was more imagined than real, but opinion was nevertheless widespread that women, particularly among the white Protestant middle classes, were growing more and more infirm.[51]

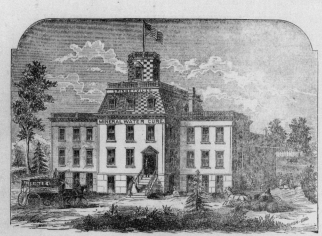

Women health reformers in the mid-nineteenth century advocated the use of water cure establishments like this one as an alternative to invasive medical therapies. Hydropathy was a major component of the medical self-help movement.
Courtesy of the Library of Congress

In some quarters, such beliefs led to a real fear about women's child-bearing abilities. "The continued production of healthy children, or any children," noted one historian about this widespread sentiment, "would be endangered [by female illness]. The invalid female unable to bear children violated the ideal of true womanhood."[52] Anxieties about both the capacity and the will of American women to reproduce were fueled by a declining birthrate. By 1850, the national birthrate had slipped from 7.04 births (in 1800) to 5.42. As historian James H. Cassedy argues, "People worried increasingly about the effects produced on 'delicate' female nervous systems by their increased exposure to the physical phases of modern living—the cacophony of city noise, the bustle of travel, the excitements produced by newspaper reading, [and] the tensions produced by their husbands' ventures and risks in business."[53]

The eventual result, many feared, would be to force the nation increasingly to rely on immigrants to populate its vast reaches. Some medical advice givers believed that contraceptive practices damaged women's reproductive systems. Popular advice-writer William Alcott was only one of a large number of medical men who castigated Americans from the 1830s to the 1850s for their use of birth control and abortion. Either practice, they claimed, could result in permanent sterility. Others, although not convinced that birth control and abortion were that prevalent, nevertheless warned women who gave in to the pleasures and luxuries of modern life that they were forfeiting their chances of parenthood. At stake was not only their marital happiness but also the nation's future.[54]

In spite of such dire forebodings, there is little evidence that wives were abandoning motherhood entirely. Bearing and rearing children remained, as Judith Walzer Leavitt has noted, "a vital component in the social definition of womanhood." It represented, in fact, women's "most valued work." In colonial America, that "work" had added to the family's and the community's economic well-being; by the middle decades of the nineteenth century, however, an unprecedented public and private glorification of motherhood suggested that bearing children constituted a woman's sole reason for existing. In middle-class America, by midcentury the mother-child bond had become—at least in theory—the most important family tie, taking precedence over the husband-wife relationship. As historian Sylvia Hoffert has argued, the "ideology of motherhood assured [women] that having children could fulfill both private and public needs. Bearing children, it promised, was certain to guarantee personal happiness because it renewed the bonds of intimacy that served as the basis of a stable marriage."[55]

This was a significant new interpretation of the place of motherhood in the culture and one that was likely to raise anxieties. The majority of colonial "goodwives," women who worked in cooperation with their spouses to sustain the household and the communal economy, had been mothers, of course, and in some ways motherhood was their most important function; but it was not the only thing that defined them as women. With the American Revolution, some historians have argued, the "goodwife" gave way to the Republican Mother. The new focus on civic virtue allowed middle- and upper-class white women to demand enlarged educational opportunities both for their daughters and for themselves. The rationale was that without educated mothers, the young Republic could not assure itself that sons would become well-informed citizens. Women did not fail to remind their husbands that in a real sense the continuation of the Republic rested on mothers' efforts.[56]

As the Revolutionary era faded into memory, however, and as women found that their new educational opportunities had not significantly enlarged their lives, many who had sought to define a new ideal for American womanhood found ways to turn their restricted roles to new advantage. As historian Nancy Cott has demonstrated, the new "doctrine of women's sphere opened to women (reserved for them) the avenues of domestic influence, religious morality, and child nurture." Out of this impulse came the ideology of domesticity, the central tenet of which was that the home, where women presided, was the central institution of American life; the domestic role—particularly the maternal role—of women became the linchpin of social unity.[57]

Indeed, by the middle of the century, it had become a middle-class article of faith that healthy family life required a woman to direct her emotional and physical energies into creating the proper home life. Domestic reformers such as Catharine Beecher made it clear that this was not a concession to male notions of women's inferiority. Rather, the reformers asserted, in order for the nation to prosper, women everywhere were *choosing* to forgo the pleasures of worldly success in favor of their higher calling: They were answerable for the nation's moral vision, and the only place to instill that vision was in the home. As domestic writer Mrs. L. H. G. Abell reminded her readers, the influence of mothers was indeed "far reaching." As a mother, she insisted, a woman had a task much more important than whatever accomplishments men may enjoy in the larger world, for "she must sow the seed, and watch with ceaseless anxiety its growth, plant the tender and delicate germs of principle, and train the young tendrils of the feelings and affections. She is set to guard, to instruct, to mould the *moral nature.*" In addition to what we might call this public function of motherhood, however, there was also woman's responsibility to make her husband happy; and marital happiness was, according to the advice givers, "a condition made possible only by the presence of a child, whose birth was guaranteed to enhance the affection that husband and wife felt for each other."[58]

Of course, it is always difficult to know how seriously readers took the injunctions of the advice givers, but several studies of mid-nineteenth-century family and community history have offered portraits of middle-class family life that conform quite remarkably to the prescriptive literature. It is not that women were real-life counterparts of fictional heroines or that people's behavior conformed exactly to the directions given in advice books; rather, they believed in the cultural values embodied in the literary material, whether or not their own lives seem to confirm those values. As historian Mary Ryan noted of the family relationships in one upstate New York city, "The bond between mother and child assumed central place in the constellation of family affection."[59]

Such veneration of motherhood united those reformers, such as the phrenologists and hydropathists, who wanted to enlarge women's educational opportunities, with those who adhered to more conventional notions. Naturally, the two groups tended to view the decline in the birthrate differently. According to some of the reformers, those women and their husbands who chose to limit their family size were not rejecting parenthood. Far from it—if women were to "mould the moral nature" of their offspring, they needed the time and the health to do so. A woman who spent her entire life pregnant or nursing, some reasoned, would have used up so much strength in childbearing as to have little left for childrearing. Although this may have been cold comfort for those who were convinced that the decline in the birthrate boded ill for American society, the two groups agreed more than they disagreed about the significance of motherhood, if not the number of children each couple should have. It was one thing to be single: Catharine Beecher, the most famous domestic reformer of her generation, and a single woman herself, claimed that the unmarried could employ their maternal instincts as teachers, nurses, and physicians. But wives were expected, by nearly everyone, to be mothers. In such a world, childlessness could be a tragedy.

Unfortunately, evidence of the ways in which women in the early to mid–nineteenth century responded to infertility in their own marriages is scarce. However, a few women have left some record both of their emotional reaction to childlessness and of the ways in which they attempted to deal with it. One of them, novelist and antislavery reformer Lydia Maria Child (1802–80), came of age before the full flowering of the cult of motherhood; the other two, women's rights reformer Amelia Bloomer (1818–94) and Civil War diarist Mary Chesnut (1823–86), became women in the midst of it and felt its full weight. Their experiences of infertility, therefore, offer some insight into both the range of individual responses and the kinds of pressures, internal and external, that childless women faced as the century wore on.

As a solitary young girl growing up in the New England countryside, Lydia Maria Francis had looked forward not to marriage and motherhood but to a literary career. By her early twenties, she had already enjoyed a taste of modest fame (at least among the Boston literati) as the author of *Hobomok,* a tale of interracial love set in colonial Massachusetts. Published in 1824, *Hobomok,* particularly when the public learned that the author was a young woman barely out of her teens, seemed both titillating and slightly scandalous. Indeed, when the novel first appeared, its subject—marriage between a white woman and an Indian—earned the writer some disparaging remarks. Within months, however, opinion had turned, and young Maria Francis enjoyed a season of celebrity in the salons of Boston, followed by a long career, first as a novelist, juvenile writer, and advice giver, later as a well-known antislavery journalist.[60]

In 1828 Maria married David Lee Child, a dreamy, impractical intellectual and a stubborn idealist. As his wife would soon discover, when David Child embraced a reform, he did so wholeheartedly, and usually in such a way that he alienated even potential supporters. When he tried his hand at business, he invariably chose the wrong time, the wrong place, or the wrong set of associates. Some of this was evident when she accepted his proposal, but its full implications took years for her to realize. Objectively, perhaps, she should have considered it just as well that no children appeared in this marriage, fraught as it was with such economic uncertainty. But in fact both she and David wished very much for children. Still, although her childlessness disappointed her, there is no evidence that she sought medical advice. Nor did she and David adopt, although apparently they considered doing so at one point.[61]

Lydia Maria Child had a rich and full career, and she also had all of the cares and anxieties of being the family breadwinner. Nevertheless, the thought of her and David's childlessness seemed never far from consciousness. In the first year or two of her marriage, she appeared relieved that there was no extra mouth to feed. Complaining to her sister-in-law Lydia B. Child about their financial woes, she suggested that, thank goodness, at least she was not yet pregnant—for the moment, there was "no prospect of anybody but ourselves to take care of."[62] But after another year had passed, and still no sign of pregnancy appeared, she wrote her mother-in-law, "I do wish I would be a mother, and that even more for my husband's sake than for my own. But God's will be done. I am certain that Divine Providence orders all things for our good." Her acceptance of the will of Providence never entirely assuaged her disappointment. In a letter congratulating her friends the Lorings on the news of Mrs. Loring's pregnancy, Child once again came face to face with her own sadness: "I never felt so forcibly as within the last year, that to a childless wife, 'life is almost untenanted.' " If in the early years of her marriage she seemed to think that fatherhood would have made David less irresponsible, she cherished no such illusions later on, tellingly remarking to her friend Sarah Shaw in 1859 that "my good David serves me for husband and 'baby and all.' " But she never ceased to regret her childlessness.[63]

Like Lydia Maria Child, Amelia Jenks Bloomer was a writer and editor, most remembered for the costume that still bears her name. Married at the age of twenty-two to editor Dexter Bloomer, she became a women's rights advocate and temperance reformer. Encouraged by a husband who admired her journalistic abilities, Amelia Bloomer, having written for several local and regional newspapers, became editor and publisher of the reformist *Lily* at its founding in 1848. She continued at this post until 1854, when she sold the paper in preparation for moving with her husband to what was then the frontier outpost of Council Bluffs, Iowa.[64]

While Lydia Maria Child either truly was rarely ill or minimized whatever health problems she may have had, Amelia Bloomer was often in what the nineteenth century referred to as "delicate health." Indeed, for the first year of her marriage she was repeatedly ill, suffering from "intermittent fever." (Intermittent fever was a general term that referred not just to malaria but also to a variety of ailments distinguished by fevers that came and went.) Whether any of her numerous trips to medicinal springs or various health resorts were related to her childlessness, neither she nor her husband disclosed. For whatever reason, for the first twenty years or so of her married life, Bloomer spent time at various health resorts; in her husband's recollections, she was often unwell.[65]

Amelia and Dexter Bloomer adopted two children—brother and sister—shortly after moving to Council Bluffs. Her husband recalled after her death that they had always had nieces or nephews staying with them from the early years of their marriage. But she, at least (he is reticent about his own feelings), wanted children of her own. When the Bloomers

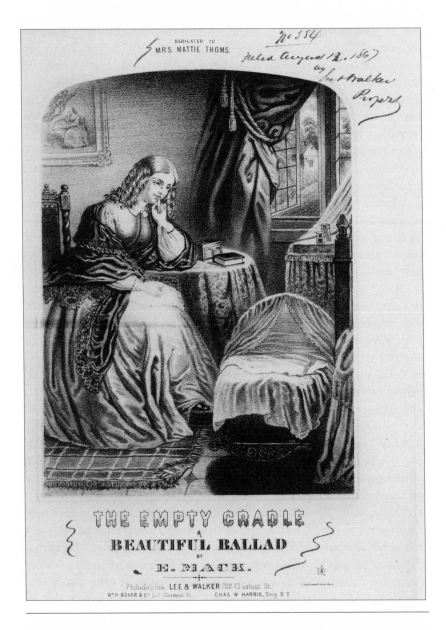

This is a sheet music cover; the lyrics that it accompanied appear to have been lost, but an "empty cradle," no matter how it came to be unfilled, evoked a poignant response. Lydia Maria Child, speaking from personal experience, told a friend that "to a childless wife, 'life is almost untenanted.' "

Courtesy of the Library of Congress

adopted their first child, she was thirty-seven and he thirty-nine. Shortly afterward, the little boy was joined by his younger sister. For the next several years Amelia concentrated most of her attention on her family and her home.[66] Upon selling the *Lily* she wrote, "Home and husband being dearer to us than all beside," her publishing career had become of "secondary importance." And although she remained involved in reform causes between 1855 and 1870, most of her activities were on the local level. Her adopted children would have been adolescents before she once again took on any major public responsibilities.[67]

Lydia Maria Child left behind professions of regret for her childlessness, but she accepted it as the will of Providence. Amelia Bloomer chose adoption as the only way to have children "of her own." Mary Boykin Chesnut did neither, but she seems to have suffered far more over her childlessness. Born into a distinguished South Carolina family—her father served as governor and later as a United States senator—Mary Boykin married James Chesnut when she was just seventeen. Her husband began a career in politics, and she herself made friends with the wives of rising Southerners, including Varina Davis, the wife of Jefferson Davis. Unlike Lydia Maria Child or Amelia Jenks Bloomer, Mary Chesnut was not a public figure during her lifetime. She became well known only after her death, as a result of her posthumously published Civil War diaries. During her own life, she was simply a childless wife in a prominent family.[68] In Mary Chesnut's world, large families were not just encouraged but expected. When she and James married, they planned for numerous children. Her failure to have any, according to her biographer, caused her "despondency." Friends apparently tried to keep up her spirits by urging her to continue to hope for a pregnancy, letting her know when friends conceived after long years of marriage.[69]

Constant remarks on her childlessness from her mother-in-law only worsened her feelings. She complained of the senior Mrs. Chesnut's "bragging *to me* with exquisite taste—me a childless wretch" of her numerous grandchildren. Even her father-in-law, "who rarely wounds me," could be insensitive, telling his wife in Mary's presence, "You must feel that you have not been useless in your day and generation. You have now twenty-seven great grandchildren." Mary was distraught. "God help me," she wrote, "no good have I done—to myself or any one else."[70]

Of these three women, Mary Chesnut seems to have found childlessness most painful, although her greater emotional expressiveness may have been as much a matter of personality as of greater depth of feeling. Mary Chesnut managed to conceive at least once and possibly more of-

ten, but she was unable to carry a pregnancy to term. Like Amelia
Bloomer, she often traveled to spas and health resorts—albeit more fashionable ones than Bloomer frequented—and she spent time in Philadelphia with her uncle, a prominent physician. Her sudden 1845 trip to Europe with James may have been as much in pursuit of pregnancy as
diversion. Alone of the three women she may have actively sought medical help, however unavailing. For her, childlessness was a tragedy, the
pain of which she tried to alleviate by "borrowing" the children of relatives for long extended visits. She may also have eased her pain through
drugs. Having suffered from what her physicians diagnosed as a heart
condition since her childhood, she continued to experience periodic bouts
of ill health that were severe enough to cause alarm in her family. Some
of her doctors prescribed opium, which it seems she took for her emotional as well as her physical pain.[71]

The experiences of these three women may be seen as emblematic of
the ways in which nineteenth-century women came to cope with involuntary childlessness. Lydia Maria Child accepted the will of the Lord with
sadness but resignation. Perhaps, having come of age nearly twenty years
before the other two women, she was the least touched by the cultural belief of the era that bearing children was the most glorious thing to which
a woman could aspire. Amelia and Dexter Bloomer chose to adopt, which
may seem like a very eighteenth-century solution to childlessness, but in
fact adoption was beginning to mean something different in the nineteenth century. The Bloomers' adopted children were not the orphans of
other family members, nor were they brought into an expansive household community. Rather, the Bloomers adopted in order to have their
"own" children, to complete their conjugal family. And Bloomer in fact
suspended her career as a national reformer until the children were nearly
grown, although she did not retire entirely into private life. Mary Chesnut probably sought medical help, having both the financial resources to
travel to the urban centers, where such help was increasingly becoming
available, and the desire, fueled by her own wishes and pressure from her
husband's family, to bear her own children.

Mary Chesnut—if she did indeed seek medical help—would have done
so just about the time that elite American physicians began to turn their
attention in earnest to the problem of infertility, influenced both by the
growing national anxiety about the fertility of American women and by

the new medical ideas making their way across the Atlantic from France. The first sign of what would become the dominant orientation among leading American practitioners was the appearance in 1844 of an American edition of a weighty French treatise, Vincent Mondat's *On Sterility in the Male and Female*.[72]

Elite American physicians, eager to discover a rational physiological basis on which to ground their understanding of the reproductive process, welcomed Mondat's emphasis on experimental science. As the first work on sterility based on the findings of Parisian anatomists and physiologists to appear in the United States, *On Sterility* exerted considerable influence on the ways in which "advanced" American practitioners began to approach the question of infertility just before midcentury. Mondat grappled with the still-controversial question of the role of ovum and semen in conception, maintaining on the basis of the physiological evidence that the ovists had been correct, because "the[ir] system . . . is more in accordance with the organic arrangement of the parts, and also with the laws of physiology." Mondat did acknowledge that it was difficult for men to accept the idea that "the man . . . co-operates in generation only in a secondary nature," but his convincing evidence against the animalculist position made it increasingly untenable. Indeed, within a few years it had disappeared from academic medicine.[73]

Mondat's principal contribution lay in his careful attempts to ground his explanations of the etiology of infertility on experimental findings in physiology and anatomy. As had generations before him, Mondat gave great weight to menstrual disorders; however, what was new was his interpretation of such disorders as manifestations of specific uterine pathology. So too with leucorrhea. Mondat, noting that this condition had been considered a cause of sterility since Hippocrates, linked it with blockages of the fallopian tubes. His therapies reflected these new ideas. Although he had not completely abandoned conventional therapeutics—he continued to recommend baths or blisters for leucorrhea—such prescriptions were overshadowed by his extensive use of instruments, the mark of a modern physician. As one of the first physicians to suggest that malposition of the uterus or cervix was a major cause of sterility, he treated such conditions with instruments placed in the uterus to realign it. These instruments were the forerunners of the modern sound, which is a thin rod inserted into the uterine cavity to measure its length.[74]

Mondat also developed instruments to treat male impotence, which he considered a rare but curable condition. Giving impotence the medical-sounding name of anaphrodisia, he diagnosed its causes as physiological ("systemic" diseases, malformations of the penis, and various disorders of the foreskin such as phimosis, which is a narrowing of the opening); psychological (excessive passion, hatred, jealousy, "violent love," and "excessive" masturbation); or intellectual (too much creative thought). To cure it he devised an instrument he called the congestor, a kind of vacuum pump used for local application of pressure on the penis. He sometimes supplemented such therapy with time-tested aphrodisiacs.[75]

The grounding of specific diagnoses for infertility in local pathologies and the use of instruments to treat such pathologies had become increasingly accepted in Europe by the 1840s. With the American publication, first, of the work of Mondat and, later, of English authority James Whitehead's *On the Causes and Treatment of Abortion and Sterility*, practitioners in the United States had access to the most advanced theoretical and practical information. In addition, as elite young American physicians increasingly rounded out their medical training with a tour of the hospitals of France where much of the new experimentation took place, they gained firsthand experience of the new methods for treating sterility.[76]

Within the next quarter of a century, these new ideas would fundamentally alter the treatment of infertility, at least among "advanced" practitioners whose careers were tied to the hospitals and elite medical schools in American cities. Infertility treatment would in fact become one way to counter the influence of the medical self-help movement, which had an especially firm hold on the women of the middle class.[77] Increasingly, as physicians began to locate the causes of infertility within the reproductive organs themselves, rather than ascribing the condition to a more general disequilibrium within the body, the efficacy of self-treatment would be called into question. Surgery and instrumentation, rather than diet and exercise, would become the dominant therapies as American physicians began one of their earliest ventures into high-technology medicine.

two

"Purely Surgical"?

*Technology, Instrumentation,
and the Redefinition of
Sterility at Midcentury*

The fact is, that most of the diseases of the uterus are as purely surgical as are those of the eye, and require the same nice discrimination of the true surgeon.

J. *Marion Sims*, 1866

A woman seeking medical help to become pregnant in almost any American city in 1850 most likely came away with advice to get more exercise and change her diet. If she complained as well of menstrual discomfort or leucorrhea, she might also receive a vaginal douche or a tonic. Almost any physician who had on hand some "nitrate of silver for ulcerations, . . . a cylindrical speculum, . . . astringent injection[s]," and perhaps a "Physics globe pessary" (used for uterine prolapse, or "falling of the womb") felt prepared to treat almost any known condition of the female reproductive system. But by 1870, should our hypothetical childless woman happen upon a practitioner who kept up with new medical developments, especially one associated with an urban voluntary hospital, she would probably find herself diagnosed with a defective cervix, for which the recommended treatment was surgery. In neither year would a physician have been likely to ask to see her husband. Although by the 1860s data on male sterility existed, physicians almost to a man (the gender-specific term is intentional) continued to believe that it was an extremely rare condition.[1]

In the course of these two decades, ideas about the proper treatment of the "diseases of women," as they were still called during the years just before the emergence of gynecology, changed dramatically. Technological developments, in the form of new instruments and surgical techniques, burst on the medical scene. Recamier's curette and the Sims speculum, as well as such exotic creations as the hysterotome, uterotome, uterine guillotine, and uterine injector provided new opportunities for seeing, and for reconfiguring, the interior of women's bodies. Controversial at first, the use of instrumentation and surgery on women's sexual organs became commonplace by the end of this period among physicians eager to establish themselves as experts in an emerging medical field. Dramatic innovations in the treatment of sterility—as elite physicians increasingly came to call the condition of involuntary childlessness—demonstrated the profound nature of the changes occurring in both the theory and the practice of physicians who treated women with reproductive disorders. Women themselves, apparently in increasing numbers, actively sought instrumental and surgical treatment, both demonstrating the existence of demand for these methods and encouraging more physicians to provide them. The "woman's surgeons" of the 1850s and 1860s, and the women who patronized them, had a profound impact on what would become the specialty of gynecology.

Few Americans could have predicted these new directions in 1850. Health reformers, many of them women, had just begun to savor what they saw as victory over the old medical establishment, with its heroic levels of bleeding and dosing. By midcentury, every state that had once instituted medical licensure had now repealed it. Anyone could call herself or himself a physician. Indeed, one of the earliest medical sects, founded by Samuel Thomson, had turned that possibility into a philosophy. Thomson had patented his system of botanical medicine in 1813, to which he sold "family rights."[2] But after his death, his followers battled over whether to hold to the founder's principles of self-education or to create Thomsonian medical schools. As the movement splintered, some Thomsonians established medical schools and institutes, as did the Eclectics, a rival botanical sect that absorbed much of the Thomsonian movement by the 1850s. As befitted their name, Eclectics incorporated noninvasive therapies from the various schools of "irregulars."[3] More prevalent than botanical medicine was hydropathy. Building on a long legacy of belief in the curative powers of health spas and incorporating a simple dietary philosophy, hydropathy had won over even a number of regular practitioners and claimed thousands of adherents among the middle-class women who, as both practitioners and patients, were the mainstay of the medical reform movement.[4]

By the 1850s, the medical self-help movement, fueled by distrust of the heroic medicine practiced by the medical establishment in the 1830s and 1840s, had become an established phenomenon itself. But at the same time that women were trooping by the thousands into the lecture halls in the name of medical self-knowledge, and institutions developing alternatives to conventional medicine flourished, a contrary trend—emanating from the clinics and morgues of Paris—gathered strength among the medical elite.

Regular medicine may have been in disfavor among large segments of the American population in the middle decades of the nineteenth century, but a corps of urban physicians, trained for the most part in Philadelphia, New York, and Massachusetts, was attempting to transform both the theory and the practice of American medicine. Beginning in the 1840s, young men from elite medical schools increasingly culminated their studies with a tour of the famous Parisian hospitals. In Paris, where the twin passions of dissection and statistics ruled, young Americans learned how physicians and surgeons, working side by side, correlated the lesions found at autopsy with the symptoms of living patients. The French had discarded classical medical doctrine for the gritty insights of clinical observation and postmortem examination, collecting and analyzing their findings statistically. It was the French who first developed instruments for examining, then probing, the body. The first stethoscope came into use in France in 1816.[5]

The young Americans who made the pilgrimage to Paris, and those who kept up with the developments abroad in the medical literature, began to question their profession's long-held belief in systemic pathology and to move toward an emphasis on the local causes of disease. Until the mid-1850s elite American physicians, in contrast to their French mentors, gave more than lip service to the value of the older therapeutic traditions; nevertheless, they welcomed the new findings as diagnostic revelations.[6] Moving in a direction exactly opposite from the currently popular trends in medicine—self-knowledge and in some cases self-treatment—these practitioners laid claim to a new professional expertise.

French medicine had a significant impact on American physicians interested in the diseases of women in this era. Free from the prudery and squeamishness that surrounded much of American and British medical treatment of women, the French proclaimed their intention to solve the mysteries of the physiological processes that governed the reproductive process. The high mortality rate in the great French hospitals gave anatomists a continuing supply of bodies. Dissecting the reproductive organs of women who died in their childbearing years, they searched for signs of ovulation. To the Americans who came to study there, some of whom might never have seen a woman's internal organs, Parisian medicine was a revelation.[7]

One such American, Augustus Gardner, would play an important role in transforming medical views of sterility. In 1856, a few years after returning from Paris, he brought out his *On the Causes and Curative Treatment of Sterility, with a Preliminary Statement of the Physiology of Generation*.[8] In Paris, Gardner had learned that local disorders of the reproductive system formed the principal impediments to conception. Among these conditions, he believed, were polyps in the uterus, lacerations and "ulcerations" of the cervix, and what he called a "stricture" of the cervix. To treat them he used invasive therapies: silver wire to ligate polyps, a procedure in which the wire was tightened around the base of the polyp; metal dilators or sponge tents to open the cervix; and occasionally the use of "a short pointed knife" to enlarge the cervical os. But Gardner did not abandon old therapeutics entirely. Like many well-trained physicians of his generation, Gardner incorporated the new insights he had gained in France with the time-tested remedies he had learned in medical school. Hence he continued to employ silver nitrate for cervical lesions; for "chronic congestion" of the pelvic organs, a term used for generalized pelvic pain or discomfort, he recommended cathartics as well as the application of leeches to the external abdominal region and sometimes to the cervix itself.[9]

Gardner was concerned with the causes and prevention as well as the cure of sterility. Drawing on a belief among some Paris-trained physicians that disorders of the digestive system lay behind a number of conditions that were seemingly unrelated, Gardner emphasized what he surmised was a physiological connection between the ovaries and the digestive system. He thereby developed an explanation for menstrual complaints that, while it relied not on classical humoral medicine but on pathologies in specific organs, nevertheless called for some therapies that his more old-fashioned colleagues could easily recognize. To treat menstrual dysfunctions that might later lead to sterility, and to prevent them altogether, he recommended a balanced diet and regular exercise. Other conditions that predisposed a woman to sterility, such as "chronic congestion of the pelvis," he believed, were due not to poor health habits but rather to contraceptive measures taken in the early years of marriage, or worse yet, an abortion. Prevention of sterility required practitioners to warn young women of the dangers of faulty diets and sedentary habits, the evil results of all contraceptive measures, and the long-term consequence of procuring an abortion in the early years of married life.[10]

Gardner's book, a good summary of the ideas about sterility current among elite American practitioners, presented new diagnoses and a combination of old and new treatments. It also refuted the idea that a woman's orgasm was necessary for conception, defining impregnation as a chemical or mechanical process that was neither enhanced nor inhibited by a woman's sexual pleasure. Nevertheless, Gardner remained dissatisfied with his inability to explain how conception occurred in the first place, knowledge that would seem to be necessary to understand the physiological basis of infertility. Most importantly, the exact manner in which sperm and ovum came together remained obscure. "The laborious embryologist," Gardner wrote, "in vain traces the spermatozoon in its path, and even when the microscope reveals him at his final entrance into the ovum—how the new creation is effected is still a mystery above the ken of ordinary mortals." On the question of whether sterility affected men as well as women, Gardner suspected, but was not entirely convinced, that it was possible, in rare cases, for a man to be sterile even if he were capable of ejaculation. Eager to know more, Gardner was nonetheless cautious not to claim greater expertise than he actually believed he possessed. As a result, his prescriptions combined the new with the old, the invasive with the benign.[11]

Practitioners such as Gardner would seem to have faced an uphill battle for the hearts and minds of America's infertile women, although if the advertisements for a plethora of proprietary "cures" are any indication, a clear demand for infertility therapies existed. Pitches of charlatans for "female cordials" or "female specifics" preyed on the childless. These drug hucksters ranged from the likes of Charles Lohman, the husband of abortionist Madame Restell, who sold both fertility pills and abortifacients by mail, to medical school graduates in search of an easy fortune such as J. A. Rose of Philadelphia. Rose, who manufactured the "Fem

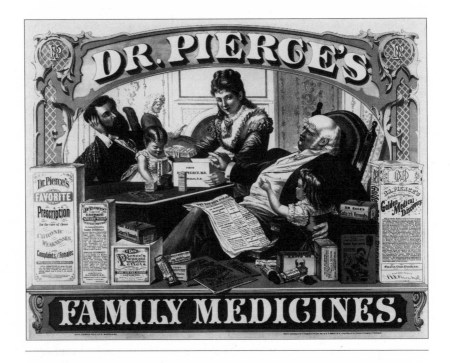

Proprietary medicines for "female weakness" and infertility abounded in the mid- to late nineteenth century; they went by the names of "female cordials" and "female specifics." Courtesy of the Library of Congress

Specific," promised his "married and barren" customers that "after a proper and regular use of this valuable compound" they would surely produce "healthy children." And if not? "As many neglect themselves until a cure is hopeless," the pills "may occasionally fail," and in that case a woman had no one to blame but herself.[12]

Besides the proprietary products hawked by hucksters, women had access to the prescriptions of medical sectarians and alternative healers, who offered variations of time-honored treatments easily comprehensible to the women who took them. Typical Thomsonian remedies for conditions causing barrenness were evan root or unicorn root tonics. Eclectics recommended a tonic of black cobosh with hartshorn and alcohol. For habitual miscarriage the phrenologist Orson Fowler, who was well known in hydropathy circles, suggested a tea made from "squaw vine, an evergreen growing in most woods." The treatment was so popular, Fowler noted, that a number of urban drug stores marketed it under the name "Mother's Cordial." Some hydropathists also recommended alternating hot and cold wraps in sheeting, along with a healthful diet that excluded alcohol, tea, and coffee.[13]

Joel Shew, one of the American founders of the water cure movement, who may have earned a regular M.D. degree before his conversion to hydropathy, warned women to be suspicious of any invasive treatment. In *Midwifery and the Diseases of Women,* he insisted that no woman suffering from any "organic disease," by which he meant a local pathology, could ever conceive; she should instead accept her childless state. But if she had an unspecified "functional" condition, she might become pregnant "by invigorating the general health" through regular use of the water cure, very moderate indulgence in sexual pleasures, and "strict temperance in all things." If such treatment did not enable her to conceive, Shew was fond of saying, she would at the very least enjoy better health.[14]

Of course, there had always been a gap between the therapies of regular physicians and alternative healers. In the colonial era, midwives and physicians alike may have prescribed herbal remedies; but in general, only physicians used the lancet. What was different in the nineteenth century was that both regulars and sectarians *defined* themselves in opposition to one another, with the sectarians laying claim to the mantle of democratic medicine and the regulars to expertise.[15] In the mid–nineteenth century, the irregulars drew much of their strength from the proposition that their therapies were milder, more effective, and more easily understood by the people who resorted to them than the "heroic" measures of the regulars. This was as true for treatments for sterility as for other conditions. But with the growing influence of anatomy among elite regulars and the advent of new instruments for probing the bodies of living patients, the regulars could begin to claim—whether accurately or not is for the moment beside the point—that they now could diagnose and treat sterility in ways that older systemic therapeutics could not, and that such treatment required specialized skills that only the professional could acquire.[16]

This new philosophy was the precursor of gynecology, which would not fully emerge as a medical specialty until the last three decades of the nineteenth century. Before there were gynecologists, however, there were "woman's surgeons." And in terms of the history of infertility, two of the most important woman's surgeons were J. Marion Sims and Thomas Addis Emmet of the Woman's Hospital in New York, the first hospital devoted exclusively to the surgical treatment of the disorders of women's reproductive systems.[17]

The Surgical Solution: J. Marion Sims and the Woman's Hospital

Although J. Marion Sims did not appear to be thinking of infertile women when he dreamed of creating a "woman's hospital," curing sterility soon became one of his consuming interests and remained at the core of his radical ideas about how to treat the disorders of the female reproductive system. In the United States, Sims—often called the father of gynecology—is the pivotal figure in the transformation of the treatment of infertility in the 1850s and 1860s. He was a controversial one as well, both in his own time and in ours. Some historians have hailed Sims as a benefactor to suffering women; others have damned him a reckless experimenter who subjected women to surgical onslaughts on what often proved to be, in hindsight, physiologically normal organs. Although his first biographer, Seale Harris, respectfully entitled his work *Woman's Surgeon,* his second, Deborah Kuhn McGregor, more pointedly called hers *Sexual Surgery.*[18]

Sims himself claimed that he became a "woman's surgeon" by accident. Born in South Carolina in 1813, he chose a career in medicine over the objections of his father, who did not consider medicine to be either respectable or lucrative enough for a young southern gentleman of extravagant habits and limited means. The elder Sims knew full well that with little family money, young James Marion would have to make it on his own. Disregarding parental desires, Sims began his medical studies in South Carolina in 1833. The next year, following in the wake of a number of aspiring southern physicians, he moved to Philadelphia to take his medical degree at Jefferson Medical School in 1835. He then returned home and married Theresa Jones, his childhood sweetheart. After having tried and failed to make a living in his native South Carolina, he moved to Alabama, settling first in the small town of Mount Meigs and later moving to Montgomery.[19]

The early years were difficult. Sims found the fierce competition among physicians unsettling and the practice of medicine both boring and unrewarding. From the outset of his career, he preferred the quick results of surgery to the tediousness of general medical practice. If an operation went well, its results were immediate and often dramatic; early in his ca-

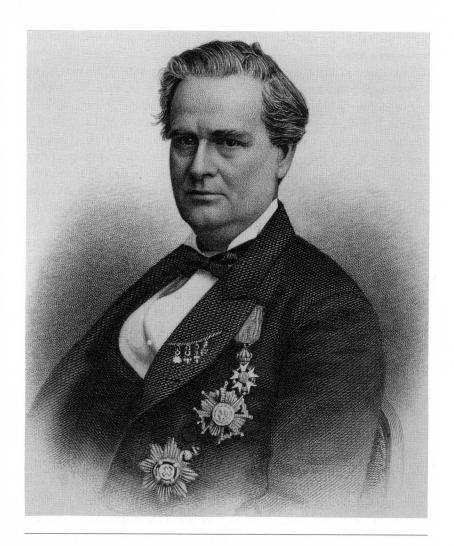

J. Marion Sims, a pivotal figure in the transformation of infertility treatment in the 1850s
and 1860s
Courtesy of the College of Physicians of Philadelphia

reer he performed a number of operations for facial deformities that
brought him considerable local reputation. At this stage in his career, he
showed a distaste not only for obstetrics (in fact, he avoided obstetrics his
entire career) but also for the very idea of concerning himself in any way
with women's reproductive organs. "If there was anything I hated," he

later recalled of his early career, "it was investigating the organs of the female pelvis."[20]

Sims's first venture into gynecological surgery came at the request of several local planters. Among the enslaved women on their plantations were a number who, having undergone very difficult childbirths, suffered from vesico-vaginal fistula. Sims agreed to treat them and soon had a number of these women in a makeshift "hospital" in his Montgomery back yard. Within a few years Sims became the first physician ever to succeed in curing this exceedingly disagreeable condition, then a rather common complication in childbirth. (A vesico-vaginal fistula, which is an abnormal passage or connection between the vagina and the bladder, results from prolonged labor that fails to progress.) This condition was no respecter of social or economic status. In Sims's case, his earliest patients were slaves, and once he moved to the North many of his later ones were poor Irish immigrants, but physicians saw fistulas in their private practices as well. Historians have suggested that rickets, a vitamin deficiency that often causes pelvic deformity, was the chief underlying culprit. In Sims's day, some physicians blamed these fistulas on excessive and inexpert use of forceps during delivery, while others claimed that an early forceps intervention could prevent their occurrence. For centuries physicians had been trying without success to cure the condition, which doomed a woman to experience constant leakage into the vagina from the bladder. (A related condition was recto-vaginal fistula, resulting in leakage of feces into the vagina. A woman might have one or both.) While not life-threatening, fistulas caused women constant discomfort and rendered normal life impossible.[21]

By his own account, Sims refused to operate on the young enslaved women until he became convinced that he could do so successfully. At that point, according to Seale Harris, creating the appropriate surgical technique became "almost a monomania with him." Repeated failure did not deter him. Without anesthesia but with a heavy postoperative use of opium, he operated over and over again on Lucy, Betsey, Anarcha, and others. In 1849, after thirty operations on Anarcha in four years, he finally succeeded in repairing her fistula. By that time, some of his neighbors and fellow physicians were expressing their horror and shock at such experimentation: "All kinds of whispers were beginning to circulate around town—dark rumors that it was a terrible thing . . . to keep on using human beings as experimental animals for . . . unproven surgical theories." But others shrugged off the suffering of the women when the operation proved successful. Sims himself, confident that he had made a major medical advance that was of benefit to women, felt assured that this operation would make both his reputation and his fortune. We have only Sims's account of the views of the women on whom the surgery was performed; they pressed him, he claimed, for relief from their condition and begged him to keep trying. In reality, of course, they lacked the power to say no, whatever they wished.[22]

When Sims published his classic article, "On the Treatment of Vesico-Vaginal Fistula," in 1852, he chose not to mention that his patients were slaves, betraying either his own misgivings or his recognition that physicians outside the slaveholding South would probably be even more appalled than his southern neighbors had been. Those historians who have retrospectively castigated him have argued that his main concern in devising this operation was to make his name (not to mention his fortune) in medicine, that he tortured the women on whom he operated by refusing to use anesthesia, and that because the women were enslaved they had absolutely no power to consent to or refuse the operation. Sims's defenders have said in response that he actually cured, through surgical ingenuity and resourcefulness, a condition that had ruined women's lives for centuries.

It is absolutely true that Sims both operated on women without the power to say no and that he adhered to the racist, and commonly held, assumption that blacks suffered pain less acutely than whites. The anesthesia issue is a little more complicated. His decision not to use it in the 1840s, when it had just been introduced into medical practice, was not predicated on the fact that his patients were black or enslaved. Sims fully intended to perform the operation on white southern women without anesthesia as well, but they found the pain intolerable. As a result, these women simply did not undergo the operation. There were two reasons for his early unwillingness to employ anesthesia. First, his operative technique in these years required the patient to be awake in order to cooperate in the surgery; second, he still believed that anesthesia was riskier than the surgery. He said later that vesico-vaginal fistula surgery was "not painful enough" for him to take either the "trouble" or the "risk" attending the early use of anesthesia. In fact, not until the late 1860s did he employ anesthesia for this operation.[23]

Sims's successful treatment of vesico-vaginal fistula led almost directly to the founding of the Woman's Hospital. There, Sims's intellectual predilection, formed in Alabama—that the overwhelming majority of the diseases of the female reproductive system were structural and therefore curable by surgery—hardened into dogma. It may seem a long way from vesico-vaginal fistula to infertility treatment. But the instruments and techniques that Sims developed as he worked his way to a cure for fistula not only provided the technical tools that he would use in his other reproductive surgery but also led him to formulate a theoretical perspective that guided his subsequent career and would have special pertinence to the treatment of sterility.

Following his surgical successes in Alabama, Sims moved to New York in 1852. Keenly ambitious, he was eager to show off his fistula cure and receive widespread acclaim. Initially, he met disappointment. Perhaps he underestimated the clannishness of the New York medical establishment; but as a southerner and a man with somewhat more than his share of pride, he found a chilly reception. Sims himself attributed the coolness to jealousy, but it was equally possible that skepticism toward his surgical claims more accurately defined the attitude of New York's elite practitioners. Sims complained bitterly that local physicians invited him to perform his new operation, observed his technique, then cast him aside. But many of them thought both that he was too free with the knife and that his claims for the success of his surgery were overblown.[24]

The upstart newcomer had an alternative plan. When his initial overtures to prominent physicians did not bring the desired results, Sims, cleverly bypassing them, turned directly to a group of women philanthropists, a few of them wealthy, and all of them well-connected. Led by Sarah Platt Doremus, the women rose to the challenge of fundraising. The moving spirit behind the hospital, Doremus counseled Sims about how to persuade prominent and influential women to serve on the Board of Lady Managers and used her own considerable influence to gain legislative and financial support for the institution. Married to a New York merchant and the mother of nine children, she was a tireless reformer and charity organizer. One physician called her a "remarkable" woman "who devot[ed] her life to the service of others." Doremus was as clever as she was good, persuading her friends and coworkers in charitable causes to join forces with her in this new venture.[25]

Doremus and her allies built the Woman's Hospital and appointed Sims its chief surgeon. The new hospital differed markedly from the "lying in" hospitals to which poor women usually turned for their health needs. Not only was there no maternity ward, but the hospital devoted itself strictly to surgical cases involving the reproductive organs. Although Sims's patrons initially had intended to dedicate the facility solely to the cure of vesico-vaginal fistula, Sims himself very quickly enlarged its scope to encompass a full range of "woman's surgery." This "afterthought," as

Thomas Emmet later called it, had enormous influence on the early development of gynecology.[26]

In theory, Sims reported to the Board of Lady Managers, who supposedly ran the hospital; nevertheless, in the early years he generally managed to get his own way. His first victory was to convince the board to reverse its ruling that he hire a woman as his assistant surgeon. The Lady Managers' choice had been Emily Blackwell, Elizabeth Blackwell's younger sister, who had trained abroad under the great obstetrician-surgeon James Y. Simpson. Sims talked the Lady Managers out of their plan. Whether he did so because he disliked the idea of working with a woman, or because he chafed at the prospect of being observed by a young doctor whose formal training was better than his, must be left to speculation. What is clear is that he persuaded the board to let him appoint twenty-seven-year-old Thomas Addis Emmet as assistant surgeon. Not until the twentieth century would a woman physician practice at the Woman's Hospital.[27]

When the new hospital opened its doors at 83 Madison Avenue in May 1855, Sims intended for it to serve both the "worthy poor," who would occupy "free beds," and middle-class paying patients. Wealthy patients, however, would receive their treatment in these early years in the more luxurious accommodations at Sims's private "hospital." (Emmet would open a similar establishment in 1862.) The women who came to the new hospital in the 1850s and 1860s, the only period for which original case records exist, suffered from a number of complaints. Complications related to childbirth, including fistulas and lacerations of various kinds, were common. Childless wives suffered from pelvic pain, sterility, and dysmenorrhea. Young unmarried women complained of menstrual disorders. Sims performed at least one clitoridectomy (removal of the clitoris) on a young single woman suffering, so her record indicated, from dysmenorrhea. The most serious cases were the women who had large ovarian tumors. Antiseptic surgery had not been adopted, and in these years surgeons usually opened the abdomen to remove an ovary only when a patient's life seemed in imminent danger. In such major operations mortality was high.[28]

Determined to showcase his surgical skills and to show up the New York medical establishment, Sims lost no opportunity to boast of his many "cures" for vesico-vaginal fistula. But what was a cure? Surely not a life free from recurrence, if the fate of Mary Smith, the hospital's first patient, is any indication. After Sims operated on her fistula, the repair held for a few years. In fact, Mrs. Smith became well enough to take a

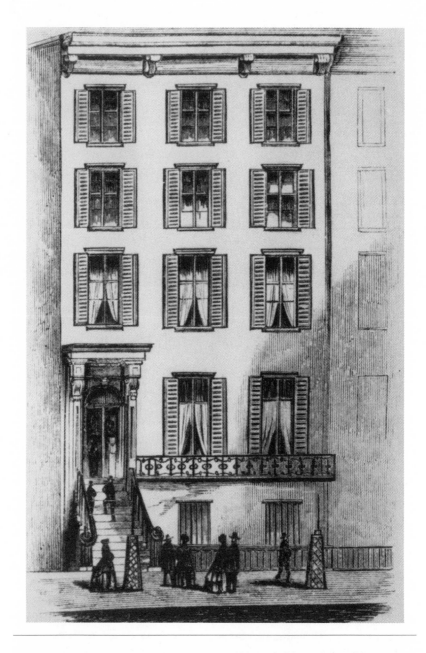

The Woman's Hospital, where Sims began his rise to prominence, opened its doors in 1855 at 83 Madison Avenue. By the 1870s, the hospital had outgrown this building, and a larger and more modern one was constructed.
Courtesy of the College of Physicians of Philadelphia

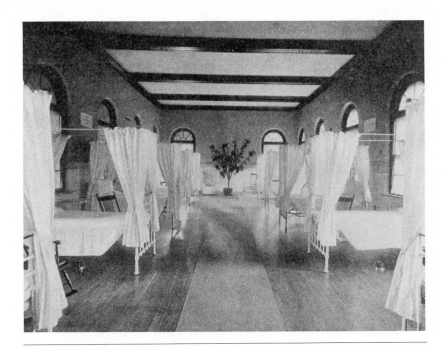

An endowed ward of "free beds" at the new Woman's Hospital, constructed in the 1870s. Women unable to pay for their medical care, including infertility patients, would occupy such beds.
Courtesy of the College of Physicians of Philadelphia

nursing job in the hospital. But her condition had been particularly severe, and eventually problems arose, leading all told to thirty operations of various kinds. Finally she refused to have any more surgery, although Emmet later tried to persuade her that he had devised a new technique that would permanently alleviate her problem. Mrs. Smith was both "cured" many times and never cured, ending her days as a street beggar, unable to work. In a tragic footnote to an unfortunate life, Emmet later recalled, she was killed in a street accident. Even though Mary Smith's case was unusual, as the very fact that her sufferings continued to haunt Emmet for decades indicates, it was not uncommon for a woman to be operated on two or three times and each time to be listed as cured. To put it mildly, the brisk notation at the end of most of the records in the casebooks, "discharged cured," cannot always be taken at face value.[29]

But to Sims, Emmet, and the young surgeons whom they trained at the

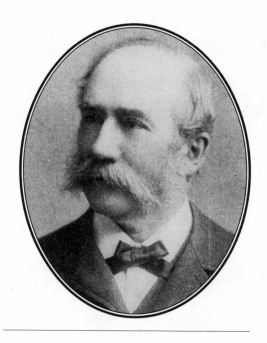

Thomas Addis Emmet, Sims's assistant and later Surgeon in Chief at the Woman's Hospital. He remained associated with the hospital until the end of the nineteenth
century.
Courtesy of the College of Physicians of Philadelphia

Woman's Hospital, relapses were in the unknown future, when new techniques would fix the problems of the old; "cures" were in the present—
cases of vesico-vaginal fistulas repaired, or severe dysmenorrhea alleviated. Sometimes a major operation even saved the life of a patient.
Confident of their abilities, they saw themselves as an innovative breed of
technologically sophisticated practitioners, using new instruments to create a window onto a malleable internal world.

Neither Sims nor Emmet ever explained how their interest in treating
sterility developed. True, they had new tools. The Sims speculum, which
he had designed and perfected in order to facilitate visual control during
surgery for vesico-vaginal fistula, had potential as a diagnostic tool as
well. Now that they could literally see into at least part of a woman's reproductive system, they may have believed that they could discover the
source of her involuntary childlessness. Given the prevalence of the cult
of motherhood, the gnawing fears about the fertility of American women,

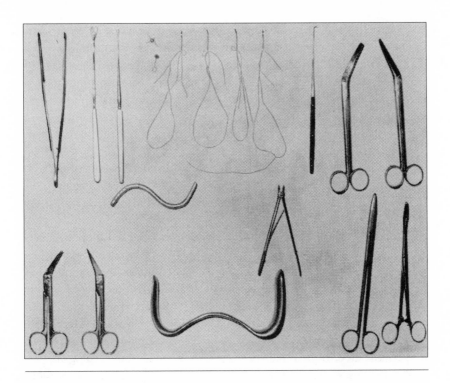

These surgical instruments belonged to J. Marion Sims. The instrument at the lower center
of the page is the famous Sims speculum, which he designed to facilitate the operation for
vesico-vaginal fistula.
Courtesy of the College of Physicians of Philadelphia

the growing interest among elite practitioners in the subject, and these
new instruments that opened up internal vistas, such a scenario is easy to
envisage. Sims said only that the plight of his childless patients moved him
to compassion. Glorying in his own large and loving family, he believed
that for both men and women, children were the greatest source of happiness. Emmet, a convert to Catholicism and a devoted family man, was
always very sympathetic to women unable to conceive. Their hospital
population, which included a number of childless married women who
came to them complaining of dysmenorrhea and leucorrhea as well as
sterility, provided ready-made opportunities for observation and experimentation. The sheer numbers of such women, in addition to their private patients, also enabled Sims to make generalizations about the causes
of infertility.[30]

It is also possible that Sims and Emmet were responding at least in part to unexpected patient demands. Although no specific data for New York City are available, in mid-nineteenth-century Boston nearly 20 percent of marriages among the city's least well-off were childless, as were some 13 percent of the marriages of the well-to-do.[31] The fact that childlessness was more prevalent among the indigent than the affluent contravenes commonly held nineteenth-century assumptions about the "overly prolific" working classes; nevertheless, if New York were like Boston, then Sims and his protégés might easily have seen substantial numbers of childless women in their hospital practice.

The philanthropic women who financed the Woman's Hospital surely were not thinking about ways to encourage the poor to have more children as they canvassed the city for funds to create the hospital, and perhaps J. Marion Sims really was thinking only of the accidents of parturition when he first turned his attention to pelvic surgery. But convinced as he had become that the vast majority of diseases of women were curable only by surgery, his conclusion that sterility required a surgical solution was probably inevitable. Sims revolutionized medical ideas about infertility, and in the process ushered in a wave of technological innovation that contributed to the rapid emergence of the field of gynecology.

Before Sims, American physicians had tended to be very cautious about treating infertility surgically, and the most ambitious surgical treatments were performed abroad. For example, in 1849 London practitioner W. Tyler Smith reported on three daring but unsuccessful attempts to open blocked fallopian tubes through dilatation.[32] Sims never attempted this particular operation, but his approach to infertility treatment clearly relied almost exclusively on surgical and instrumental therapies, and he consistently asserted the superiority of these techniques to all others. "The fact is," he insisted, "that most of the diseases of the uterus are as purely surgical as are those of the eye, and require the same nice discrimination of the true surgeon."[33]

In his early years in New York, Sims varied his surgical techniques constantly. Emmet once protested that no one could learn from Sims, since he operated so quickly, never explained what he did, and never performed the same procedure in the same way twice.[34] But if his techniques varied, his basic ideas did not. To him, a woman's reproductive system was a machine; if it failed to function properly, then a surgeon was needed to repair—or in some cases rebuild—the malfunctioning part. Sims was not alone in his observation that severe dysmenorrhea seemed to accompany sterility, but he was the most absolute in his conviction that its cause almost invariably was a mechanical defect in the cervical canal.

The cervix is the passageway to the uterus. Its opening to the vagina is called the external os; that to the uterus, the internal os. The cervical canal lies between each os. As Sims saw it, in cases of dysmenorrhea either the canal was "flexed" in such a way as to cause a backup in the passage of menstrual fluid or the cervical os was too small to allow its free passage. "I lay it down as an axiom," he proclaimed in his major treatise, "that there can be no dysmenorrhea, properly speaking . . . [without] some mechanical obstacle to the egress of the flow at some point between the os internum and the os externum, or throughout the whole cervical canal." And the most common conditions, he was sure, were "a contracted os and a narrowed cervical canal or a flexed one."[35]

And if the menstrual blood had difficulty flowing outward, Sims argued, then sperm would have equal difficulty entering the uterus. The idea of obstruction was not particularly novel in itself. But many of Sims's colleagues in elite medical circles, who agreed that obstructions might sometimes exist, nevertheless disagreed both with the idea that they were the principal cause of sterility and with the conclusion that surgery was the proper way to treat infertility in general. Dilatation with sponge tents or steel dilators, many argued, worked equally well and was less dangerous. If they did resort to surgery, it was in the context of a philosophy of treatment that accorded the knife simply one role—and often a small one—in their overall practices. Although Sims appears to have won Augustus Gardner to a belief in the superiority of surgery over dilatation by 1860, others were not so easily persuaded. Sometimes the fact that they had technologies of their own to protect conditioned their views. Hugh Hodge, for example, who invented one of the nineteenth century's most popular pessaries, understandably remained convinced that such devices offered the best cure for "sterile dysmenorrhea." And when pessaries failed, Hodge turned next to gradual dilatation.[36]

Sims and Emmet did not agree with this school of thought. Cervical incision, and sometimes amputation, were called for whenever they discovered, by peering at the cervix with the aid of the Sims speculum, conditions that they called the conoid cervix, anteflexion of the cervical canal, or a "pinhole os."[37] To a modern practitioner, what Sims called a conoid or conical cervix looks perfectly normal anatomically, and a diagnosis of cervical anteflexion might be insignificant. The "pinhole os," however, may be normal in a woman who has never borne children, or it may have resulted from repeated pelvic infections. Some of these women probably did have true cervical stenosis, which could have been brought on by infection. They may have had gonorrhea.

Indeed, judging from the symptoms described by a number of Sims's sterile patients, a modern physician would most likely suspect the gonococcus. Time after time the case records reveal a young married woman, perhaps in her twenties or early thirties, who had always been in excellent health, with regular and painless periods, until the time of her marriage. Within a few months of their weddings, these women suffered at least one instance of crippling pelvic pain, followed by months or years of persistent discomfort; many also complained of chronic leucorrhea; and they were childless. In such cases, examinations usually disclosed "chronic inflammation" and an "indurated cervix uteri." By the 1890s many physicians would have diagnosed gonorrhea, but in the 1850s and 1860s virtually no doctor believed that an asymptomatic man could transmit gonorrhea, or that the disease had long-term medical consequences.[38]

When he first began to incise the cervix, Sims tried a variety of methods. Sometimes he removed the posterior lip of the cervix, sometimes the anterior. In later years, he, Emmet, and the young surgeons at the Woman's Hospital most often performed a bilateral incision using new instruments that Sims had devised—special scissors used for snipping away at the cervical tissue, and the angle-cutting uterotome.[39] Sims sometimes amputated the cervix. He might have done it more often, he later reported, but apparently his patients balked, especially when they learned that one woman had died after having the surgery. Altogether he performed only fifty amputations compared to "hundreds" of incisions. His colleagues, he said, expressed disapproval of amputation, warning him that it was more likely to prevent than to enhance the chances of pregnancy. (It would, of course, make a miscarriage more likely if a patient did conceive.) Sims held on to his own opinion, however, refusing to accept the criticism of "my medical friends," although he had only two cases of pregnancy to cite in rebuttal. In spite of his own lack of success, he remained convinced "that if amputation had been performed in many cases in which I simply cut the cervix open, conception might have occurred where it has not."[40]

Sims and Emmet had begun to treat sterility both at the Woman's Hospital and in private practice as early as 1856. Their patients were immigrants and native-born Americans, middle class and working class. Some came from a considerable distance to be treated by Sims, and one physician's wife came from New England specifically to be under Emmet's

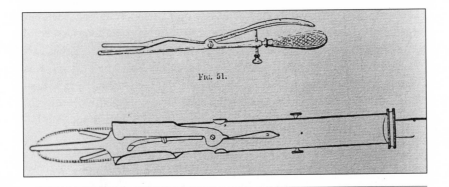

Two versions of the uterotome, which was used to incise the cervix. The original, shown above, could incise only one-half of the cervix at a time. The modified instrument, below, had double blades.
From *Clinical Notes on Uterine Surgery*, 1873 edition

care. Sims's southern connections brought him at least one patient from Georgia.[41]

Thirty-year-old Mary Boyle was a typical hospital case. An Irish immigrant, she had been married for six years when she sought treatment for dyspareunia (painful intercourse) and "sterile dysmenorrhea" in 1858. The case records do not show who admitted or first treated her, the flamboyant and self-assured Sims or the more solemn and circumspect Emmet. The doctors performed the common procedure of cervical incision in order to make its opening into the vagina larger.[42] Mrs. Boyle did not receive anesthesia for this procedure. Until after the Civil War, Sims and Emmet remained doubtful of the safety of anesthesia, using it only for extraordinary procedures such as ovariotomy (one of the two nineteenth-century terms for removal of the ovaries). After her surgery, the doctors kept her at the hospital for a month, when they sent her home to await her next menstrual period. She returned on March 19, "having," according to Emmet's notes, "just menstruated almost entirely free from pain for the first time in her life."[43]

If it were true, as Sims believed, that most dysmenorrhea and sterility resulted from a mechanical blockage of the cervix, this operation to widen the opening should have been enough both to alleviate Mary Boyle's pain and to enable her to conceive. However, even though upon examination the doctors were able to pass "the largest sound" into her uterus "without difficulty," they could not assure her that the opening had been enlarged enough to enable her to conceive. She decided to undergo a second operation "in order to facilitate conception." This time, "the canal was more freely dilated by a lateral incision on each side and [the incision] was extended well up into the body of the organ." Her second stay in the hospital lasted eleven days. On March 30, she was discharged with this notation: "Cured. Dr. Sims." The records do not tell us whether she ever became pregnant.[44]

Some patients underwent preliminary procedures prior to operations on the cervix. In December of 1856, Canadian-born Josephine Walker, twenty-nine years old, came from Connecticut to consult Sims for her infertility. Married since the age of seventeen, she also complained of dysmenorrhea, headaches, and back pains. On December 5, Sims dilated her os and used Recamier's curette to scrape out her uterus. Two weeks later, when they examined her again, her os remained closed. Next, he or Emmet incised her os on one side. Mid-January found her still in the hospital, her os still "not sufficiently dilated." So, Sims "redrilled the opening."[45]

Mrs. Boyle and Mrs. Walker were not the only women subjected to more than one operation. It was possible for a patient to spend the better part of a year either undergoing surgery or recovering from it. Annie Tyler, for example, one of Sims's private patients, had a complete cervical incision in February 1858 at his personal "hospital." In March he moved her to the Woman's Hospital, where she underwent a lateral incision. Despite being "discharged cured" at the end of March, she returned in November, still not pregnant. This time, Sims "divid[ed] the posterior lip directly backward toward the union of the vagina and neck." Once more, she was discharged "cured."[46] Some women received surgical treatments even when they had no obvious symptoms, such as dysmenorrhea or chronic pelvic pain, that might account for their sterility. Lydia Miller, for example, the thirty-six-year-old wife of a New England physician, childless after fourteen years of marriage, complained of nothing but her inability to conceive. Emmet noted in his case report that "her chief desire is to become a mother, . . . and . . . an operation was her only hope of relief."[47]

The medical complaints of the patients offer no clues about why Sims or Emmet chose one type of incision over another in these operations. It is possible that, believing as they did that there existed a uniform correct appearance of the cervix, their goal was to reshape each woman's cervix by altering or removing whatever caused the deviation from that appearance. Or they might simply have been engaging in a trial-and-error process. After Sims returned from Europe with considerably enlarged experience, the operation became more standardized. All told, Sims reported, he had performed hundreds of cervical incisions at the Woman's Hospital and many more than that in his private practice. They were not all done to cure sterility, of course; some young unmarried women underwent the operation for dysmenorrhea. Sims remained convinced, however, that dysmenorrhea invariably signaled impaired fertility. It may well be that a diagnosis of dysmenorrhea simply masked an actual complaint of infertility. Many women, after all, considered their childlessness a bitter misfortune; to have a painful physical condition as its cause might have eased their emotional burden.[48]

At the close of many of the files of infertility cases at the Woman's Hospital Emmet or one of the other surgeons made the notation, "discharged cured." This did not mean that the patient had become pregnant, but only that the os was opened, the cervical canal straightened, and any of the infections that the surgery itself often generated had been alleviated. A number of the women were "cured" several times. We did not see a resultant pregnancy mentioned anywhere in the case notes. One might legitimately wonder, therefore, on what empirical basis the confidence of Sims and Emmet rested. Neither of them was ever concerned with obstetrics. They appeared never to have done any follow-up. If a patient conceived, they would know about it only if she informed them. But there were obviously some pregnancies. In the *Clinical Notes,* Sims often concluded a case discussion with mention of a successful pregnancy. And since modern infertility practitioners well know even today that they may have as many cases of unexplained pregnancy as they do of unexplained infertility, such results in Sims's practice should come as no surprise.[49]

Nevertheless, it is impossible to say why Sims did not attempt in any systematic way to analyze his patients' success either in conceiving or in giving birth. Since he did statistical studies of uterine fibroids, it cannot be argued that he never thought in statistical terms; for whatever reason, however, he left behind no quantitative data to confirm his confidence in his procedures. And, in fact, much of Sims's surgery for infertility was performed to correct what seem to have been perfectly normal organs. It would certainly be understandable if anyone skeptical of the motives of these mid-nineteenth-century surgeons agreed with Sims's medical detractors, who condemned such cervical surgery as a harmful fad.[50]

However, the conclusions drawn by Sims and Emmet were not necessarily unreasonable. In the Woman's Hospital they saw young woman after young woman suffering from severe dysmenorrhea accompanied by infertility. Thanks to the autopsies performed by the French anatomists and the passion of French medicine for keeping records, they had an idea, so they thought, of what normal female anatomy should look like (although why Sims, who insisted that there was no such thing as a normative vagina, should be convinced that every cervix should be alike remains a mystery). They could also make their own observations. The Sims speculum facilitated easy visual examination. The ovariotomies performed sometimes by Sims and Emmet but more often by their colleague T. Gaillard Thomas provided them with additional information about the appearance of the reproductive organs. And because of their absolute faith that a women's reproductive system was like a machine, either functioning well or in need of repair—a mechanical way of thinking that was at least far less mired in cultural conventions about women's roles than the soon-to-be fashionable views of conservative medical men in the 1870s and 1880s who argued that a woman's reproductive organs were connected to her brain—they gravitated toward surgical treatment.[51]

The Doctor-Patient Relationship

As interesting as it is to speculate on whether any of these treatments "worked" in a modern sense, it is perhaps more fruitful to ask how it was that Sims and Emmet persuaded women to undergo such surgery. This question gets at the heart of a controversial issue in women's history: to what extent were women victims, and to what extent were they exercising choice or control in their relationships with male figures of authority? It also speaks to an often-discussed issue in medical history: how, and to what extent, did physicians exercise professional authority before the era in which such authority had become institutionalized?

Sims and Emmet, of course, attempted to make use of the reputations they were acquiring at the Woman's Hospital to build up their private practices, a common course of action for elite hospital-based physicians, and one reason why it was so crucial to Sims that he establish the Woman's Hospital. Sims was more open about his ambitions than Emmet, boasting that after his successful operations at the hospital became known, "very soon my private consultation rooms were filled." The voluntary hospital, indeed, served as a discreet form of advertising.[52] But if the hospital brought them visibility, they still had to convince women that they could treat them successfully.

Both Sims and Emmet, as Sims's assistant and later his successor, evinced an incredible self-confidence in their work at a time when many of their fellow physicians still expressed a sense of uncertainty because old therapies had been discredited and new ones seemed as yet unproven. These two men were able to impart this confidence to their patients, even at times when such confidence was entirely unwarranted. Unlike later generations of physicians who could rely on the institutional authority of the profession itself, Sims and Emmet relied on the power of their personalities, although in very different ways.

On the face of it, Emmet was more authoritarian. In his private practice, he once claimed, he isolated each patient in order to make her behave "as a child in my hands." Once he had gained the upper hand, he said, he easily convinced his patient to follow his advice, imbued as she was with "the desire to please me and to merit my approval." But if he seemed like a tyrant in private practice, in the hospital he carefully preserved the dignity of the women whom he treated. The hospital case records for the early years, all either taken personally by him or at his direction, carefully listed a title for each woman and not simply her name. At a time when poor and immigrant women rarely rose to the dignity of a surname when dealing with their "social betters" in their daily lives, let alone the title of Miss or Mrs., his careful notations demonstrated genuine sensitivity.[53]

Many, perhaps most, of Emmet's hospital patients were Irish Catholic immigrants. Emmet too was Irish-American and a Catholic. Although born in the United States into a prosperous family and brought up as a Protestant, Emmet descended from Irish patriots, and he boasted at least one martyr to the cause of Irish independence on his family tree. He married a Catholic, adopted her church, and became an active and zealous believer. And so fervently was he committed to the Woman's Hospital that when Sims decamped for Europe in 1862, apparently leaving the institution in such disarray that closure seemed imminent, Emmet persuaded a number of his private patients to become paying patients at the hospital. This meant, of course, that revenues that would have gone to him personally went instead to the hospital, which, by then, had become his passion as well as a place of work.[54]

Sims held quite different attitudes, generally drawing a much sharper line between his private patients and those he treated at the Woman's Hospital. Deferential to his wealthy patients, he treated them in his private "hospital" or in their own homes. Only a few of his private patients seem to have ever spent time at the Woman's Hospital. Emmet's authoritarian streak perhaps paradoxically led him to treat his patients more evenhandedly. He did not see his wealthy patients as being in any way either more entitled to make decisions about their own care or more deserving of dignity than his poorer ones. Sims's sense of social distinction, in contrast, meant that in his private practice the wishes of the patient might overrule his own judgment, thereby giving at least some women a considerable measure of control. That does not mean that Sims approved when his patients insisted on a particular kind of therapy, simply that he often felt compelled to go along.[55]

A number of these women, Sims complained, insisted on treatments at variance with his recommendations. Complying reluctantly, he then laid the blame for any failures on his independent-minded patients. In 1859, when a colleague referred a young married woman suffering from "sterile dysmenorrhea" to him, Sims immediately diagnosed, not surprisingly, a disorder of the cervix—in this case, a conical cervix with a very small os. He recommended a cervical incision. Dr. Metcalfe, the patient's primary physician, concurred. But the patient refused, insisting on gradual dilatation instead. Sims grudgingly began a course of opening the cervix gradually with larger and larger dilators called bougies. But at her second dilatation, several days after the first, the patient complained of considerable pain. That evening, "she had a rigor, followed by fever, and a most intense attack of metro-peritonitis, which lasted many weeks, and from which she barely escaped with her life." Before this, he had on other occasions consented to use this treatment for other equally determined patients, although it had always been against his own judgment. Never again, he resolved. "This," he concluded dramatically, "was my last bougie case."[56]

Sims's experiments in artificial insemination offer another, albeit more ambiguous, example of the ways in which some patients determined their treatments. As the first physician of high standing in the regular medical profession to admit to performing artificial insemination in the nineteenth century, he considered it an experimental method that would test his theories of conception. It was never, he made clear, a treatment of first resort for him. In every case in which he tried it, he noted, "the operation of incising the os and cervix would have been the proper course to pursue." Some patients who refused to have surgery were willing to agree to what Sims told them was "the uncertain alternative of uterine injection." For two years Sims explored this technique. To obtain the sperm, he waited in another room while his patient had intercourse with her husband. Entering the room immediately afterward, he withdrew the semen from her

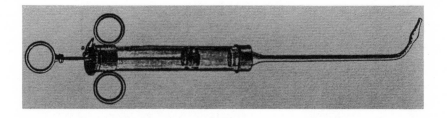

J. Marion Sims used this instrument for uterine insemination. Many of his colleagues were appalled at his experiments in artificial insemination.
From *Clinical Notes on Uterine Surgery,* 1873 edition

vagina with an instrument he had specially made for the purpose; then, carefully calculating the amount, he injected the fluid into the uterus.[57]

His first inseminations caused intense cramps ("uterine colic," as it was then called), which is not surprising, since he injected several drops of semen directly into the uterus. (He did not fail to remind these patients that surgery would have been less painful.) Even after he arrived at a level that the patients could tolerate—"half a drop"—success eluded him. Only one conception resulted, and that, sadly, ended in a miscarriage. Altogether the half-dozen patients involved tried the experiment over a two-year period, with a total of fifty-five inseminations. Although Sims said he had no desire to repeat these attempts, he was convinced that if physicians had a better idea of the ideal time to perform the insemination, they would have more success than he had. "I have very little doubt," he concluded, "that we shall learn more about embryology; and . . . if we understood more about the proper period for conception, this mechanical fertilization might become exact enough to depend upon it."[58] These cases of artificial insemination differ from the other cases in which he used a nonsurgical therapy because in the first instances discussed here he actually opposed, but bowed to, his patients' wishes. Here, although he thought surgery would be more effective, he was clearly eager to see if artificial insemination would work. Nevertheless, he only performed it in instances in which women refused to consent to surgery. Among both groups, choice was involved, but the nature of the choice was different.[59]

The case records of the Woman's Hospital indicate that some hospital as well as private patients were able to negotiate some aspects of their treatment. Occasionally, a woman would present herself at the hospital and then adamantly refuse to be examined, but more often women simply refused treatment after discovering what the doctors had in store for them. A number of patients in fact appear to have demanded, and received, treatment other than that preferred by the physicians. For example, there were several women whose diagnoses—an inflamed and "strictured" cervix, or a contracted os—were identical to those of women who did undergo surgery. But these patients instead were fitted with pessaries, or simply given medication. At least one such patient underwent surgery only after two years of trying other therapies.[60]

One thing seems clear from this discussion of the relationship between these doctors and their patients. At least some of these women, somehow, learned about different treatments for infertility and attempted to make their own decisions about their treatment, and the doctors took their wishes into account. These women were not unlike the pregnant women whom historian Judith Walzer Leavitt has studied, who negotiated the circumstances under which they would invite male doctors to deliver their children. But two things were different: First, women in the nineteenth century gave birth in their homes; the doctors were in their space. Although it was sometimes true that Sims operated on wealthy women in their homes, for the most part their surgery took place either in his private "hospital" or the Woman's Hospital, and this was even more often the case for Emmet. Second, unless a woman suffered from severe menstrual pain as well as infertility, she was seeking treatment for a condition that was neither physically debilitating nor life-threatening. A woman in the ninth month of pregnancy was going to give birth; the only questions that remained were who would attend her and under what circumstances. An infertile woman—if she lived in a community with a number of practitioners holding different opinions—had greater choice. And increasingly, women seemed to be choosing invasive treatments. In the words of one Buffalo physician, such therapies had even "become very fashionable."[61]

But how did women know what treatments were available and from whom to get them? Paradoxically, on at least one level the medical self-help movement appears to have led women straight to the expert's consulting rooms. American women had been learning a great deal about their bodies. Frederick Hollick, probably the best known of the popular health lecturers of the nineteenth century, lugged his anatomically correct papier-mâché models—crafted in Paris, of course—from city to city on his acclaimed lecture tours, and made more women familiar with the functioning of their reproductive systems than any other single individual in the mid-nineteenth century. His crowds often numbered in the hundreds for a single lecture, and his medical advice books could be found in log cabins and miners' camps as well as on the private bookshelves of middle-class urbanites. Hollick urged his readers to avoid the "cordials" or other "specifics" advertised as never-failing cures for sterility. "The only treatment likely to succeed," he advised bluntly, was "that which first ascertains the cause, and if possible, removes it."[62]

In addition to Hollick, women also could turn to another widely read popular medical advice giver during the third quarter of the nineteenth century, Edward Bliss Foote, an 1858 graduate of the University of Pennsylvania Medical School. Foote, like Hollick, gave out advice by mail; he also kept up a New York practice. Birth control advocate, friend to radicals and free-lovers, Foote was hardly a conventional physician. But a large sector of the American public apparently found his advice useful. His first advice book, *Medical Common Sense,* was popular enough that he soon brought out *Plain Talk,* a much enlarged, and somewhat revised, edition.[63]

In some respects, Foote kept very up-to-date. In spite of his general skepticism about the efficacy of surgery, for example, he reminded his readers that in cases of pelvic "tumor or dropsy" it was necessary that "every vestige . . . be removed before conception is allowed to take place." And whether he got the idea for his "impregnating syringe" from J. Marion Sims or not, he nevertheless was familiar with artificial insemination. He recommended its use not only in cases where the cervix was "long, slim, and contracted, pointing . . . to the side, . . . upward, or downward" (or, as Sims would have put it, a conoid cervix with a small os and anteflexion of the canal) but also in cases where the problem rested either with lack of sperm production or an unexplained sterility. In the case of the malformed cervix the husband's semen was to be used, which was controversial in itself. But Foote went further than Sims, who performed inseminations *only* using the husband's semen. Foote explicitly informed his readers that if the husband's semen were found to be devoid of spermatozoa, "the male germs must be obtained" from someone else. An outside donor was also required, he said, in cases of sterility due to what some physicians called "temperamental inadaptation," a diagnosis which in some ways prefigured our modern one of "unexplained infertility." Foote sold his impregnating syringe, with complete instructions, through the mail for $5.00, and if his readers lacked the money, they surely would have picked up the principles of using the syringe from the book itself.[64]

E. B. Foote never mentioned J. Marion Sims, but he lived in New York and kept current on medical matters. His impregnating syringe was for

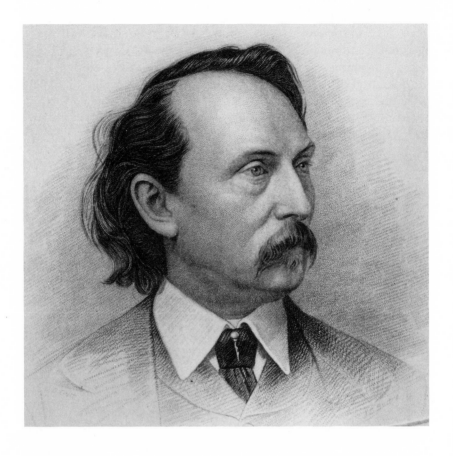

E. B. Foote, popular mid-nineteenth-century medical advice giver and promoter of the "impregnating syringe," which couples could use themselves for artificial insemination.
Courtesy of the College of Physicians of Philadelphia

vaginal, not uterine, insemination, yet his description of the cervical conditions that might call for its use mirrored in nonmedical language Sims's and Emmet's own diagnoses.

Sims and Foote, in fact, had more in common than they would have acknowledged. Both endorsed mechanical models of conception; both practiced artificial insemination. And the radical Foote had in common with the social-climbing Sims a refusal to bow to Victorian notions of what was moral. That is not to say that Sims was not in his own behavior a model Victorian paterfamilias, but that he believed that simple and plain explanations of reproductive functions benefitted patient and physician alike. Foote, in contrast, was a genuine sexual radical. Still, both of them believed in the importance of children to the happiness of men and women alike, and considered it their mission to help women conceive. If for Sims this meant artificial insemination, so be it. If for Foote it meant the additional step of giving couples the option of what we now call donor insemination, then that too could be morally justified. Any woman who attended health lectures, for example, or dipped into either Hollick's or Foote's widely available works, would have learned a great deal about some of the possible causes of infertility and the kinds of treatment available. It is entirely possible that having done all they could to restore their own health, if they had access to a willing physician, women chose to go another step and seek surgical treatment.

Women in New York could easily have known about Sims from their friends or family. Among the wealthy and socially prominent, Sims had had his champions since the 1850s. And working- and middle-class women could have heard from friends who had been treated at the Woman's Hospital. Other physicians also referred patients to him, in spite of his controversial reputation. After he returned to New York in 1868 from a stunningly successful European sojourn, during which time he also published his masterwork, *Clinical Notes on Uterine Surgery, with Special Reference to the Management of the Sterile Condition,* he had become even more prominent.

Although Sims developed many of his surgical treatments for infertility during his early years at the Woman's Hospital, he earned his international reputation as an expatriate in Paris and London. Sims had left New York in 1862. An outspoken Confederate sympathizer, he found both his practice and the numbers of his friends dwindling. In debt and unhappy, he sailed for France, eventually sending for his family and extending his stay for six years. It was on the Continent that Sims wrote the *Clinical Notes,* which began as a "pamphlet on the subject of sterility" but soon grew into a volume of several hundred pages, published in 1866 both in England and in the United States and later translated into several languages.[65]

Knowing, or so he claimed, "more [about sterility] than anybody else," Sims ridiculed most of his colleagues as old-fashioned in their attitudes toward its diagnosis and cure. Advising them to discard old notions such as a belief in "constitutional" factors in cases of involuntary childlessness, he insisted that in the end, the various causes of infertility entailed "but so many mechanical causes of obstruction, which must be recognized and remedied." If physicians failed to cure women's reproductive difficulties, he went on, it was their own fault, "for of all organs the uterus is now most subservient to the laws of physical exploration; and in every case of diseased action, if we cannot map out accurately the peculiar condition of the uterus producing or accompanying it, it is simply because we do not apply our knowledge of those physical laws to its investigation."[66]

Sims's insistence on the superiority of his views was often too much for his colleagues to bear in silence. W. D. Buck complained in the *New York Medical Journal* about the "cutting and slashing, and gouging, and split-ting, and skewering" that surgeons "anxious for notoriety" performed on women's reproductive organs. President of the New Hampshire State Medical Society, Buck was an outspoken critic of Sims, as was Samuel D. Gross, the eminent Philadelphia surgeon who frequently denounced his colleagues who were attempting to create a specialty in the diseases of women. "Doctors and patients alike have womb on the brain," he grum-bled. "At present diseases of the uterus are the fashionable disorders," he insisted, accusing women of inciting physicians to perform unnecessary procedures. "Not to have an ulcer upon the womb is to be beyond the pale of the sex."[67]

Even more than his radical views on the role of surgery in treating in-fertility as well as other diseases of women, Sims's disregard of sexual pro-prieties outraged many of his colleagues. Even though he wrote *Clinical Notes* for fellow physicians, Sims eschewed the common practice of shift-ing to Latin whenever he discussed an explicitly sexual matter. He wrote in plain and unembarrassed English and justified himself on the grounds that the importance of the service he was rendering to infertile couples ex-cused any lapses in propriety.[68]

Sims was candid about his visits to his patients' bedrooms, and what he found there. Perhaps most shocking, Sims described how he had "over and over again examined the condition of the uterus after coition, and of-ten in four or five minutes after it, [and] I have also frequently removed the mucus of the cervical canal immediately after sexual intercourse," in order to discover whether active spermatozoa were present. (Sims was one of the few physicians who believed—and frequently reiterated his belief—that potent men could be sterile.) When one considers that in the 1860s even to use a speculum to conduct a pelvic examination engendered considerable controversy among physicians, that practitioners found such frankness scandalous is no surprise. The editor of the *Medical Times and Gazette* of London expressed the distaste of many when he said that he would rather leave the profession than follow Sims's path: "If such practices were to be considered the business of the Physician there are a good many of us who would quit [medicine] for some other calling that would let us keep our sense of decency and self-respect."[69]

Despite his having earned an international reputation in Europe in the 1860s, becoming physician to the wealthy and titled, in the United States Sims continued to be a controversial figure. When he returned to New York and the Woman's Hospital in 1868, new doctors with views of their own had been added as consulting surgeons, and Emmet had become a powerful force in himself, no longer the respectful young protégé. Arguments ensued over medical decisions among the doctors, and over policy between the consulting physicians and the lay Board of Governors. Sims, now accustomed to international acclaim, was even less willing to take instructions from a group of nonphysicians. After a particularly bitter dispute in the early 1870s, he offered his resignation. To his great surprise and anger, the board accepted it. Deprived of his principal institutional base, for the rest of his career Sims divided his time between his private practices in Europe and the United States. He produced no new theoretical or therapeutic ideas in the last decade or so of his career.[70]

In spite of the opposition of his colleagues in the 1860s to his single-minded emphasis on surgery, however, within a decade or so his views would come to prevail. One reason was that his ideas seemed to "work," perhaps not in the sense that he made the sterile fertile (although apparently enough of his patients conceived to enable him to develop a reputation for success), but that he convinced his patients that his instruments and his surgical expertise provided them with more hope of relief—from their pelvic pain, their dysmenorrhea, and their sterility—than any dietary prescriptions, gradual instrumental therapy, or self-help could do. The fact that he actually had been the first to cure vesico-vaginal fistula, an accomplishment of genuine significance that had released many afflicted women from a lifetime of suffering, gave credence to his less well-substantiated claims. With the Woman's Hospital as an institutional base, and ably assisted by the more administratively inclined Thomas Emmet, Sims had created a small corps of "woman's surgeons" who became identified with the cure of women's reproductive disorders just as physicians were seeking to reclaim the authority they had lost during the era of medical democratization.

The lesson was not lost on Sims's colleagues. By the time he came to write his autobiography in the early 1880s, just before his death, he could boast that he had outlasted his critics. When Sims first began to treat sterility surgically, few beyond his patients and immediate circle of medical colleagues were aware of what he was doing. With the appearance of the *Clinical Notes* in 1866, any practitioner who read a medical journal became familiar with his name and his views, could buy the book, and could try his techniques. And although he was still a controversial figure, especially within what we might call his own medical circle of elite hospital-based practitioners, their criticism of what they considered his radical wielding of the knife and scissors did not contravene their agreement with his principal premise that mechanical "obstructions" caused most infertility.[71]

By around 1870, Sims found himself part of a medical movement. The elite hospital-based physicians of Emmet's generation and somewhat younger saw in surgery and specialization a way to position themselves professionally and to develop a field of expertise that would set them apart from ordinary physicians.[72] One does not need to argue that sterility treatment became a rationale for the development of gynecology in order to understand that the emergence of such a specialty enabled physicians to claim an expertise in all aspects of the reproductive process. The work of J. Marion Sims and his cadre of reproductive surgeons at the Woman's Hospital, in fact, helped to set the tone for gynecology in every way but one. The next generation of emergent gynecologists, unlike Marion Sims, would show no reluctance in prescribing behavioral norms as well as promoting surgical techniques. This fallout from nineteenth-century "sexual science," to borrow a term from historian Cynthia Russett, would for the next several decades guide the development of gynecology and shape the profession's developments of new treatments for infertility.

three

The "Degeneracy of American Womanhood"

Gynecology Redefines Infertility, 1870–1900

The present system of girl cramming and college forcing of women is accountable for much of the sterility and of the physical degeneracy of American womanhood. . . . Restless activity, a dissatisfaction with her duties and calling, and a want of reverence for her special vocation, go hand in hand with sterility.

Horace Bigelow, M.D., 1883

The reproductive behavior of American women came under even greater scrutiny after the Civil War than it had in the heyday of the health reform movement. As the marriage rate among highly educated women dropped and the birthrate among the white Protestant middle classes continued its sharp fall, discussions and arguments over the significance of these changes became an important part of the nation's public discourse. Women seemed to be rebelling against conventional ideas of their appropriate roles. In the final analysis, most women did not turn their backs on matrimony and maternity, seeking instead to make room in their lives for outside interests in addition to their domestic responsibilities. Nevertheless, a noticeable minority explicitly chose to seek higher education and productive careers rather than marriage and family life. Debates raged within individual families, in popular and serious periodicals, and among public figures over the best methods of either encouraging—or stifling—the changes that were taking place.

Among those attempting to take a leading role in defining the terms of the discussion were physicians interested in the diseases of women, who considered themselves well placed to provide explanations and solutions to what many viewed as an increasing problem. Now calling themselves gynecologists, during these decades they set themselves the task of monitoring and regulating women's reproductive behavior. Bolstered by a new science, ensconced in a new setting, and armed with new diagnostic and therapeutic tools, they formed a vanguard of experts on the process of human reproduction. Because the fertility of American women was a major social concern in the late nineteenth century, the problem of infertility, while it by no means dominated the field of gynecology, held an important place in its early development. Although they were only a minority of the physicians who treated women in this period (most Americans received their care from generalists, many of whom may have trained decades earlier in proprietary medical schools or as apprentices), gynecologists established the intellectual infrastructure that made new research into fertility possible. They disseminated their findings in new journals and societies and also trained the next generation of physicians, who would apply that new knowledge.

Historians are familiar with the attempts of physicians to influence women's behavior during the post–Civil War era; as historian Regina Morantz-Sanchez has noted, "doctors found themselves the spokespersons for the affirmation of traditional verities."[1] The subject of "sterility," now the preferred medical term for involuntary childlessness, provided numerous opportunities for the assertion of conventional values, as physicians articulated an explanation of its etiology that centered on women's inappropriate behavior. Such confident pronouncements about the root causes of infertility, designed to advance the claims of gynecologists to authority in both reproductive and behavioral matters, nevertheless masked an underlying uncertainty about their ability to treat the condition effectively. This chapter focuses on the delineation of such views, and the challenges to them, during the early decades of the development of gynecology.

In the years after the Civil War, increasing numbers of women began to range farther from the confines of home and family. A number of factors, from the great surge of immigration, which provided a domestic labor force for middle-class households, to the more subtle impact of women's growing social influence as they became the acknowledged custodians of the nation's moral values, fueled changes in their attitudes and behavior. Middle-class women went off to seminary or college, joined women's clubs, became social purity or temperance reformers. Some of them, their ranks swelling as the century came nearer to its close, worked for the suffrage cause; others became settlement house workers; an even larger number volunteered for various charities. Married women, to be sure, did not usually hold down paying positions. To do so was considered exceedingly daring and radical. In general, women who contemplated professional careers recognized that they were making a choice between work and marriage. Until after the turn of the twentieth century, fewer than 5 percent of married women—the overwhelming majority of them working class—held jobs outside the home, most of them because their families required their income. But many wives, whether through social activism or social activities, nevertheless had come to define themselves to varying degrees as individuals with interests separate from, although often connected to, their day-to-day domestic responsibilities.[2]

It was not so much the actuality of wives neglecting their domestic duties in order to challenge their husbands' positions in the outside world that set Americans to debating what they invariably called the "Woman Question." Rather, it was a confluence of women's demands for education, for opportunities for professional careers, and for access to the political system, combined with what seemed to be their declining capacity or inclination to raise large families, that raised anxieties for the future. Social progressives responded to these fears by insisting that giving women the rights to which they were entitled would neither destroy the family nor depopulate the nation, but social conservatives saw things differently.

As family size continued to drop, reaching an average of 3.56 children by 1900, the marriage rate was also declining to the lowest level ever attained in American history. Moreover, the fertility rate was lowest among urban native-born whites and highest among immigrants and African Americans. The closing years of the nineteenth century brought this country its greatest "extremes of differential fertility," as one demographic historian has expressed it.[3] Many of the most prominent gynecologists lived and worked in New York, Philadelphia, Boston, Chicago, and Baltimore. They could not help but be aware of both the nation's changing demographics and women's growing aspirations, and many of them were increasingly distressed by the ways in which the nation's population was being transformed.

To highlight such cultural attitudes among members of the medical profession is not to deny the medical advances that undergirded the new field of gynecology. New developments in anesthesia had made surgery a somewhat less terrifying prospect for patients. By the end of the 1860s, surgeons at the Woman's Hospital, for example, routinely anesthetized their patients, and by the 1880s, new forms of general and local anesthesia made it possible for surgeons to tailor the anesthetic to the procedure. Antiseptic techniques came into use in the 1870s, although considerable controversy raged over their effectiveness. By the end of the century, aseptic techniques would replace antisepsis—at least among elite hospital-based gynecologists. Asepsis, and the bacteriology that undergirded it, would make it possible for gynecological surgeons to perform major operations with both greater technical proficiency and increased confidence that their patients would survive. By the turn of the century, sterilization of instruments, x-rays, and the creation of pathology laboratories all served as essential adjuncts to gynecology, which took its place within an increasingly sophisticated hospital setting.[4]

In some respects, therefore, the development of gynecology paralleled the growth of other specialized fields in medicine during the same era.[5] But in one fundamental aspect, gynecology was different: Women's reproductive organs have a symbolic significance that other parts of the body do not possess. The early gynecologists were influenced not simply by new developments in science but also by a more overarching set of beliefs within the scientific community that related much of human behavior to biology. As applied to gender, historian Cynthia Russett has called this paradigm, which dominated American science for most of the late nineteenth century, "sexual science." The core principle of sexual science was that the differences between male and female reproductive organs signified equally fundamental differences in their intellectual and moral capacities and their social responsibilities. A corollary followed—that women had a biological mandate to marry and bear children. If they failed to do, so they not only outraged social convention but also contravened scientific laws. Women's health, therefore, required both childbearing and conventional social behavior.[6]

"Sexual Science"

Eager to be seen as scientific in an age when science seemed to hold out the "dazzling promise of certain knowledge," gynecologists quickly embraced these explanations of sexual difference. In the early 1870s one work, because it was so widely read and talked about, came to define the parameters of this discussion for the public. *Sex in Education,* written by Harvard physician Edward H. Clarke, argued that young women were educating themselves into sterility. Although historians have no doubt tired of reading about this book, which appears in nearly every discussion of medical attitudes toward women in this period, it would be a mistake to believe that simply because it seems trite to late-twentieth-century minds, late-nineteenth-century Americans did not study it with deadly seriousness.[7]

Widely reviewed and praised, *Sex in Education* made Clarke an instant celebrity, going through eleven printings in its first year. Lectures followed, as did a self-promotional sequel a year later, called *The Building of a Brain.* Invoking "the law of science," Clarke argued that advocates of educational parity between the sexes stood for nothing less than the destruction of the race. Young women from high school through college age, he insisted, should not be putting in long hours studying difficult academic subjects. They should learn slowly; and during their menstrual periods, their minds required absolute rest. Middle- and upper-class parents did neither their daughters nor the nation a favor when they sent their female offspring to college. A rigorous education, he claimed, had a "sterilizing influence" on young women, and in another generation "the race will be propagated from its inferior classes."[8]

The fact that his argument rested on fewer than a dozen cases did not give Clarke a moment's pause; his colleagues soon weighed in with their one or two, or half-dozen confirmatory stories. Limited evidence notwithstanding, he had the weight of medical prejudice on his side. *Sex in Education* did not prevent women from attending college, but it did cause women's college presidents and trustees to give special attention to exercise, physiology, and hygiene programs for their students so as to counter Clarke's arguments. M. Carey Thomas, later the president of Bryn Mawr College, remembered that in the early days of women's education, she and others "were haunted . . . by the clanging chains of that gloomy little specter, Dr. Edward H. Clarke's *Sex in Education.*"[9]

If Clarke's ideas did not always prevail, they nevertheless set the terms of the debate over the relationship between women's aspirations and fertility for at least the next twenty years. Woman, most physicians appeared to believe, had a particularly "sensitive organization"; her reproductive system dominated every aspect of her being, and as a consequence society had a duty to restrict behavior that might put her ability to reproduce in danger. Or, as Horace Bigelow put it in 1883, education "is accountable for much of the sterility and physical degeneracy of American womanhood. . . . Restless activity, a dissatisfaction with her duties and calling, and a want of reverence for her special vocation, go hand in hand with sterility."[10]

But as Bigelow surely realized, women rejected their biological mandates in other ways as well. About 75 percent of the fertility decline in this era, demographers have estimated, was voluntary. Historians have amply documented the use of contraception among the middle classes in the latter half of the nineteenth century, and abortion also remained a viable alternative when birth control methods failed. Although antiabortion laws appeared on the books of many states in the 1870s, local courts remained lenient in enforcing them until the 1880s and 1890s. Even after that, many illegal abortionists were able to operate with relative impunity. Gynecologists responded to the widespread use of abortion and contraception by warning couples that either practice would eventually result in permanent sterility.[11]

These ideas came to bolster explanations of the causes of reproductive disorders, including infertility, in the 1870s, as gynecologists solidified their organizational base. Creating new societies and journals allowed them both to meet with like-minded colleagues and to publicize their own work. Local gynecological societies proliferated soon after the founding of the first in Boston in 1869. The first national journal to devote sustained consideration to gynecology, the *American Journal of Obstetrics and the Diseases of Women and Children,* began publication in 1868. From its inception, it devoted about half its space to gynecology; a regular feature was its annual "Report of Progress in Gynecology."

The exclusive American Gynecological Society, which limited the number of its fellows to sixty, was founded in 1876 and was the first national organization of gynecologists. Its charter members included nearly all of the eastern seaboard's luminaries—J. Marion Sims, Thomas Addis Emmet, Robert Battey, Alexander J. C. Skene, Emil Noeggerath, and T. Gaillard Thomas were founding members—with a sprinkling of practitioners from other areas of the country. A decade later, physicians from cities and small towns beyond the East Coast created a more inclusive organization, the American Association of Obstetricians and Gynecologists, which gave less well-connected physicians their own national organization. By the early 1890s, in addition to the *Transactions of the American Gynecological Society,* there were at least five journals that listed gynecology in their titles, with a circulation of well over eighteen thousand.[12] These journals provided physicians with information on new techniques and surgical methods and offer historians a means of tracking the major concerns of practitioners as the specialty developed.

In terms of infertility treatment, two things stand out in the journals: First, therapies for sterility—as practitioners now almost always called what once was known as barrenness—in the 1870s and 1880s were based on the ideas and specific techniques developed by Sims and reflected his growing influence. Most practitioners continued to believe that a mechanical obstruction caused by a small cervical os accompanied by anteflexion of the canal or uterus was the commonest proximate cause of sterility. Some continued to prefer the more gradual instrumental treatments; however, cervical incision became much more common as journal articles declared it to result in greater numbers of pregnancies. The only "new" diagnosis to appear frequently was of "uterine catarrh" (for a range of vaginal discharges), but this term was simply a new designation for leucorrhea. Although more attention from the 1870s onward was given to the deviation of the uterus from what doctors insisted was its normal midline position, such a diagnosis also was a variant of Sims's mechanistic approach. For treating these malpositions of the uterus, physicians resorted to uterine "adjusters" (instruments placed in the uterus for the purpose of manipulating its position) and pessaries to put the uterus back in place and keep it there.[13]

But if treatment followed the mechanical model popularized by Sims, it cannot be denied that explanations of the causes of infertility had changed significantly. In place of Sims's obvious unconcern about how women seemed to develop these retroflexions and anteflexions—if anything, he appeared to think they might have been congenital—gynecologists who came after him found the origins of such conditions in women's behavior. Beginning in the 1870s, gynecologists routinely made women's roles a subject of discussion at their annual meetings. John P. Reynolds, for example, in his presidential address to the American Gynecological Society in 1890, took it upon himself to remind his colleagues not to shirk their responsibility to attempt to regulate their patients' behavior. A woman, especially a mother or mother-to-be, he exclaimed, "cannot—nay on every ground must not—do the work of a man."[14]

The idea that inappropriate behavior causes infertility, or in other

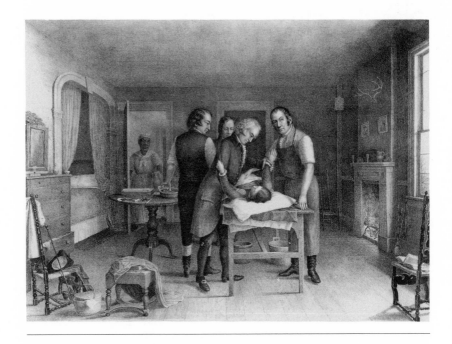

Ephraim McDowell, a Kentucky practitioner, performed the first recorded successful ovariotomy in 1809. His patient suffered from a life-threatening ovarian tumor. Neither anesthesia nor antiseptics had been discovered, yet the patient recovered to live some thirty-five more years. Ovariotomy became the signature surgery of gynecology in the last third of the nineteenth century. This interpretation is by artist and engraver George Dasson Knapp (1833–1910).
Courtesy of the Library of Congress

words, that the inability to conceive is in some way volitional, was dominant in this era and has recurred periodically ever since.[15] It was every doctor's duty, insisted one physician, to instruct patients to abandon "all those ambitious outreachings of the modern woman, which unfit her for her duties as wife and mother." The young woman who failed to heed such advice and who sought a college education—or worse, a career after she earned her degree—would most likely find herself suffering from sterility brought on by "uterine inflammation." And if she had not studied too much or aspired to a profession, she and her husband possibly engaged in "excessive coition" in the early months or years of marriage, which could lead to another cause of sterility, "uterine catarrh." Even without too frequent intercourse, contraceptive use alone could cause later sterility. A woman who had used any form of contraception would realize "too late," when "the desire of motherhood becomes strong within her," that she faced "the affliction of being childless."[16]

These attitudes derived from an approach to women's reproductive health that emphasized the direct relationship between a woman's emotions and behavior and her reproductive system. The surgical procedure most prominently identified with this model of reproductive disease in the historical literature is not surgery for sterility but ovariotomy, the nineteenth-century misnomer for a bilateral oophorectomy, or excision of the ovaries. The so-called normal ovariotomy was performed for a range of conditions having nothing directly to do with the reproductive organs. Perhaps the most frequently performed gynecological surgery of the 1870s and 1880s, the procedure was generally called "Battey's operation" after the Georgia gynecologist who popularized it.[17]

Even though technological advances gave them the tools to perform such surgery, technology cannot explain gynecologists' willingness to extirpate the ovaries of women suffering not from life-threatening tumors but from a variety of other symptoms. Even a woman afflicted with painful menstruation, which was more commonly treated by analgesics, narcotics, pessaries, or operatively by cervical incision, might now undergo ovariotomy. A diagnosis of "nervous disease," severe headaches, "hysteria," or "nymphomania" also found gynecologists reaching for their instruments. Only the new belief that all of the diseases of women, whatever their nature, originated in their reproductive organs can account for it. In the name of reproductive health, thousands of women underwent premature menopause.[18]

Ovariotomists claimed that the ovaries they removed were all "pathological." It nettled them to read that the distinguished J. Matthews Duncan contemptuously referred to their operation as "spaying." T. Gaillard Thomas, one of the foremost American gynecological authorities and an experienced ovariotomist himself, was reluctant to criticize his colleague Robert Battey directly, but he noted pointedly that the "procedure . . . may be greatly abused."[19]

Such criticism, however, was rare in the 1870s and 1880s. J. Marion Sims himself, never one to miss an opportunity to perform any new kind of surgery, not only lent his approval to his fellow southerner but assisted him at several operations, although Thomas Addis Emmet was critical. Paul Mundé, editor of the *American Journal of Obstetrics,* asserted in 1876 that ovariotomists exhibited no tendencies toward abusing the procedure, nor did he "think it likely" that they ever would.[20] Ovariotomy at that time symbolized surgical advancement; it was important to gynecologists not simply for its own sake but also for its testimony that the risks of invasive surgery had greatly diminished. There is some irony in this. Members of a profession that opposed every form of birth control except abstinence, that had led the fight to outlaw abortion, and that stood on the front lines in the battle to keep women from straying from their domestic roles nevertheless sanctioned the performance of numberless surgeries that made it impossible for these women ever to conceive.

However, the analysis of the causes of infertility and the indications for Battey's operation were but two sides of the same coin. Many of the patients who underwent ovariotomy did not seem fit, in their doctors' eyes, to be mothers. They were hysterical, or mentally ill (a number were in institutions), or sexually promiscuous.[21] Ovariotomy was related to the treatment of infertility in another, perhaps less obvious way as well. The widespread practice of this operation had one practical effect for the treatment of infertility by enabling practitioners to gain both surgical proficiency and a better understanding of the internal structure of women's pelvic organs. Even though it was possible to perform most of the "normal ovariotomies" vaginally, operators increasingly preferred abdominal surgery (called laparotomy). As gynecologists became more skillful at laparotomy, they also developed greater knowledge of such pelvic pathologies as adhesions and blocked fallopian tubes. By the time Battey's operation had sunk into disgrace in the 1890s, practitioners were using the knowledge they had gained performing it to develop new surgical techniques for restoring fertility.[22]

The confidence of the ovariotomists in the 1870s and 1880s seems especially astounding in view of their own recognition that they had only a vague understanding of the cycle of ovulation and menstruation, the physiological process that served as the linchpin of gynecological theory, whether the issue was the diagnosis of sterility or a decision to remove the ovaries. In spite of assertions by gynecologists that they understood the connections between a woman's mental state and her reproductive system, however, doubts about their ability to explicate the physiology on which they based their surgical feats had existed as early as the 1870s. Some physicians, for example, insisted that when they removed a patient's ovaries the expected menopause did not always occur. (Surprisingly, it did not occur to them that their operations might have been incomplete.) This "finding," as well as evidence contrary to the prevailing belief, which was that ovulation occurred during menstruation, also cast doubt on accepted ideas about this function, which is, after all, the bedrock of the female reproductive process.[23]

Earlier in the century, physicians had thought the issue settled. Reasoning from the animal to the human procreative process, scientists equated estrus in mammals to menstruation in women. Since animals ovulate during estrus, it seemed logical to assume that women ovulate during menstruation. This idea, most prominently associated with German medical science, now came under attack, as postmortem examinations on women who had died while menstruating failed to indicate the presence of a matured ovum. By 1876, a full-blown controversy had emerged and formed the major topic of discussion in the annual "Report on the Progress on Gynecology" in the *American Journal of Obstetrics*.[24]

Acceptance of the animal analogy had directly influenced practical advice given to patients in such cases as the timing of intercourse to facilitate the possibility of pregnancy. "Conception," nearly all medical authorities agreed, "was thought to be most probable immediately after the cessation of the flow, [and] this period of special susceptibility was supposed to last from ten to twelve days after the cessation of the catamenia." New evidence, it appeared, cast doubts on the validity of this as well as other aspects of the animal model. As the editor summarized several recently discovered "incontrovertible facts":

1. If a Graafian follicle ruptures during every menstruation, we should find evidence of that rupture at the postmortem of every women dying during or soon after the flow. But that is not universally the case. . . .

2. Ovulation frequently takes place without menstruation, as when conception takes place during lactation, or in women who have never yet menstruated. . . .

3. Of late years the cases have been increasing in number, in which, after the operation of double ovariotomy, menstruation continued regularly for years.

Although most gynecologists continued to believe that there must be a direct relationship between ovulation and menstruation, a number of them began to acknowledge that the new data left the nature of that relationship more obscure than ever.[25]

Beyond the obvious scientific and clinical reasons that led gynecologists to search for the key to understanding the relationship between menstruation and ovulation, among male gynecologists there also seemed to be an outright fascination with menstrual blood as representing the essence of female "difference." This was a relatively new phenomenon. Up through the eighteenth century, menstruation had been viewed not as a peculiar process that made women men's opposites but instead as another piece of evidence that the health of the body required the constant intake and outgo of fluids and solids to keep it in balance. Men sometimes underwent venesection in order to get rid of the "plethora" of blood that women evacuated more naturally, for example. And nosebleeds in some adolescent boys, one eighteenth-century authority noted, served to rid the body of extra blood that in girls found "a more easy vent downwards." But in the course of altering their ideas about the nature of men's and women's reproductive organs, male physicians enshrined menstruation as the principal marker of woman's fundamental difference. No longer an analogue to the male (if inferior and less perfectly formed), woman had become the opposite.[26] George Engelmann, president of the American Society of Gynecologists, insisted as late as 1900 that menstruation invariably rendered women unfit for the demands of a competitive profession. A woman could not, he insisted, think and reproduce at the same time.[27]

Male physicians' preoccupation with menstruation was accompanied by an interest in female sexuality that one can only describe as prurient, although they disguised their curiosity with expressions of concern over women's reproductive capacity and mental health. Staid and respectable journals carried articles about sex-obsessed young women brought to the point of paralysis, "aggravated" instances of masturbation, and the female sexual response.[28] The *American Journal of Obstetrics,* for example, published an innocuously titled article purporting to explain how sperm and ovum connected; in reality, it detailed how the author, with the consent of the patient's husband, brought a female patient to orgasm with manual stimulation. His goal, he claimed, was to test his theory that a suctionlike action on the part of the cervix during orgasm facilitated conception. While it is true that physicians also discussed some aspects of male sexuality, especially masturbation and its relationship to impotence, there was nothing quite like this in the medical literature on men![29]

Gynecological interpretations of the causes of infertility in these two decades were intimately connected to the popularity of Battey's operation, the definition of menstruation as a fundamental marker of women's intellectual inferiority, and the almost obsessive fascination with female sexuality among members of a profession that only recently had shrunk from conducting pelvic examinations. What many practitioners considered to be a growing infertility problem provided one more arena in which gyne-

cologists used their new organizations to stake out positions on major social issues. Physicians who claimed to serve as "priests at the altar of
woman's health" believed they had a moral obligation to speak out
against anything that infringed on such health. On subjects from education to bedroom intimacies, they did so, announcing that the use of birth
control and abortion, as well as demands for higher education and access
to professional careers, were having a detrimental effect on the family and
the nation.[30]

This is not to say that opposing views did not exist, both inside and
outside the profession. A group of Boston women, soon after the publication of Clarke's book, denounced it and encouraged physician Mary
Putnam Jacobi to write an article in rebuttal for Harvard University's
1876 Boylston Essay competition, which was on the subject of menstruation's effects on women. Using case studies and statistical analysis, Jacobi's essay argued that normal women had no special need to stop their
activities during menstruation. The judges (who could have had no idea
the writer was a woman, since all essays were submitted anonymously)
awarded her the prize. Even though it did not immediately change the
minds of a majority of her male colleagues, women practitioners took
heart from such research. Clelia Mosher, the Stanford physician whom
most historians recognize for her pioneering survey of female sexuality,
spent most of her career in trying to demonstrate that menstruation did
not incapacitate women for careers or profound intellectual work. Such
studies of healthy as well as infirm women were designed to shift the basis on which the discussions of reproduction were conducted—to move
toward an empirically grounded resolution of questions about the effects
of menstruation on women's intellectual lives and their overall health.[31]

Women practitioners could become intensely exasperated with their
male colleagues' views. At the Woman's Medical College in Philadelphia,
which sent a significant proportion of its graduates to India, China, and
the Middle East as medical missionaries, reports from the field indicated
that treatment for sterility formed a considerable part of these doctors'
practices. In 1886, Sarah Weintraub reported from Syria that fully two-
thirds of her patients sought treatment for sterility, prompting Mary Putnam Jacobi to remark that she would like to have the letter published in
order to debunk male physicians' insistence on a connection between education and sterility.[32]

Such ideas, however, appeared to have little impact on the thinking of
the profession as a whole before the 1890s (and some prominent practitioners refused to alter their beliefs well into the twentieth century). Male

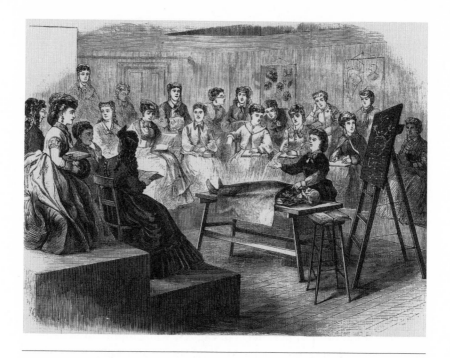

These women medical students at the New York Medical College for Women were shown in *Frank Leslie's Illustrated Newspaper* learning anatomy using a male cadaver. Most of them, however, would end up treating women and children.
Courtesy of the Library of Congress

gynecologists resisted dealing with these questions at such a concrete level in large part because giving up both the belief that education resulted in sterility and the idea of menstruation as the defining womanly process—not simply physically but also intellectually and emotionally—might have forced them to rethink their positions on the social roles of women. And in fact many gynecologists rarely had to confront directly as colleagues the women who made such arguments. Although some of the local gynecological societies admitted one or two women into their ranks, the American Gynecological Society would not elect its first woman member until 1921 (and not until 1970 would it elect its second). The physicians who dominated gynecology in most of the late nineteenth century and therefore the discussion of sterility were almost all men.[33]

New Ideas

By the end of the century, a number of factors caused a small but important sector of the gynecological elite to challenge several of the basic tenets upon which the reproductive theory developed in the 1870s and 1880s rested. Some prominent infertility experts, among whom George Engelmann was perhaps the most vocal, continued to hold to older views, but unanimity no longer prevailed. New ideas and new evidence began to suggest that infertility, rather than resulting from women's refusal to bow to conventional behavior, could be accounted for by more specifically physiological disorders, particularly of the ovaries and fallopian tubes. Perhaps the most important single factor in accomplishing this change was the dramatic alteration of medical views of gonorrhea.

Readers will recall that a number of sterile patients at the Woman's Hospital had conditions that a modern physician would readily identify as pelvic inflammatory disease, which can result from untreated gonorrhea. The common diagnosis of "uterine catarrh" in the 1870s was congruent with the same cause, as were the symptoms of severe and continual pelvic pain that brought many a young childless married woman to the doctor's office. Indeed, it is entirely possible that significant numbers of working- and middle-class women risked exposure to gonorrhea in late-nineteenth-century urban America. Considered a minor and self-limiting form of venereal disease, gonorrhea was generally associated with prostitutes, and commercial sex was widely available in the late nineteenth century. When infected, men routinely turned to both regular and homeopathic physicians, as well as to cures by mail and shady practitioners who promised instant panaceas. In point of fact there was no cure, nor would there be until the availability of penicillin in the 1940s. But neither the young single men who contracted gonorrhea and later became engaged, nor the married men who engaged in commercial sex, and certainly not their doctors, suspected that an asymptomatic man could still have gonorrhea.[34]

When Emil Noeggerath suggested to the contrary in the early 1870s, and further maintained that gonorrhea was a major cause of sterility in women, many of his colleagues dismissed his conclusions as absurd. To have accepted Noeggerath's views would have required them to reverse totally the prevailing etiological model that blamed a woman's behavior for her infertility. To implicate a specific disease, and especially one that incriminated husbands, was too great a leap for most gynecologists, particularly since Noeggerath did not at first seem to have the scientific evidence to prove his theory.[35]

Noeggerath had first publicly proclaimed in 1872 his idea that gonorrhea could linger in men for months or years, despite having ostensibly been cured. Four years later, after collecting more cases, he presented further findings at the first meeting of the new American Gynecological Society. Having treated hundreds of women for sterility, he remarked, he was puzzled that he could successfully treat some cases of uterine catarrh or cervical abnormalities, whereas in other cases presenting what seemed to him the same symptoms, the patients' sterility proved totally intractable. He began, he said, to suspect gonorrhea and thereafter made it a practice to interview the husbands of all his sterility patients and to require a semen analysis, both very uncommon practices. When he discovered that half the men were azoospermic (that is, their semen contained no sperm), he was so startled that he had a colleague replicate his experiments. When the results were the same, Noeggerath concluded that the husband was often responsible for a couple's inability to conceive. Some men had azoospermia. Others, even though their sperm appeared to be normal, had infected their wives, who suffered from stubborn "catarrhs" and recurrent or constant pain, and who remained sterile.[36]

Noeggerath's colleagues were incredulous, firmly believing that a man pronounced cured of gonorrhea could safely marry or resume sexual relations with his wife. Now they were being told that these "cured" men transmitted the disease to their wives, who at the least suffered severely and often were rendered sterile. According to Noeggerath, nearly two-thirds of his patients with what he called "latent gonorrhea" were completely sterile; another 18 percent experienced impaired fertility. His fellow physicians found his case reports completely unconvincing; as far as they could tell, indeed as far as he admitted himself, he had no direct evidence for his conclusions. Instead, he had reasoned inductively from the cases of numerous women who married men who had once had gonorrhea, or whose husbands contracted it through extramarital sex. These women, previously healthy, all began to suffer similar symptoms, which varied in some particular or other, but to him seemed remarkably alike. The one thing all these women had in common, he discovered, was that their husbands had been "cured" of gonorrhea.[37]

When his hearers scoffed, Noeggerath retorted, "After the gentlemen have given five years or more of careful study to this question, I shall expect to hear more approval than I have done today." He was prophetic; within a few years Albert Neisser isolated the gonococcus, one of the first

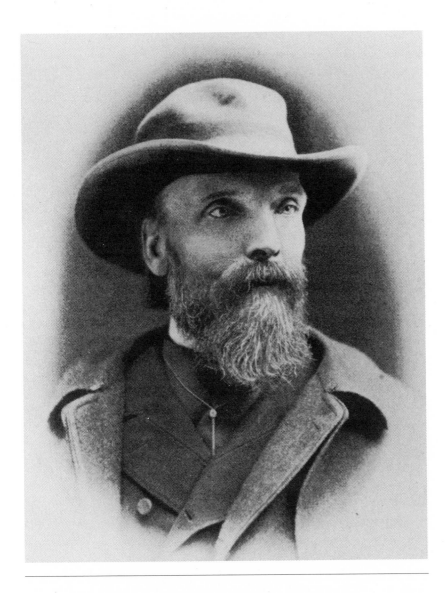

Emil Noeggerath. Until the late nineteenth century, gonorrhea was considered a relatively minor and self-limiting venereal disease. When Noeggerath, a German-born New York practitioner, suggested in the 1870s that the disease was not only more long-lasting than they believed, but was also a major cause of sterility in women, many of his colleagues dismissed his conclusions as unfounded. Within a few years, however, Albert Neisser isolated the gonococcus, one of the first disease-causing organisms to be identified.
Courtesy of the College of Physicians of Philadelphia

disease-causing organisms to be identified. Although many gynecologists did not accept Noeggerath's findings until the 1890s, a few of them as early as the 1880s began to argue, in the face of enormous social opposition, that preventing gonorrhea was important enough to justify the medical inspection of prostitutes and the licensing of their trade.[38]

Between the 1870s and the turn of the century, sterility took on greater importance within the gynecological profession, as gynecologists claimed that their concern over infertility resulted from an increasing incidence of it. Most practitioners in Europe and the United States relied upon the statistical studies of the rate of infertility compiled by Edinburgh's J. Matthews Duncan, who had begun studying the issue in the 1850s. In the early 1880s, after reviewing his own work and surveying the studies of others, Duncan concluded that "estimates [of the proportion of sterile marriages] from various sources give an amount varying from one in seven to one in twelve—one in ten being nearer the true amount." In addition to what Duncan called "absolute sterility" (what physicians today call primary infertility), other couples suffered from what was called "one-child" sterility, and they numbered about 8 percent of all families.[39] Most American practitioners were convinced that Duncan's statistics confirmed their own more impressionistic observations. Baltimore gynecologist Thomas Ashby, for example, as certain as he was that sterility was a serious and increasingly common medical problem, admitted that "it would be extremely difficult to prove these assertions by statistical evidence." Instead, he drew his conclusions mainly from "individual experience."[40]

Because the data are so impressionistic, because so much historical attention has been given to family limitation, and because much of the medical profession gave way to hysteria over the fact that American women were having fewer children, it would be very easy to dismiss these observations about increasing sterility as simply more hyperbole. But perhaps we should not be so hastily dismissive. In fact, the proportion of childless couples, and not simply smaller families, was on the rise in the late nineteenth century. Among white women born in 1835 who had ever married, just a little over 7 percent were childless. Within the next twenty years, there was a slow increase in childlessness, followed by a very sharp jump. Of white women born in 1870, nearly 16 percent remained childless. Black women's fertility showed a similar pattern. Among African American women born in 1835, the proportion who had no children had been about 5 percent. For those born in 1870, it was about 13 percent, and one prominent physician noted that about 24 percent of his African American patients experienced sterility. Of course, there is absolutely no way to know how much childlessness was intentional and how much imposed. But given the prevailing ideology, it is hard to imagine that all these couples chose not to have any children. It is in fact entirely possible that in the closing decades of the nineteenth century physicians were seeing an increased number of infertility problems in their own practices.[41]

As practitioners began to accept gonorrhea as a cause of sterility, they were forced to give more attention to the existence of infertility in men. During the 1860s, Sims, drawing on the findings of English researcher T. C. Curling as well as his own experience, was virtually alone among American physicians in arguing that male sterility could exist even when a man exhibited sexual potency. But the idea gradually gained more credence. William Goodell, who held the Chair in Obstetrics and the Diseases of Women at the University of Pennsylvania, dramatically told the story of his own conversion to this view to a group of his colleagues in 1877. He owed his change of heart, he said, to the loving husband of one of his patients. The woman, severely unhappy over her childlessness, wanted an operation that Goodell was not sure she required. While Goodell was trying to decide what to do, the patient's husband came to him and confessed his fear that his decade-old gonorrhea was responsible for their childlessness. Goodell had his semen examined twice, and found the husband to be azoospermic. As a result, he exhorted his colleagues "in the interest of science . . . as well as humanity" to examine the husband before treating the wife. His fellow physicians, however, remained reluctant, and even Goodell admitted, "such a diagnostic procedure is . . . repulsive to make." By the end of the century, however, the idea of semen examination did take hold among a number of the field's prominent practitioners.[42]

Recognition of the existence of azoospermia, which can result from a number of causes besides gonorrhea, may have led one of the most eminent Philadelphia gynecologists to resort to a clandestine donor insemination. In 1884, according to the later account of a physician who claimed to have been present, William Pancoast, professor at Jefferson Medical School, had been unsuccessfully treating the wife of a Quaker merchant for sterility. After all his treatments failed, he persuaded the husband to allow his semen to be analyzed; there were no spermatozoa. Pancoast, under the pretext of performing some minor surgical procedure, chloroformed the patient and inseminated her with the semen of one of his medical students. (Apparently, he told the husband.) She conceived, and doctor and husband kept the truth from her. When the story came out some two decades later, Pancoast had died and so could neither deny nor confirm what had happened. Whether apocryphal or not, the story was widely believed; physicians did not consider it implausible either that it happened or that it remained a secret. Robert L. Dickinson began performing donor inseminations in the 1890s, although he did not publicize the fact that he had done so until the 1930s. These examples notwithstanding, the extent to which practitioners engaged in donor insemination in the late nineteenth century is impossible to measure. Given how roundly practitioners condemned Sims, who had used only husbands' sperm, it is not surprising that donor insemination remained shrouded in secrecy.[43]

The recognition of the existence of sterility in men helped to create a specialty in male "genitourinary" diseases, the forerunner of urology. A number of new works on impotence and male sterility made their appearance in the 1890s. Respectable professors at major medical schools, in addition to the mail-order quacks and shady back-street operators, were now on hand to answer the questions that many a nervous young man on the brink of matrimony brought in to their consulting rooms. Is my penis too small? (If so, there were means to enlarge it, claimed the physicians.) How often can I have sexual intercourse without damaging my reproductive capacity or my mental powers? (The doctor could not only tell him how often—an average of twice a week for a healthy man under fifty—but also how long: three to five minutes.) But the major fear among the young men who consulted University of Pennsylvania professor Edward Martin and his counterparts elsewhere was impotence.[44]

In Martin's view, given the hysteria over youthful masturbation (which, he noted, nearly every boy indulged in at least once in a while), it was no wonder men worried. Martin, an authority among physicians on the treatment of impotence, urged doctors to prescribe tonics, pass a sound or two into the meatus (that is, insert a thin metal probe into the urethral opening at the head of the penis), and recommend a course of exercise. Actual deformities, of course, required surgery.[45]

By the 1890s, a few elite physicians had come to ascribe anywhere from 20 to 30 percent of infertility to inadequate sperm. If azoospermia resulted from gonorrheal infection, mumps, or some congenital malformation, they agreed, it was incurable. However, some doctors believed that a goodly proportion of the cases of azoospermia resulted from masturbation, morphine use, "sexual excess, [and] ungratified passion," and those cases were, they insisted, curable.[46]

The realization that men could be sterile marked an important shift in attitudes among gynecologists, but even more significant was the repudiation by a number of the field's leading practitioners of the radical reproductive surgery that had been developed in order to control women's behavior. There are several possible explanations for this change, in addition to embarrassment among elite practitioners over the operation's "almost wholesale use," in the words of Lawrence Longo, "for the cure of convulsive disorders and insanity." First, toward the end of the century, major hospitals acquired pathology laboratories. The discovery through pathological analysis that no disease existed in ovaries excised for behavioral problems shattered the rationale for performing such radical operations. By the turn of the century, sanity had at last come to reign on the ovariotomy issue. While such radical surgery for neurosis or dysmenorrhea still had some defenders, for the most part gynecologists seemed so ashamed of the excesses of the 1870s and 1880s that they often omitted in their public discussions any mention of what used to be known as "normal ovariotomy." Robert Battey's name did not cross the lips of Alexander J. C. Skene once in his retrospective of the field of gynecology in 1900.[47]

Second, as gynecologists, with the aid of better forms of anesthesia and more familiarity with asepsis, became more skillful surgeons they had less need to resort to more radical procedures for actual diseases. By the close of the century, elite American gynecologists had gained considerable technical proficiency. Thus, the lessons practitioners had learned earlier from ovariotomy could be applied to more complex and sometimes less mutilating procedures. Gynecologists had by now learned how to perform hysterectomies with safety, and the more conservative among them were also performing myomectomy (removal of fibroids from the uterus). By this time conservative surgeons, who went to great lengths to avoid removing any woman's reproductive organs except in cases of extreme exigency, had come to dominate the field. A number of them, most prominently Skene and Howard Kelly, introduced the term "medical gynecology" in the 1890s to encourage the development of nonsurgical treatments for a number of women's disorders.[48]

Conservative surgery did not mean a practice of watching and waiting before recommending an operation. In fact, these surgeons often performed daring feats. Their goal, however, was the improvement (or retention) of a woman's ability to conceive. The difference between radical and conservative surgeons was not in the amount, but in the kind, of surgery each group advocated. Radicals had argued that by extirpating diseased organs, they cured the patient and obviated the need for further surgery. The conservatives, some radicals continued to claim as the controversy heated up in the early 1890s, simply delayed the inevitable. For their part, conservatives insisted that premenopausal women should have their capacity for motherhood retained; or, if a hysterectomy was necessary, the surgeon should retain the ovaries if at all possible.[49] American physicians for the most part in the 1890s remained skeptical about the idea, just then gaining credence in Europe, that the ovary was a gland of internal secretion. Instead, the conservatives rested their claim on the notion that since menstruation and ovulation distinguished women from men, unless menopause were completed, a woman should keep her ovaries.[50]

Before laparotomy became a safe procedure, pathologists had documented in countless postmortem examinations that women in their childbearing years often had adhesions, cystic ovaries, and other signs of pelvic disease. By the last decade of the nineteenth century, the ovaries and the fallopian tubes had replaced the cervix as the principal culprits in cases of sterility, and conservatives increasingly recommended diagnostic laparotomy. Distinguished physicians now disparaged cervical incision as "the womb splitting delusion"; articles about reopening blocked fallopian tubes, removing ovarian cysts instead of extirpating the ovaries, and surgically excising pelvic adhesions now dominated the discussion of infertility treatment. In spite of the disrepute into which cervical incision had fallen, doctors had not recovered from their conviction that any deviation from the so-called normal midline position of the uterus needed to be corrected. But now many doctors rejected the idea of pessaries and "uterine adjusters," and instead surgically attached the recalcitrant uterus to the abdominal wall.[51]

Such changes did not mean that these gynecologists were becoming feminists, but rather that some of them, at least, were willing to question the idea that women's behavior resulted in reproductive disorders. Their surgical practice and new scientific discoveries had helped to push them toward this view. Their experience with infertile couples may also have contributed to their changing attitudes.

Experiencing Infertility

The dramatic demographic and social changes of the late nineteenth century notwithstanding, the overwhelming majority of women expected to marry and bear children. Even among highly educated women who had the opportunity to seek a career, in late-nineteenth-century America the choice was almost never whether to marry *and* have a career, but whether to marry *or* have a career. With the exception of women physicians, fewer than 10 percent of professional women in the late nineteenth century ever married. As historian Nancy Cott has argued, "Nineteenth-century advocates of women's right to equal work had . . . seen paid employment as alternatives to marriage." And in fact, women who could choose freely, that is, women with enough education that they could reasonably hope to have a satisfying career, were a rarity. In 1890 only about 2 percent of American women attended college, and the proportions of women graduating from high school were not substantially higher. Very few married women worked unless economic circumstances forced them to do so. Once married, a couple expected to bring children into the world. Until well after the turn of the century, even among women's rights advocates there lurked the idea that motherhood and a full-scale career were incompatible. Only the most radical of feminists before the turn of the twentieth century were publicly willing to assert otherwise. Those who did so, however, such as Charlotte Perkins Gilman, argued that such a change would require a restructuring of cherished traditions of family life as well as a radically new domestic architecture.[52]

The fact that the overwhelming majority of women married and that most married women expected and desired to be mothers does not mean that women's roles—and the roles of men as well—were not undergoing significant changes. Those middle-class women whose vision of their own roles had expanded to include social service and club membership increasingly urged their husbands to share more intimately in their domestic lives. In the middle of the nineteenth century, as a number of historians have documented, the most important bond in the family was between mother and child. In Mary Ryan's words, it held "the central place in the constellation of family affection."[53] By the end of the century, women advice givers were urging men to educate themselves for fatherhood. Within a decade, their male counterparts would be urging men to seek greater emotional closeness to their wives and to spend companionable time with their children. Indeed, as women were making incursions into the public realm, their husbands began to take a greater interest in the domestic one. One should not go too far with this; men were not sweeping and dusting, or making the family dinner. But among the middle classes, they were increasingly more involved in what one of Harriet Beecher Stowe's male characters called "the minutiae of domestic life."[54]

In fact, the transformation of the intimate familial relations among husbands and wives is one of the most significant factors for understanding the emotional dimensions of infertility in the late nineteenth century. It is true that among the middle classes, children had ceased to be an economic necessity. Americans, however, still reserved their highest approval for mothers, who were celebrated in essays, fiction, and verse for their wisdom and devotion. Women who were not mothers, unless they were single and exhibited devoted self-sacrifice in some other capacity, were viewed with suspicion. The culture labeled married women who chose not to have children as selfish and cold. According to popular writer Jennie June (who was actually women's rights advocate Jane Cunningham Croly), only a wife whose "heart and brain" were "deformed and misshapen" would make the choice to have a marriage without children.[55] Among the immigrant poor, where children *were* needed to contribute to the household income (although too many children too quickly became an economic burden), to be unable to conceive was also considered a failure of one's womanhood. One woman physician who treated poor immigrant women for sterility in Philadelphia remarked on the "ignominy" faced by women "among the lower classes when they do not bear children."[56]

For most women, children had long been the focus of family life, and it now appeared that for men as well parenthood was taking on new meaning. Couples were not having fewer children because they considered them less important. Clearly, many were using some means of birth control to limit the size of their families, but relatively few desired to opt out of parenthood altogether. To the contrary, historians of the middle-class family have found that stronger affectional ties between parents and children accompanied the decline in family size. For both parents, over the course of the nineteenth century, children developed an ever more central place in the emotional life of the family. They had more rights and privileges than the children of the antebellum era, and conversely, less responsibility for their own shortcomings, the weight of which, if we can believe the advice givers, rested on their mothers' shoulders. That burden, in turn, made the practice of childrearing all the more crucial to a family's view of its own success.[57]

Historians know a great deal about the importance of children within the society as a whole and within individual families. It is much more difficult to find direct evidence about the emotional impact of infertility in this era. The extraordinary reticence of late-nineteenth-century Americans when they were unable to have children cannot be accounted for simply

by reference to Victorian sensibilities. The freely shared confidences between sisters and mothers and daughters about their hopes and fears in
pregnancy, or between brothers about their wives' confinements, which
historian Judith Walzer Leavitt has so poignantly delineated, had no parallel among the infertile. And yet a few women have left behind some evidence, however indirect, of their feelings.[58]

Kate Douglas Wiggin, Margaret Deland, and Ella Wheeler Wilcox
were three late-nineteenth-century writers who were involuntarily childless. Wiggin was the popular author of *Rebecca of Sunnybrook Farm* and
one of the early leaders of the kindergarten movement in the United
States. Nora Smith, her sister and biographer, claimed that Wiggin continued her commitment to the kindergarten movement, even after she became famous, because it enabled her to assuage her sadness over her inability to bear her own children. It is unclear whether Wiggin ever sought
infertility treatment, although Smith referred delicately to "a serious surgical operation" (a widely used euphemism for gynecological operations)
that Wiggin underwent, that might either have accounted for her childlessness or have been in pursuit of pregnancy.[59] The novelist Margaret Deland also was veiled in her expressions of regret for her childlessness. As
her biographer noted, Deland was not given to talking about her personal
problems, even to close friends in her personal correspondence, informing them "briefly" that she had undergone surgery. Among the childless
late-nineteenth-century writers, only Ella Wheeler Wilcox openly wrote
about her anguish, and with her the situation was somewhat different; she
had borne one child, who lived less than a day.[60] It is possible, of course,
that these women's expressions of regret were merely concessions to a culture where motherhood virtually defined womanhood. However, their
lifelong commitment to children's issues suggests some depth of emotion.

In contrast to the women, men were almost uniformly silent; as a result, their feelings are even more difficult to grasp. Such reticence makes
it seem even more remarkable that Henry Adams, whose published autobiographical work was devoid of any mention of his intimate life, should
be one of the few men who spoke—even indirectly—about his infertile
marriage. Both he and his wife, Clover, expressed their unhappiness over
their childlessness. When they married in 1872, she was twenty-nine, he
thirty-four. By all accounts, their early years of marriage were emotionally close and mutually fulfilling, in spite of her occasional periods of
melancholy. They had hoped to have a family, but no children arrived. She
coped with her childlessness sometimes by feigning disinterest in the nu-

merous births among her family or friends, sometimes by giving way to outbursts. As she told her cousin Anne Lothrop, any woman who proclaimed disinterest in motherhood was lying. "It isn't true," she cried. *"All women want children!"*[61]

Henry's library contained a copy of J. Marion Sims's famous work on sterility; if he and Clover consulted either Sims himself or another physician about their problem, it was to no avail. Patricia O'Toole, an Adams biographer, has said that Henry had married "with the hope of having children, but by 1876 had realized that his desires might go unfulfilled. In answer to news of a birth and a death, his normally fluid pen developed a stammer. 'I wish—wish—wish—well, I wish various things, but among others that the mystery of Birth and the Grave were either less important to us, or more encouraging.' " Apparently he gave up hope soon afterwards, and in later years remarked testily that if it were not for the impertinent inquiries from family and friends about his and Clover's continued childlessness, "I should never think about the subject." Perhaps. As for Clover, the extent to which their inability to have children contributed to her periodic depressions or to her eventual suicide is impossible to determine, but that it caused her disappointment in her lifetime is clear. After her death, a close friend remarked that she had everything she could have wanted, except children.[62]

Clover and Henry Adams cannot have been the only couple in late-nineteenth-century America to face the veiled or open inquiries of family members, the curiosity of friends and acquaintances, "half the world not letting the other half alone," as the nettled Henry Adams put it. If so articulate a man as Adams, who was rarely at a loss for words, found his pen faltering when he tried to express his desire for children, perhaps other men had even greater difficulty in giving voice to their own emotional longings. Their silence may not have reflected lack of feeling.[63] If men did not talk about their childlessness, however, it does appear that at least some of them were taking an interest in their wives' medical treatments. As limited as the data are, there is no doubt that the husbands of infertile women were more visible in the late nineteenth century than they were in the 1850s and 1860s. A number of physicians began to note the presence of husbands during consultations. And some of them were now advocating semen testing, an early step toward viewing the infertility as a couple's, and not a woman's, problem.[64]

Seeking Medical Treatment

The numbers of women, with or without their husbands, who sought infertility treatment in this period cannot be counted with any accuracy. H. Marion Sims, son of J. Marion, claimed in 1888, "Probably the gynecologist of today is consulted more often in regard to the sterile condition of woman than for any [other] disease."[65] Articles in the gynecological journals demonstrate that practitioners' interest in new treatment techniques and the effectiveness of existing ones did not abate, and hospital-based gynecologists appear to have had substantial practices in infertility treatment. Exploring the interaction between these physicians and their patients allows historians to make a distinction between the rhetoric of medical understandings of infertility and the reality of treating it.

Women who decided to consult a physician for sterility in this era were setting out on an uncertain course. In our own day, visits to the gynecologist are far more commonplace, but a century ago people rarely saw doctors for anything less than a serious condition. Those women who took themselves to clinic or consulting room in search of solutions to their childlessness, therefore, clearly assumed that they were suffering from a treatable medical condition and believed that such a condition was serious enough for medical intervention. Physicians increasingly had the upper hand in this interaction because they asserted their mastery over the mysteries of science and technology. This did not mean, however, that women were willing to accede to everything the physician said. Indeed, some women, who seemed to be quite well informed about their medical options, were not reluctant to say what therapies they would or would not tolerate. Gynecologists might have denominated themselves "priests" of women's health, but women did not simply play the role of a passive icon. The interaction between physician and patient was fraught with ambiguity. Doctors had something a woman did not, access to diagnostic and therapeutic tools to provide her with a reason for her childlessness and perhaps an alleviation of it. Women could choose to accept or refuse treatment, or to persuade the physician to try something else. And when their husbands became involved, the situation became even more complex.[66]

That women often insisted on having their own way is clear from the numerous complaints of practitioners, who expressed considerable annoyance at their patients' refusal to take their advice. As gynecologist Paul Mundé grumbled, "In quite a large number of cases . . . the unwillingness of the patient to submit to the use of the knife, has restricted me to tents and dilators."[67] But some women demanded operations in such a way that conscientious physicians had difficulty dissuading them. Gynecologists regularly noted the presence of women who made the rounds of their consulting rooms, demanding surgery from a new doctor when the former one refused. One of William Goodell's patients, for example, "so begged and so urged me to perform any operation which would be likely to make her fruitful," that in spite of his belief that the surgery was uncalled for he came close to agreeing.[68] Other women refused to wear a pessary, or would wear one only if they could take narcotics for the discomfort. Some demanded general anesthesia before they would undergo dilatation, in spite of physicians' belief that the pain was slight and the danger from the anesthesia too great. (Most doctors did use a topical anesthetic, but this was not enough for some women.)[69]

Gynecologists had mixed reactions to dealing with their patients' husbands, as well. By the 1890s, as elite gynecologists argued for the need to analyze seminal fluid, the recalcitrant husband who refused semen testing became a staple of doctors' anecdotes. For every loving husband who wished to spare his wife unnecessary surgery, there were more who took umbrage at the imagined insult to their virility. One outraged husband knocked his wife to the floor in the doctor's office and loudly proclaimed that the physician himself was "insane" to suggest he might be sterile. Such attitudes on the part of husbands led many physicians simply to give up on the idea of demanding sperm samples. Indeed, in spite of the fact that husbands were more in evidence than ever, male involvement was by no means universal. Some women seemed unwilling even to tell their husbands that they were seeing a physician for an infertility problem. Max Huhner, the early-twentieth-century pioneer of postcoital testing, noted that one of the difficulties of attempting to test a husband for infertility was that he might not even be aware that his wife was seeking treatment. Outside of the practices of eminent gynecologists, semen analysis did not become a routine part of arriving at a diagnosis of infertility until the 1950s; and even today many physicians remain very sensitive to male anxieties about the relationship of their sperm count to their sexual capacities.[70]

The most common type of doctor-husband interaction came in the context of a wife's medical treatment, and it took the form of conflicts over surgery. One physician, who diagnosed a diseased ovary as the cause of a patient's infertility, informed her that her chance of pregnancy would be enhanced if she had it removed. Her husband, who feared she might die as a result of the surgery, talked her out of it.[71]

Although men had become a more common presence in physicians' consulting rooms, it remained true that *wives* continued almost always to be the focus of medical intervention. Infertility treatment was most often a female experience, even if sometimes mediated by a husband's involvement. It was also an experience that cut across ethnic, racial, and class lines, as women who could not afford private care took advantage of the services of free clinics in large northern cities. Max Huhner found that in a sample of one thousand gynecological cases treated at his free clinic, a full 70 percent, most of them immigrant wives and many married for a year or less, had come in specifically for treatment of their infertility.[72]

The scene of women's interactions with practitioners varied—paying patients waited their turn in physicians' consulting rooms, and the poor lined up at hospital outpatient clinics—but the recommended course of treatment was generally the same. The difficulty, of course, was that poor women rarely had the leisure to devote to an extensive period of treatment, which might involve days of bed rest or a series of operations.

Some practitioners, it is evident, had little sympathy for their clinic patients, valuing them principally as case material for experimental treatments to be presented at meetings or published in journal articles. Annoyance and irritation appeared to constitute the whole of their attitude toward these women, who, these unsympathetic doctors complained, rarely bothered to complete their treatment. As one New York gynecologist snapped, his clinic patients "underrate[d] the value of medical services which cost them no money."[73] However, it is important not to rush to the conclusion that working-class women were invariably shortchanged. At the Woman's Hospital in New York, Thomas Addis Emmet continued to treat women of all social classes with care and dignity until he retired at the close of the century. Other practitioners followed suit. In Baltimore, Thomas Ashby recalled with sympathy one of his patients, an African American domestic worker, who underwent two surgeries in the 1890s for pelvic adhesions that Ashby believed were causing her infertility. Although she was able to conceive, he recalled, because her life was a round of unending hard labor, she was unable to carry a pregnancy to term.[74]

The evidence presented here suggests that at least some women from all walks of life—middle and working class, black and white, native-born and immigrant—were seeking infertility treatment by the turn of the century. Patients, their husbands, and practitioners did not necessarily behave in class- or ethnically stereotyped ways. For example, the loving husband who in order to spare his wife an operation was willing to confess, after a decade of silence, that he had contracted gonorrhea was an Irish immigrant. Class and ethnicity do not seem to have determined women's deci-

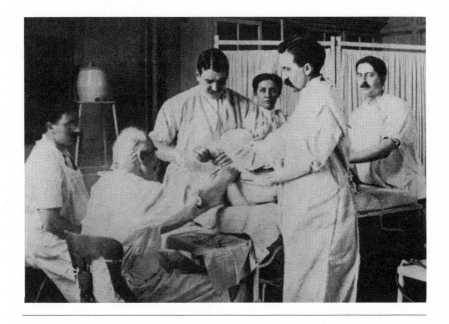

Gynecological surgery at the end of the nineteenth century. Thomas Addis Emmet performs his last operation at the Woman's Hospital.
Courtesy of the College of Physicians of Philadelphia

sions to seek out infertility greatment or the kinds of treatment they received. Geographical factors were probably much more influential. Up-to-date treatment was much more readily available in large urban areas in the north for all women.[75]

One might wonder whether women were seeking treatment in greater numbers out of any sense that therapies were becoming more successful. This is a difficult question to answer. Only a few gynecologists in the late nineteenth century gave success rates for their treatments, although they all had success stories. Joseph Kammerer's statistical study, in which he reported 25 pregnancies out of a group of 176 women, was unusual. In spite of the fact that the profession as a whole was moving toward a statistical model in reporting operative results in other kinds of surgery, the treatment of sterility was different. It often took a long time, and follow-up was difficult. Not until around World War I would physicians make any sustained attempts at determining the efficacy of their infertility treatments. That said, it is probably also true that physicians continued to use the anecdotal model of reportage because they did not have very many successes. T. Gaillard Thomas spoke for most of his profession when he noted that treating sterility brought him "the least satisfaction and the most disappointment" of anything in his gynecological career.[76]

Most women treated for sterility in the late nineteenth century left their doctor's care without a pregnancy. Indeed, even Kammerer's figures, drawn from his private practice because he had so little success with his clinic patients, represented a cure rate of under 15 percent. And even this figure overstates the numbers of infertile couples overall who were able to have their own biological offspring. Most women with infertility problems did not consult a physician, although that does not necessarily mean that they passively accepted their fate. The success of Lydia Pinkham's tonic, which for a while was advertised as having "a baby in every bottle," attests to the strength of popular faith (or hope) in home remedies. Pinkham's tonic, the formula of which was based on the botanical medicines of the previous generation, contained some of the same roots and leaves that Eclectics and Thomsonians would have given women who had come to them with an infertility problem in the 1840s and 1850s. Lydia Pinkham's elixir and others such as Dr. Pierce's Golden Medical Discovery in some ways replaced the medicines that previous generations of "barren" women had concocted for themselves.[77]

Adoption: Another "Cure" for Infertility?

At the risk of stating the obvious, it seems evident that most infertile couples had to live with their condition. In some cases, however, they were able to find another "cure" for their infertility through adoption. Evidence suggests that increased numbers of childless couples in this period decided to provide themselves with a family through adoption when biological parenthood eluded them. Unfortunately historians, noting the fact that there were few *legalized* adoptions, have generally concluded that until the twentieth century couples who took unrelated children into their households did so more for economic than emotional reasons. But recent research by Julie Berebitsky has shown that a considerable number of childless couples in this period sought infants and young children to "raise as their own." While few of these couples utilized the legal system to formalize the adoptions, most of them gave the children their surnames, chose infants whenever possible so that it would be easier to conceal from the children the fact that they were not the biological parents, and often waged guerrilla warfare when a charity society or a biological parent tried to regain custody.[78]

The late nineteenth century seems to have provided a unique opportunity for both formal adoption and these adoptionlike practices as well. By the early twentieth century, changing notions of the rights of biological parents would make infants more difficult to come by (although paradoxically, just as adoption was becoming more difficult, it would become touted in popular magazines as the most sensible solution to involuntary childlessness). The evidence concerning adoption for the late nineteenth century is fragmentary but suggestive. Laws governing the practice proliferated in this period. Massachusetts passed the country's first adoption law (in 1851), Wisconsin came next in 1853, and Pennsylvania followed suit in 1855. In the quarter-century after the passage of the Massachusetts law, more than twenty states passed some sort of adoption law. Elsewhere, formal adoption required special action by the legislature.[79]

In Massachusetts, the Temporary Home for the Destitute directly influenced the passage of that state's adoption law, and in the words of two scholars, "became the earliest known proponent of welfare adoption." By the early 1870s, in fact, the Temporary Home had evolved into a de facto adoption agency. For over a decade, the institution had been encouraging childless couples to adopt its youngest charges; in 1871, it opened a Baby Department and began actively seeking out infants in the city's poor neighborhoods. The Temporary Home sought out unwed mothers and sometimes coerced them into relinquishing their babies; occasionally, the managers initiated guardianship actions in court when poor parents refused to part with their children. In deciding which children to admit to the Home, the managers deliberately looked for so-called adoptable children—white, seemingly healthy, and intelligent infants.[80]

The Temporary Home kept up this policy, in the face of criticism from Boston's other charitable societies, until the early 1890s. Until then, while a majority of the babies were the offspring of immigrants, over 65 percent of the adopting parents were native white Protestants. During these years, volunteers from the same social group as the adoptive parents controlled the institution and actively participated in its day-to-day management. By the turn of the century, paid agents had replaced the volunteers. These professionalized workers brought a new philosophy to their work, one that encouraged unwed mothers to keep their children, perhaps not so much out of a sentimental vision of the mother-child bond, but because such women should be made to "bear rather than escape" their maternal duty.[81]

In other cities, children's welfare societies were not so eager even in the latter half of the nineteenth century to break up poor families or to remove babies from their unmarried mothers. Whether from an understanding that parents wanted to be with their children or from the idea that the poor should be forced to take "responsibility," such agencies were often reluctant to force parents into relinquishing their rights. Even parents who did sign away a child sometimes found ways of having their children returned. Still, determined childless couples—white and African American, working-class and well-to-do—sought out infants to raise as their own, whether or not they adopted them legally. After the turn of the century, when social welfare agencies created more explicit policies that encouraged unwed mothers to keep their babies, adoption became an ever more complicated option for the childless. (Although such agencies strongly promoted foster parenthood as an alternative to institutionalizing homeless but not orphaned children, childless couples preferred to adopt.) But for the moment, an untold number of couples found one solution to their childlessness.[82]

Adoption was not a universal panacea. Some feared a hereditary taint in an illegitimate baby or the child of poor immigrants; in others, the yearning for biological parenthood was so strong that no alternative would compensate. Still others feared that relatives or neighbors might stigmatize the adopted child. Some, of course, had no access to infants to adopt, but there were childless women who actively participated in organizations similar to the Temporary Home for the Destitute who decided that adoption was not a solution for them. Prominent Kentucky social reformer and suffragist Madeline McDowell Breckinridge, for example, wife of Lexington newspaper publisher Desha Breckinridge, devoted considerable energy to the Kentucky Children's Home Society, the letterhead of whose stationery featured an engraving of a small child, its arms outstretched, with the words, "Please Help Me Find a Home." But she and her husband never adopted.[83]

The writer Margaret Deland, orphaned herself as an infant and adopted by an aunt and uncle, also chose not to adopt. By her own account, even though her adoptive parents always treated her as they did their biological children, once Deland became an adolescent, she began to feel less and less a part of the family. For several years, in fact, she estranged herself, although she later repaired the relationship. As a young matron, before her writing career became successful, Deland actively participated in the effort to redeem "fallen" women by hiring unwed mothers as domestics. (The young women brought their babies with them when they took a position, and upper-middle-class women who hired such domestic help considered themselves to be performing a noble service.) Deland's reluctance to adopt may have been shaped by her own not very happy experience as an adopted child; in addition, her work with unwed mothers and their children regularly brought babies into her life.[84]

These two "cures" for infertility—medical treatment and adoption—began to acquire their modern trappings in the late nineteenth century. Adoption laws proliferated, and social agencies began to take on the responsibility of making the policies that would guide placement agencies into the twentieth century. Within the medical profession, treatment for sterility had become an important part of gynecology, and gynecology itself had become a recognized specialty. Whereas in 1875 medical schools had limited their gynecological instruction to a few lectures, now there were entire courses devoted to the subject. And the increase in the journal literature, with its detailed descriptions of how to recognize gonorrhea in a patient and exactly how to perform a surgical procedure, allowed gynecologists to read about new developments. Although elite medical practitioners were only a small part of the medical profession, they wrote the texts and taught the courses on gynecology and genitourinary surgery, and most medical students in the last twenty years of the nineteenth century had exposure to the new ideas.

Of course, not every involuntarily childless woman who went to her family doctor was told to bring in her husband for a semen examination (indeed, the constant exhortation in the journals by the very few eminent practitioners who did so suggests the reverse) or that cervical amputation came to a halt. And for every ovary resected or fallopian tube unblocked that resulted in pregnancy, there were numerous failures. Many urban as well as rural women either chose not to or were unable to consult a physician and continued to rely on Lydia Pinkham's tonic, Dr. Pierce's Golden Medical Discovery, or mail-order electrotherapeutics.

But by now treatment for sterility had become a routine service offered by gynecological specialists as well as by some general practitioners who had been trained in regular or homeopathic institutions. As the twentieth century opened, physicians expressed confidence that their increasing operative skills would enable more women to conceive, and that those skills would be in great demand. Within the larger society, questions were forming about men's sexual responsibility and about the role of the state in encouraging or discouraging reproduction. These questions helped to shape the attitudes toward infertility that would permeate the twentieth century's response to involuntary childlessness.

Entr'acte

four   # Framing Infertility

Sexuality, Marriage, and
Parenthood in Twentieth-
Century America

Love and nothing else ... very soon is
nothing else.

Walter Lippmann, 1929

Toward the end of the nineteenth century, as the last chapter revealed, increasing numbers of women in America's cities, sometimes with the involvement of their husbands, actively sought to alleviate their involuntary childlessness by seeking medical treatment. Gynecologists based in urban voluntary hospitals, who stood at the forefront of this emerging specialty, took the lead in diagnosing the condition and providing new surgical treatments. These practitioners were the key providers of services; however, medical advances were not the only force behind the determination of these women to become mothers, as suggested by the emergence of what sociologist Viviana Zelizer has called "sentimental" adoption during this period.[1] By the second decade or so of the twentieth century, medical treatment and sentimental adoption had become accepted ways for couples to fill their "empty cradles." In the mid–nineteenth century, when Mary Chesnut, as it appears, sought medical advice for her infertility, and Amelia and Dexter Bloomer adopted two children largely because she craved the experience of motherhood, they were among a small number of women who took active measures to end their childlessness. By the early twentieth century, they would be joined by thousands of others. Medical therapies and adoption would go hand-in-hand over the course of the twentieth century. From the 1930s to the 1950s, adoption would even be touted as a medical therapy, as many physicians began to argue (wrongly) that couples who adopted enjoyed greatly increased odds of conceiving their own children.

This "entr'acte" is designed to serve as a guide to the social and cultural changes that became central to the growing willingness to pursue parenthood aggressively in the twentieth century. It is not so much about infertility as it is about its cultural "frame"—transformations that took place in the ways in which Americans thought about sexuality, marriage, and parenthood. In understanding how these institutions were changing, the cultural dimensions of Americans' experience of infertility in the twentieth century become more comprehensible.[2]

By the early twentieth century, the Victorian consensus about sexuality, marriage, and the proper roles for men and women had become battered by birth control advocates, mocked by prostitutes and their clients as well as by the lure of working-class "charity girls" who bartered sexual favors for gifts and good times, challenged by middle-class "New Women," and subverted by married couples who demanded intimacy in their relationships and who divorced when marriage failed to live up to their expectations. By the 1920s, the now shaky edifice had buckled and finally given way.[3] Marriage and family life came under increased pressure to satisfy an ever-expanding array of emotional needs. Whereas nineteenth-century domestic reformers had enshrined the role of women within the home as the linchpin of social cohesion, twentieth-century social "experts" claimed that children provided the raison d'être for both family and community life. Prospective parents now weighed the value of children on a different scale; the result was, as Zelizer has put it, the "sacralization" of children.[4]

By the 1920s, as a result of a combination of the enforcement of child labor laws and the restriction of immigration, children had virtually ceased to be necessary contributors to the family income, even among the working classes. Nearly all youngsters stayed in school at least until the age of fourteen or sixteen; high school attendance had become an American commonplace. Although without a recognizable economic value, children had become "priceless." For some couples, indeed, they were be-

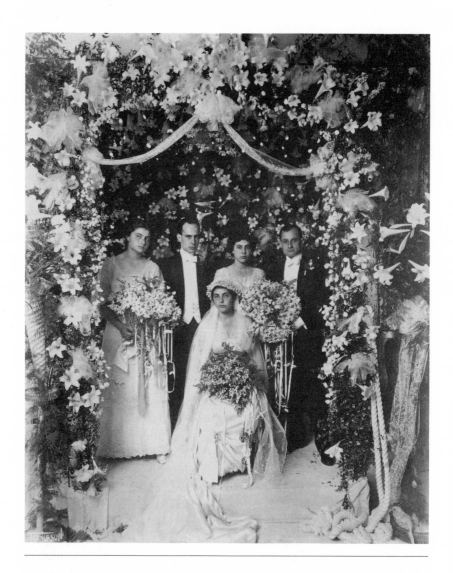

A wedding party. In spite of the new freedoms many middle-class women seemed to enjoy in the early twentieth century, the overarching message of the larger society was that the ultimate goal of every "normal" woman was marriage.
Courtesy of the Library of Congress

coming almost a commodity, a kind of consumer good that symbolized family completion and marital success. In this period, exemplified most clearly in the way in which the society dealt with adoption, we can see the insidious beginnings of what we might call in the late twentieth century the commodification of children.[5]

The involuntarily childless couple of the new century had to contend with changing attitudes toward marriage and the family as they attempted to cope with their situation. Over the course of the first third of the twentieth century, Americans worked out a new consensus on the nature of sexuality, marriage, and parenthood, the implications of which would continue to reverberate throughout the century, and indeed would not face a significant challenge until the 1970s.[6] In the early twentieth century, such issues as birth control, sexual intimacy, and divorce became subjects of open debate. As a part of this process of airing formerly proscribed topics in the public arena, the issue of infertility for the first time appeared in the popular press. Ironically, women with infertility problems first began to speak out as a defense against being labeled as participants in what had come to be called "race suicide."

In 1903, President Theodore Roosevelt introduced the idea of "race suicide" to an American middle class already uneasy about the implications of unrestricted immigration. The term, coined by sociologist E. A. Ross, referred to the drastic decline, discussed in the last chapter, in the birthrate among native-born white Protestants of English descent. Roosevelt hinted darkly of the causes of that decline, continuing to return to the subject throughout his presidency and beyond it. As he declaimed in 1911, "The greatest of all curses is the curse of sterility; and the severest of all condemnations should be . . . visited upon willful sterility." Couples unable to have children, he conceded, faced "a great misfortune." Voluntary childlessness, however, came from a shameful desire for a life "of ease and self-indulgence."[7]

Roosevelt's speeches on race suicide eerily echoed Edward Clarke's warning to an earlier generation that the United States would soon have to rely on its "inferior classes" to populate the nation. The prophecy, many believed, had come true. In sociological journals, popular magazines, and medical literature, writers came to terms with the ever-declining rate of reproduction among middle-class Americans. For the most part, they seconded Roosevelt's denunciation of birth control. Ethel Wadsworth Cartland, a minister's wife and mother of four, wailed in the pages of *Outlook* that "the old stock, the grand old stock, the fine, cultivated, progressive, loyal, Puritan stock, is dying out . . . a passing suicidal!"[8] Conventional wisdom, she told her readers, held that a couple should have four children "for the upbuilding of the race," if they expected to compete with the prolific immigrants. As she and other opponents of birth control complained, however, the "fine . . . old stock" Americans were at best having one or two. They were correct. Family size continued to fall, and by 1910 fully a quarter of all completed urban families had only two children. In the Middle Atlantic and Great Lakes regions, the proportion of two-child families rose to 40 percent. But not everyone agreed that the sole culprit causing the decline in family size was birth control. E. A. Ross himself came to believe that "much of the childlessness of native wives is due to little-understood physical causes."[9]

Many physicians, particularly in the early years of the twentieth century, were inclined to agree that although smaller families of two or three children bore the imprint of contraceptive practices, absolute childlessness and the one-child family usually were the result of infertility. In spite of the admission by a number of prominent gynecologists that education had not rendered American women sterile, some of their colleagues continued to insist that higher education lowered women's reproductive capacity. George Engelmann, a nationally known infertility expert, remained convinced that "college work" with its accompanying "nerve exhaustion" remained a major cause of sterility in women.[10]

Women, too, were most often held responsible for the use of contraception, which most doctors agreed often led to infertility. Exactly how birth control was supposed to cause infertility was unclear; the problems, physicians agreed, developed no matter what the method. Even withdrawal, a technique completely free from chemicals or foreign substances, was said to cause "passive congestion" in women. Gynecologists complained that women who eventually came to regret the "nefarious practice" of contraception and felt the pull of motherhood by their late twenties or early thirties were "tedious and trying" to treat, because their infertility was "self-inflicted." Men, however, came in for an increasing share of blame, either because they strayed from the path of chastity and contracted venereal disease or because they persuaded their wives to overindulge in sexual intercourse.[11]

The idea that every form of contraception could cause sterility did not come under sustained attack until the 1920s and 1930s. Until then, most doctors considered it their "duty to point out" to any patient who had practiced birth control that "her sterility and her suffering" were her own fault.[12] Such views had clearly made their way into the popular press by the early part of the century. Blaming women for infertility might seem

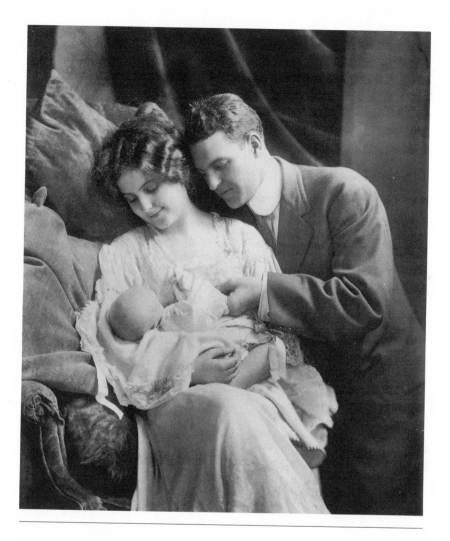

The new baby. The expectation of marital intimacy did not diminish the significance of children, who remained an essential element in the new definitions of marriage and family life that emerged in the early twentieth century.
Courtesy of the Library of Congress

like familiar territory, a holdover of late-nineteenth-century attitudes, but in fact no general circulation magazine in the late nineteenth century would have handled such a subject. In the early twentieth century, in contrast, such discussions would become a staple of women's magazines. One remarkable group of letters written to *Good Housekeeping* magazine in 1911 and 1912 resulted from a reader's bold announcement that she and her husband had chosen to remain childless until they could comfortably afford a baby. Subsequent issues fairly crackled in response, as letters poured in from mothers, childless wives, and one (male) physician, all denouncing her as unspeakably selfish. Several readers, including the physician, warned that when she tired of her childlessness, as they were sure she would, she would find herself unable to conceive.[13]

More significant in terms of bringing topics of sexuality and infertility before the public, however, was the widespread discussion of men's responsibility for inflicting sterility on their wives as a result of acquiring gonorrhea from prostitutes. In the late nineteenth century, this had been a subject for discussion only among physicians. By the early twentieth century, venereal disease was openly discussed in the popular press, as an influential group of physicians and antivice reformers attempted to convince the public that gonorrhea was perhaps the most important cause of both absolute and "one-child" sterility in the United States.[14]

In 1904, Prince Albert Morrow, a New York practitioner who became the nation's foremost expert on venereal disease, claimed in *Social Diseases and Marriage* that gonorrhea was "the most widespread and universal disease in the adult male population"; among the men of New York, 75 percent "or more" had been infected. Other physicians acclaimed his work, rushing to give their own statistics, which were just as shocking. They were also based on equally suspect data, since, like him, his supporters extrapolated their figures from urban hospital patient populations, not from the public at large. In fact, no systematic nationwide study of venereal disease appeared in these years. Nevertheless, unlike Emil Noeggerath, whose similar—although less overwrought—statements a generation before the Progressive Era were initially disbelieved, Morrow spoke to a receptive audience of practitioners and the public.[15]

Claims that at least 50 percent of gynecological surgery performed on women was the result of untreated gonorrhea became a medical commonplace and easily passed into popular belief. After all, the antivice crusade was at high tide, and the idea that prostitution was as much a physiological crime as a moral outrage provided ammunition for the reformers. In 1906, the American Medical Association held a symposium to educate its members on the subject. Practitioners' guides—pocket-sized handbooks that the family physician often carried around as aids to diagnosis and treatment—began to reflect the belief that gonorrhea caused a high proportion of infertility. A few voices rose to protest that, in the absence of credible national surveys, estimates of infection rates of from 50 to 75 percent in men were simply too high to be believed. But they were drowned out, for the moment, by the rush to believe that there was a relatively simple solution to the declining middle-class birthrate: Outlaw prostitution and ostracize the men who patronized the prostitutes, this scenario went, and race suicide will no longer be a problem.[16]

Putting together in one frame an image of depravity implied by a sexually transmitted disease with a portrait of idealized purity suggested by an innocent bride provided sure-fire sensationalism in the early twentieth century, allowing Americans to talk openly about sexuality under the guise of safeguarding the health of future mothers. This is not to say that Americans initially welcomed such talk. The 1906 decision of the *Ladies Home Journal,* which had a circulation of over a million, to discuss venereal disease brought howls of protest. But Edward Bok, the publisher, stood firm, and hundreds of thousands of women learned from physician Abraham L. Wolbarst that the chief destroyer of marital happiness was the idea that young men had a right to "scatter a supply of 'wild oats' before they settle down and marry." According to Wolbarst, "the highest authorities in medical investigation" agreed that these "wild oats" accounted for "at least fifty percent of all childless homes in this country."[17] Such articles soon became commonplace. *Good Housekeeping*'s discussion in 1911 of the importance of sex education for adolescents as a way to prevent venereal disease raised hardly an eyebrow among the magazine's readers.[18]

Male sexual behavior came under increasing scrutiny, as medical and social authorities shifted a considerable degree of the responsibility for infertility from women to men. In a brief period of reckless sexual indulgence, young men doomed themselves to childless homes and their future wives to chronic invalidism. Or so said the physicians and the reformers in the early years of the twentieth century. But was gonorrhea responsible for as much childlessness as they claimed? It is difficult to know. We can never definitively calculate the role of gonorrhea in abetting the fertility decline in the early twentieth century, but that the decline was real and dramatic is not in question. About 16 percent of the married white women who were in their childbearing years during the first two decades of the twentieth century, and about 18 percent of their counterparts among women of color, remained childless, and those who became parents had fewer children. George Engelmann attributed the high rate of infertility among his African American patients to gonorrhea, but there is no way to determine the accuracy of his etiological explanation. Others

insisted, without citing numbers, that patient after patient from every ethnic background and social class had had her health ruined, her chances
for motherhood destroyed, and her reproductive organs removed as a result of the irresponsible behavior of fiancés or husbands.[19]

On the one hand, figures on infection rates were unreliable and impressionistic, and the belief that every woman who developed gonorrhea
would suffer severe inflammations of the fallopian tubes or ovaries was
erroneous. Nevertheless, gonorrhea was not curable in the early twentieth century, and surely did cause a substantial amount of infertility. The
case reports of the Woman's Hospital, discussed in Chapter 2, and Emil
Noeggerath's research, detailed in Chapter 3, both revealed numerous instances of what we now call pelvic inflammatory disease, a common se-
quela of gonorrhea in women, as well as patient histories that conformed
to symptoms of gonorrheal infection. But in fact, since everyone appeared
to be convinced by the first decade of the twentieth century that gonorrhea had reached nearly epidemic proportions, no one at the time attempted to demonstrate otherwise.[20]

The public campaign against venereal disease led to legal action. By
1913, seven states had barred men with venereal disease from marrying.
After 1910, a new drug, Salvarsan, provided an effective treatment for
syphilis, but a cure for gonorrhea remained elusive for another generation. (Sulfa drugs became available in the 1930s and were used to treat
gonorrhea, apparently with some success, but not until the development
of penicillin in the 1940s was it truly curable.) World War I brought venereal hysteria to new heights and the diseases to greater public attention.
Despite a wide range of public action, however, gonorrhea remained an
important factor in infertility into the 1920s, when it was estimated that
there were 700,000 new cases a year. It continues to be significant today.[21]

As this emphasis on contraception or gonorrhea as causes of childlessness might suggest, by the early twentieth century authorities were focusing more on the sex organs and less on the brain in searching for etiological explanations for infertility. By World War I, virtually no credible
authority attributed sterility in women to college work. To some extent,
the pioneering work of women physicians such as Mary Putnam Jacobi
and Clelia Mosher, together with their counterparts in England, had convinced their colleagues that menstruation did not prevent women from
studying, and that studying did not render them sterile. Women physicians
and educators on both sides of the Atlantic, frustrated by the oft-repeated
late-nineteenth-century charge that education rendered women sterile,

produced a number of studies suggesting that social standing rather than education determined how many children a woman bore.[22]

More important than these studies, however, was the realization among observers during the first two decades of the twentieth century that these young college women, unlike some of the pioneering graduates of a generation earlier, were not turning their backs on conventional roles. As historian Sheila Rothman has suggested, "the notion that a college education was actually an advantage to would-be mothers gained popularity" in the first two decades of the twentieth century, making it more "socially acceptable for women to enter the university." By the 1920s, although the birthrate itself had not risen, it finally became clear that women in general had not abandoned family life for careers. The marriage rate rose, and the 1920s witnessed, as John Modell has noted, a "slightly more rapid move into parenthood," a trend that cut across racial and socioeconomic lines.[23]

The public discussions of such heretofore taboo subjects as birth control, under the guise of deploring "race suicide" and commercial sex, through the vehicle of the campaign against venereal disease, brought sexual topics into public life in a way that would have seemed unthinkable in the late nineteenth century. Although repression of inappropriate sexual behavior, rather than expression of new attitudes toward sexuality, was the goal of those who brought these issues before the public, the very fact of such open discussion marked the beginnings of a new era. By the 1920s, as historians of sexuality John D'Emilio and Estelle Freedman have demonstrated, a "shift toward a philosophy of indulgence marked the demise of nineteenth-century prescriptions about continence and self-control."[24]

Of course, historians have long questioned the alleged antisexuality of the Victorian period. Carl Degler's interpretation of Clelia Mosher's sex survey has suggested that many late-nineteenth-century women took considerable pleasure in sexual activity, a view confirmed by Peter Gay's studies of bourgeois Victorians. Nevertheless, the Victorians retained their public reticence. Women might have talked about sex to women physicians, written about it in their diaries, or whispered intimately to their husbands. They did not express their views in the popular press. When a popular magazine claimed in 1913 that "Sex O'Clock" had struck in America, it was the open discussion of sexuality to which it referred, what we might call the bells on the clock at city hall tower. It had already chimed in the bedroom. But even if the Victorians were not so "Victorian" in private as convention would have it, the end to public reticence marked an important cultural change. In part because of an urban working-class youth subculture that flaunted sexuality, in part because of the glamour of the bohemian lifestyles adopted by young (and some not so young) middle-class rebels, in part because of feminism's new direction, and in part because of the aggressive frankness of the antivice movement, sexuality emerged as a subject of widespread discussion in the years before World War I.[25]

At first, some discretion prevailed. The middle-class couples who, comfortable in their cozy domesticity, went about planning separate child-oriented spaces within their houses did not emphasize the fact that in setting aside space for their children they were also providing distinct intimate spaces for themselves. But the next generation was less inhibited in its public willingness to insist that sexual satisfaction should play a large role in marriage. Indeed, they were almost obliged to do so, since the most up-to-date psychological thought enjoined women to enjoy sex or be labeled "frigid." It was not enough to take pleasure in sex, however; one must do so in the approved manner. The new experts labeled homosexual experience as either deviant or a juvenile phase that one could be expected to outgrow. Heterosexual experience that never eventuated in motherhood, they further asserted, retarded a woman's fullest emotional development and made it impossible for her to feel complete sexual satisfaction.[26]

Thus, in spite of all the changes, in one respect the expectations about proper family life remained the same: Having children was one of the principal reasons most people married, and within marriage a woman's principal role was to be a homemaker and a mother, a man's to be a provider. The expectations were couched in different tones from the stern warnings of two decades before, but the meaning was clear all the same. In 1912, readers of *Good Housekeeping* had warned one proponent of birth control that if her marriage remained childless, her husband would lose interest in her.[27] Fourteen years later, birth control was on its slow way to becoming family planning, an acceptable means of timing births.

Voluntary childlessness among the married, however, continued to evoke dire predictions. In the 1920s, sociologist Ernest Groves warned childless Americans of the risks to their marriages: "With only sex and comfort as motives, and no functioning of parental love, there is little to protect restless couples from divorce." The influential writer Walter Lippmann expressed the same feeling even more succinctly. In a lengthy essay on the meaning of morality in modern society, in which he demonstrated his "advanced" thinking by supporting birth control, Lippmann argued that a couple who *never* had children would find their love for each other fading. "Love and nothing else," he claimed, "very soon is nothing else."[28]

In spite of the outward trappings of sexual freedom, in reality the overarching message of the larger culture was that the ultimate goal of every "normal" woman was motherhood. The newest "evidence" from psychology, whether Freudian or behaviorist, insisted that only a romantic, sexually satisfying marriage brought a woman fulfillment. (For Freudians, the achievement of complete adult sexuality in a woman required the experience of childbirth.) Also, as the next chapter will reveal, the discovery of the sex hormones would provide a new scientific basis for emphasizing the differences between men and women. If a woman attempted to contravene the experts, she paid a stiff price.[29]

Young women felt the pull of conventional roles everywhere, even from some of the very women who had rebelled against convention a generation before them. Clelia Mosher, single and childless herself, reminded the women she taught in the 1920s of their "racial obligation," informing them that "no woman reaches her fullest development who is not a wife and mother." In the home economics courses ubiquitous in high school and college alike, young women learned that while a career was appropriate for exceptional women, it was a mistake for most. Popular magazines reinforced what instructors taught in school. Without denying the achievements of women, magazine articles relentlessly conveyed the message that a woman remained incomplete without a happy marriage and children. From teachers, physicians, and popular media, young women of the 1920s received a mixed (although not literally contradictory) message, which ran something like this: The suffrage movement was victorious, and now women enjoyed the same rights and freedoms as men. Nevertheless, in order to be truly fulfilled as women, they should use their freedom "correctly," by marrying, having children, and keeping a home. As Nancy Cott has summarized the new role of women: "Women's household status and heterosexual service were now defended—even aggressively marketed—in terms of women's choice, freedom, and rationality. . . . Feminist intents and rhetoric were not ignored but appropriated."[30]

If Cott is correct in her assumption that by the 1920s feminism had been appropriated to serve the goal of ensconcing the erotically charged—and fertile—marriage as the preferred mode of existence, the concurrent taming of the controversies surrounding birth control and women's work outside the home seem entirely understandable. They now could serve or complement the family, rather than threatening it. The risk of a massive uprising of women against the family, of course, had always been over-stated. Even at the height of alarm over the divorce rate, race suicide, and the idea that women in ever greater numbers would choose careers over marriage and motherhood, the dangers had been greatly exaggerated. As Claudia Goldin has remarked, American women throughout the nine-teenth and early twentieth centuries always married at a greater rate than their European counterparts. "Marriage in America," she notes, "was al-most a universal institution." The proportion of white women who mar-ried at least once has never dropped below 90 percent in the United States, and that was during the forty years just preceding the 1920s. For most of the country's history, the percentage has been much closer to 95 percent, which Goldin calls "exceptionally high."[31]

The experience of at least one group of married women seemed to re-inforce the ideas of the experts. Of the thousand wives surveyed in the early 1920s by social scientist Katherine Bement Davis and her team at the Bureau of Social Hygiene, almost 90 percent declared their marriages happy or extremely happy. These highly educated women for the most part did not hold jobs (indeed, Davis claimed that employment after mar-riage was "not conducive" to a woman's happiness), their sexual relations were usually "pleasurable" or "satisfactory," and although more than 70 percent of them readily admitted to using birth control, only fourteen of the thousand intended to remain childless. Davis had an interest in find-ing the practice of birth control harmless; the Rockefeller Foundation, which funded her research, supported contraception, and one goal of her work was to convince the public that birth control was not a threat to morality.[32]

Davis seemed relieved to discover that knowledge of birth control had apparently not tempted many women into sexual experimentation. True, 7.1 percent of her sample had had sexual relations before marriage, but half of them only with a fiancé. A tiny 1.6 percent of the married women had been involved sexually with more than one partner. Most of the happy women had children, and those who had used birth control, ac-cording to her data, actually had a higher pregnancy rate than those who did not, leading Davis to suggest that perhaps those who rejected contra-ception may have had less need for it. Many of the women in her sample were still in their childbearing years, and among the women over thirty only sixteen were still childless.[33]

A Culture of Matrimony

The Davis study revealed the continued pull of what we might call a culture of matrimony, of which children formed an integral element. Now, women unable or unwilling to marry and bear children found themselves labeled abnormal. In the eighteenth century, the childless woman could use the "putting out" system to add to her household, just as a family with too many children could find a respectable way to provide for them in this manner. In the mid–nineteenth century, spinsterhood gained increasing respectability as the ideology of domesticity enfolded single women who worked as teachers or took on the tasks of domestic reform under its voluminous wing. In the late nineteenth and very early twentieth centuries, revered single women who devoted their lives to humanitarian reform—women like Jane Addams—were praised as saints. Even the medical profession's castigation of women for educating themselves into sterility did not dim the public's regard for married women without children who took up the cause of children's rights, as Kate Wiggin did, or participated in the child rescue movement. But by the 1920s the tide had turned. Unmarried women were snickered at as old maids, whispered about as lesbians, or in the most positive construction of their state, praised as exceptional beings who were somehow set apart from the general run of womanhood by their talents. Married women without children, regardless of whether their childlessness was voluntary or involuntary, were considered somehow "deviant" as well in this new Freudian age.[34]

Men without children not only might find themselves suspected of having inflicted a sexually transmitted disease upon their wives, but they also faced new social expectations. Although they continued to derive much of their masculine identity from their role as breadwinners, in the 1920s, as Robert Griswold has argued, the new social science "experts" decreed that a man's personality development was dependent on the quality of his family life. Middle-class men, in particular, became "increasingly concerned about the quality of their private lives . . . [and] fatherhood became part of this growing emphasis on personal life."[35]

For unhappily childless couples, all of these changes were a mixed blessing. On the one hand, society's open scrutiny may have made involuntary childlessness more difficult to bear; but on the other hand, greater public openness about sexuality and reproduction also made it easier to find resources that might provide a solution. It was not until the second decade of the twentieth century, after the airing of the race suicide question and the antivenereal disease warnings of antiprostitution reformers had made the discussion of reproductive questions possible in mass circulation periodicals, that practical, if still sentimentalized, discussions of how women coped with childlessness appeared in the public press. Clearly, the race suicide issue caused severe anxiety among involuntarily childless women. As one of them wrote to *Good Housekeeping*, "a serious surgical operation" after several years of an involuntarily childless marriage destroyed her hopes for childbearing. Desolate herself, she had the additional burden of knowing that her friends thought of her simply as a leisured and unencumbered woman. While not denying that her childlessness allowed her to do what she wanted—she chose involvement in church and charity—she would have much preferred to be " 'tied down at home' by the sweetest ties in all the world."[36]

Several readers advised her to adopt; only one suggested that she simply enjoy the opportunities that her childlessness had provided, something that society made it difficult for any childless woman to do. The popular press produced article after article on women's responsibility to reproduce, or if that were not biologically possible, to take in a homeless waif. To those who were using birth control, Laura Richards, a daughter of Julia Ward Howe, warned, "while . . . many . . . intelligent and educated women postpone or refuse motherhood, . . . the ignorant, the feeble, [and] the vicious bring forth their young at Nature's call." The larger community did not distinguish between an involuntarily childless woman and her deliberately childfree counterpart. Unless a woman in some way demonstrated her maternal instinct, by bearing children, adopting them, or, in the words of Julia Ward Howe herself, "win[ning] to her arms some motherless child," she left herself open to the charge of unwomanliness.[37]

Maternalism transcended politics. The radical Emma Goldman, who ultimately decided not to have the operation that doctors told her might alleviate her infertility, nevertheless expressed ambivalence about her decision; she believed that by not experiencing childbirth she had missed out on a quintessential experience of womanhood. Feminists influenced by the sex radical Ellen Key, although they found husbands expendable, were intensely pronatalist. Very few Americans agreed with Key that every woman had a right to bear children, whether married or not, and that the state should support unmarried women and their children; still, those who condemned women for shirking their maternal duty believed that childlessness had political dimensions.[38]

But if unwed motherhood gained little support in the United States, single women here nevertheless felt compelled to demonstrate that they possessed the maternal instinct, as stories such as Grace Ellery Channing's "Children of the Barren," about a spinster who cares for a brother's children during the parents' extended stay abroad, demonstrate. The children's mother (who left them behind for years), upon her return, dismisses her sister-in-law's care as adequate but somehow lacking the ingredient of mother love. Channing's spinster gets her revenge, however. As young adults, the children clearly prefer her to their biological mother. Channing's story was not entirely devoid of autobiographical content. Married to Walter Stetson, whom historians will recognize as Charlotte Perkins Gilman's first husband, Channing never had children of her own. She and Walter had primary custody of Walter and Charlotte's daughter. Whether she was fictionalizing her own history or not, Channing in this story was determined to show that biological parenthood did not make a woman a "true" mother.[39]

Outside the realm of fiction, kindergarten teachers, many of whom were single, rushed to defend their maternal instinct against the onslaughts of those who insisted, in the words of one writer, that their lack of biological parenthood made them less able to understand the needs of children. Their typical rejoinder, however, only demonstrated how powerfully women were constrained by social convention. "Why must a woman be a mother," one of them asked, "in order to understand children and to deal lovingly and wisely with them. Is not sex alone responsible for this instinct? . . . are not true women always mothering somebody?"[40] Claiming to share equally in the maternal instinct, however, was at best a short-term success for single women who did not wish to have their identities as women impugned. By the 1920s, vicarious maternal experiences no longer made a woman eligible for inclusion in the maternal club. Social pressure to marry had escalated, and only about 5 percent of American women did not do so.

Children were an essential element in the new definition of marriage and family life, and if a couple was unable to have them biologically, the thinking went, then adoption could alleviate their unhappiness. Escalating divorces and decreasing rates of childbirth notwithstanding, a number of contemporary observers called attention to the growing public interest in adoption. What Viviana Zelizer has termed "sentimental adoption," whereby couples chose infants that they could rear as their own children, had begun to be formalized toward the close of the nineteenth century, as readers will recall from the last chapter. While the adoption of older children who could contribute economically to the household had not ceased entirely, the records of children's homes suggest that increasing numbers of couples preferred the economically "useless" young child over the more productive older one.[41]

This trend accelerated in the early twentieth century. In spite of the eugenicists' hereditarian warnings, the ever-present threat that a biological parent would turn up and demand the child's return, and a residual sense that to acquire a child in the face of a clear decision of Providence that a couple not have one was in some way tempting fate, thousands of couples sought out infants and toddlers to adopt. Some wrote pleading letters to children's bureaus, often attempting to obtain a child from another part of the country in order to minimize the possibility of being found by birth parents; still others put advertisements in newspapers.[42]

By far the greatest outpouring of public adoptive fervor came as a result of a widely publicized campaign by the popular periodical *The Delineator,* which began in 1907 and continued for several years. Featuring photographs of winsome and healthy children, the magazine gave the impression that there were thousands of bright and charming young children readily available for adoption. *The Delineator*'s children came from a selection of public and private charitable institutions and orphanages, and the magazine assured eager would-be parents that the children were physically sound. As a study of one of the institutions indicates, however, the magazine did not reveal all it knew about the children to prospective adopters. It identified at least one sickly child of an alcoholic mother, for example, as healthy and wellborn. Both in this campaign and with other high-profile adoption placing agencies such as that run by Texas humorist and versifier Judd Mortimer Lewis, those wishing to place children emphasized their beauty, intelligence, or personality. *The Delineator* went so far as to assure couples that if the child failed to please, he or she could be returned.[43]

Women apparently took the initiative in most cases of adoption. Often they had to overcome the objections of husbands who feared hereditary evils. But there were some women who, satisfied without children themselves, sought adoption because their husbands wanted children. In a few cases, husband and wife wrote jointly to an orphanage; as one couple who affectingly promised a child the "love of *good parents*" noted, "We feel greatly" that "no children have come to us."[44] Many of these couples were doomed to disappointment. In fact, by the early twentieth century there were more couples seeking to adopt than there were so-called adoptable children. Although there were indeed thousands of homeless children, most of them had at least one living parent. Workers in the new field of social welfare had become much more reluctant to encourage unmarried mothers to relinquish their children. Their motives were mixed. Charity workers suspected that an unwed mother who gave up her child would sink further into a life of iniquity, but one who kept her child, they believed, had a greater chance for a "respectable" life. In other instances, regardless of what the social workers wanted, parents themselves adamantly refused to relinquish permanent custody.[45]

Although *The Delineator* and other child rescue publicists gave the impression that most of the children in institutional care were orphans, foundlings, or the offspring of deceived young girls who were unable to provide care and so gave up their babies, in reality the demand for children under the age of five who were legally available for permanent adoption far outran the supply. Indeed, as early as 1910 articles with such titles as "Not Enough Babies to Go Around" warned prospective adopters that children whom they could literally make their own were not so easy to come by. The more pressing need was for foster homes, but most childless couples wanted children they could either adopt legally or rear as if they had. Parents often kept a child's adoption secret; several couples noted that they moved to a new neighborhood after bringing their child home. Some women who acquired infants clandestinely—a black market in babies had begun to flourish in the early twentieth century—even apparently fooled their husbands into thinking they had borne the babies themselves.[46]

The adoptive fervor did not abate in the 1920s, nor did the supply of adoptable babies become greater. Adoption alone could never solve all the problems associated with involuntary childlessness. Birth control had made voluntary childlessness possible, and some couples clearly took advantage of the freedom to be childfree. But most middle-class couples wanted to have at least one or two children, and others wished for larger families. Among some ethnic groups, as well, the inability to produce children was a source of shame as well as sorrow. As the following chapters demonstrate, ethnic Americans both black and white, as well as native-born white Protestants, sought medical help for infertility in the twentieth century. In spite of declining fertility, rearing children remained one of the most valued tasks that a woman could perform. And for men, children provided a sense of continuity and identity; men came to judge their worth as men by their ability to provide for their children.[47]

By the 1920s, the decline in public reticence about sexual and reproductive issues brought infertility, as well as more commonly discussed issues such as birth control, out into the open for public discussion and debate. The emphasis on consumption, which contemporaries and historians alike have documented as the hallmark of modern America, encouraged such couples to believe that parenthood could be purchased in one way or another, either through treatment or through adoption. When those attitudes combined with the new sexual openness, advances in scientific knowledge about reproduction, and new medical techniques that took advantage of that science, profound changes in the perception and treatment of infertility resulted. Those changes are the subject of Part 2.

Part II

five

Degrees of Infertility

From the Sterile Woman to the Infertile Couple, 1900–1945

The usual clinical problem is . . . not that of one definitely sterile partner mated with one who is unqualifiedly fertile, but rather that of two individuals of whom both exhibit some degree of infertility.

Samuel Meaker, M.D., 1934

In 1895, the American surgeon Robert Tuttle Morris, highly respected for his expertise in what was then the dangerous operation of appendectomy, reported to his colleagues a series of "ovarian transplants." Outraged by what he considered the wholesale destruction of women's reproductive capacities by indiscriminate ovariotomy, moved by the desire of a number of women whose ovaries had been extirpated to bear children, and intrigued by intimations from European scientists that the ovary, like the thyroid and pituitary, was a "gland of internal secretion," Morris engaged in a course of experimental surgery remarkable in its time.[1]

For more than a decade, Morris implanted sections of the ovaries of fertile women into other women who had either lost their own ovaries through surgery or who had never developed mature reproductive systems. He performed these operations nearly thirty years before scientists discovered the existence of estrogen, which is one of the two hormones that control the female reproductive cycle, and a decade before the term *hormone* had even been coined. Inspired, he claimed, by the "known fact that a segment of thyroid gland will continue to do its functional work after transplantation to a remote part of the body," he reasoned that the same process might work for the ovary.[2]

In 1891, English physician George Murray had described the cure of a woman suffering from myxedema (a severe thyroid deficiency) with injections of sheep's thyroid. Few English or American scientists were persuaded at the time that the ovary possessed the same properties as the thyroid. But Morris disputed this conventional wisdom. He first applied his theory and surgical skills in the case of a twenty-six-year-old woman with severe pelvic adhesions and diseased fallopian tubes. Suffering intensely, she required radical surgery, Morris believed; but she also wanted to bear children. In order to relieve her severe pain, he removed her ovaries and most of the fallopian tubes; in hopes of retaining her ability to bear children, he left a stump of the right oviduct, to the interior of which he transferred "a small piece of the patient's diseased ovary." After returning home from a month-long stay in the hospital, the patient soon became pregnant; however, she miscarried after about three months. The cause, according to Morris, was "persistent pelvic adhesions."[3]

In this instance, Morris used the patient's own ovary for the "transplantation," as he called his operation. Soon he began to use donor ovaries. In 1906, he claimed his only success when a woman in whom he had implanted a section of another woman's ovary in 1901 succeeded in conceiving and carrying the pregnancy to term. Childless wives who had been subject to ovariotomy, upon hearing of this successful outcome, besieged Morris, and for a few years he continued to perform the operation. His technique involved simultaneous surgery on donor and recipient, and the removal from the donor of a section of ovary about the size of a pea. Keeping the excised segment in saline solution, he either divided the uterus of the recipient and implanted the new ovarian tissue into it or sutured the section of ovary to the fallopian tube. But no other patient ever conceived, and Morris eventually abandoned the operation.[4]

Foreshadowing the late-twentieth-century debates over surrogate motherhood and egg donation, Morris reflected on possible ethical and legal objections to his procedure. Recipients might, he speculated, "object to the idea of carrying a piece of ovary from another woman, as the child would have treble parentage." Nevertheless, he claimed (accurately enough, in view of the response to the one reported full-term delivery),

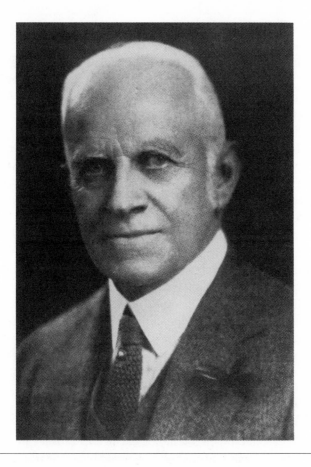

Robert Tuttle Morris, the surgeon who began in the 1890s to perform what he called "ovarian transplantations," using donor ovaries, in the hopes of enabling women whose own ovaries had been surgically removed to conceive.
Courtesy of the College of Physicians of Philadelphia

"there are many women . . . who [would] grasp at an opportunity for bearing children, and whose minds are much relieved by the possibility of such a prospect." Surprisingly, he foresaw no problems among potential donors, women of proven fertility who were undergoing gynecological surgery for a variety of conditions. Morris did not say whether these women, or only their doctors, consented to the "donations" in the surgeries he performed. But he did not believe the women would object. A woman, he said, could "spare for the other woman a segment of ovary as large as a pea without suffering any real loss."[5]

Morris, in fact, found the ethical and legal issues more intriguing than troubling: "It will be interesting," he concluded, "to know which half-mother the child from an ovarian graft will resemble." He cautioned that "there may be legal difficulties involved in questions of inheritance," but he did not hesitate to declare the woman who carried the child "the real mother." After all, "she furnished the nutrition" during pregnancy. A century later, we struggle with some of the very issues that for Morris appeared relatively easy to resolve.[6]

Morris's approach to female sterility was unique in his day, but his experiments foreshadowed the future. In the twentieth century, hormonal discoveries would revolutionize the ways in which scientists and clinicians understood infertility, and the availability of new treatments would present practitioners and childless couples alike with new medical choices and moral quandaries. This chapter explores the origins of these issues, from the discovery of the hormones and the subsequent rise of endocrinology, through the development and later widespread availability of a nonsurgical test to determine how well the fallopian tubes functioned, to the great wave of popular interest in artificial insemination in the 1930s and 1940s.

The roots of reproductive endocrinology, which had its beginnings in the 1920s with the discovery of estrogen, extended back nearly three-quarters of a century to the medical pursuit of the significance of what were called the "ductless glands." In 1849, Arnold Adolph Berthold performed his now-famous experiment of castrating roosters, then implanting the testicles in their abdominal cavities to see whether the secondary sex characteristics would reemerge. They did. That same year, Thomas Addison presented his first paper on the adrenal disease that would come to bear his name. Just six years later, his classic monograph, *On the Constitutional and Local Effects of Disease of the Supra-Renal Capsules,* described primary adrenal insufficiency, or Addison's disease. (The adrenal glands, located above the kidneys, produce essential steroid hormones, such as cortisol.) A year later, in France, Charles E. Brown-Sequard's animal adrenalectomies confirmed Addison's theory.[7]

Brown-Sequard would soon become a controversial figure in the history of endocrinology, but not for these adrenal experiments, which had been widely praised. As a result of his accomplishments, by the close of his career he had become a respected Fellow of the Royal College of Physicians and Professor of Medicine at Paris's College de France. In the 1880s, however, when he was in his sixties, Brown-Sequard began a series of rejuvenation experiments involving testicular extracts. In 1889, at the age of seventy-two, he announced that he had successfully restored his own strength, energy, and sexual vitality using injections of animal testicular extracts. There was some skepticism, but respected physicians, particularly in France and the United States, gave him a hearing and eagerly anticipated further confirmation of his results. Alas, to the dismay of men everywhere, the effects of his extracts turned out to be ephemeral. But his assertions, coming at the same time as the legitimate proof of the clinical efficacy of thyroid extracts, promoted both research on, and clinical use of, various organ extracts.[8]

Brown-Sequard was one of the earliest experimenters to argue that the testicle and ovary produced internal secretions; most of his fellow researchers in the late nineteenth century expressed doubt that these sexual organs demonstrated the same properties as the thyroid, pituitary, and adrenal glands on which scientists initially focused their attention. Thus, most researchers greeted with skepticism Emil Knauer's 1896 publication of his experiments on rabbits, in which he demonstrated that castrated female rabbits did not develop castrate atrophy when he regrafted their ovarian tissue. But when other scientists replicated Knauer's results within the next few years, the majority of researchers came to agree that the sex glands did in fact share the properties of the thyroid and were indeed glands of internal secretion.[9]

The fact remained, however, that scientists were still unsure what these properties were in *any* of the organs they had observed. By the early twentieth century, they had neither isolated any substance except epinephrine nor agreed on what to call such secretions. But in 1905 British scientist Ernest Henry Starling began to call them "hormones," a term invented by his friends Sir William B. Hardy and the classicist W. T. Vesey. The term derived from the Greek "hormao," which means "to put into quick motion, to excite or arouse." The name found favor among Starling's fellow researchers and quickly became standard. In the years before World War I, experimental scientists attempted to isolate the hormones and to confirm their findings by extensive animal experimentation.[10]

But if scientists urged caution and certainty, clinicians expressed impatience with the idea of waiting for conclusive findings. London practitioner Harold Shaw, for example, widely circulated his notion that "organotherapy," as it was then called, was clinically effective if not scientifically demonstrated. Shaw and others recommended the use of "ovarian extracts" for amenorrhea, dysmenorrhea, and even obesity. Because of this view, reputable clinicians were easy marks for charlatans. They embraced, for example, the claims of Aleksandr V. Poehl, who found his way into early-twentieth-century clinical literature as an expert on testicular extracts. Poehl today sometimes receives passing mention in the standard histories of endocrinology. Many observers in his own day viewed Poehl's claims as similar to those made for sheep's thyroid, which had in fact proved effective. In reality he was little more than a huckster, who marketed his "spermin" to treat anemia, restore potency to men and sexual desire to women, prevent miscarriages, and cure neurasthenia.[11]

Scholars have noted that after the demonstrations of the efficacy of thyroid treatments, "organotherapy in general became much more respectable," even though, as one of them noted, "looking back, thyroid extract was the only one of the tissue extracts that really worked." However, the clinicians witnessing that success were not "looking back"; particularly the more adventurous among them wanted to produce other successes to match George Murray's. Brown-Sequard's lecture tours in the United States had brought him considerable attention. Americans, partly as a result of his influence, became some of the foremost advocates of "empirical" organotherapy.[12]

Robert Morris had been one of the early believers, and as a surgeon he was convinced that the future of organotherapy would lie in its surgical applications. So sure was he in these early years that he had urged his colleagues to "hunt up some of our old patients whose adnexa have been removed, and give them the benefit of a graft of new ovary, in the possibility of relieving them from the condition of barrenness." He had also reasoned by analogy that if ovarian transplants might work, so might testicular ones, and he performed at least three such surgeries, two of which he claimed resulted in restored sexual potency, although not fertility, and the third of which failed entirely. Robert Morris's proposed marriage of surgery and organotherapy (which was just beginning to evolve into endocrinology) would not be consummated until the days of in vitro fertilization. Indeed, Morris himself abandoned his flirtation with the glands of internal secretion and returned to the more familiar gall bladder and appendix by the 1920s. Although his memoirs give no hint of the reason behind this decision, perhaps as a surgeon Morris began to feel out of place among the advocates of hormonal therapy, most of whom pinned their hopes of devising successful therapies on the medical rather than surgical use of hormonal extracts.[13]

Henry R. Harrower, the driving force behind the creation in 1916 of the Association for the Study of Internal Secretions, later the Endocrine Society, is a case in point. Harrower, a California practitioner who wrote extensively on hormonal therapy for a readership of fellow physicians— two of his early works were called *Practical Hormone Therapy* and *The Internal Secretions in Practical Medicine*—urged his colleagues to take an "empirical" approach. The word *empirical* has a special meaning to clinicians that dates back to the days when "empirics" rejected the systemic philosophies of regular physicians. By the twentieth century, it connoted a therapy for which there was no clear experimental justification. As Harrower argued, even if scientists did not yet know why organotherapy would work, it seemed clear to him that it did work. Or, as he put it in 1917, "The method of treatment inaugurated by Brown-Sequard is rational because it is resultful [*sic*]." These therapies were, he argued, "unscientific" but "nevertheless useful," even if their "basis" was "not yet wholly explainable." Harrower provided practitioners with a table of hormone extracts listing their possible uses for different conditions. He urged them to use his guidelines loosely, adding, "This table is neither arbitrary nor exact, but merely suggestive." The table contained both preparations of a single organ, such as ovarian or thyroid preparations, as well as "pluriglandular" ones. Harrower's philosophy, in short, was that physicians should rely on the trial-and-error method; the implication was that much good might be accomplished, with little or no risk to the patient.[14]

In infertility treatment as in other areas, as organotherapy evolved into endocrinology its medical applications overshadowed surgical ones. This had implications for the gynecological profession. In the late nineteenth and early twentieth centuries, gynecology was almost entirely a surgical field. Surgery was especially important in infertility treatment. Innovations in the wake of the adoption of anesthesia and asepsis had rendered laparotomy comparatively safe, and laparotomy, in turn, enabled physicians to treat some of the ovarian and tubal pathologies that prevented pregnancy. Many physicians expected in the early years of endocrinological discoveries that applied endocrinology would become a surgical field.

Because early animal experimentation had involved glandular implantation rather than the use of extracts, it was natural for surgeons to see a future for such implantation in humans. Robert Morris, for example, had acted on his belief that such implants should work. When they did not, the focus of endocrinology shifted from surgical implantation to pharmacology, and the surgeon had a smaller role to play in the developing field. In fact, after the great flurry of what Harrower called empirical organotherapy in the first two decades of the twentieth century, a number of eminent physicians advised caution in the administration of hormonal therapies. The extent to which the general practitioner heeded such advice is unclear, but elite practitioners began to look to the research scientists, be they M.D.s, chemists, biochemists, or biologists, to delineate more clearly the functions of the various endocrine glands, before advocating their wholesale use.

By the second decade of the twentieth century, scientists no longer doubted that the ovaries and testicles had properties similar to those of the other glands of internal secretion. And within the American scientific community, although a few researchers focused on the male reproductive organs, by far the greatest number were lured by the hope of at last deciphering the mysteries of the female reproductive system. Whether the early discovery of estrogen stimulated or resulted from that interest is not entirely clear, but it was this discovery that marked the beginning of a journey that led to both the creation of the birth control pill and successful in vitro fertilization. Over the course of the next several decades, scientists and clinicians pieced together many of the details of the process of ovulation and embryo implantation, beginning with the function of the ovaries.

Scientists already knew that ovaries contained ova, and that they released at least one ovum in some cyclical pattern. Between the 1920s and the 1940s they discovered how that process worked, learning that ovaries produce estrogen and progesterone, both of which are necessary for ovulation and for implantation of the fertilized egg in the uterus. Researchers in that period also began to speculate upon the role in ovulation of the hypothalamus and the pituitary, both of which are located in the brain. We now know that the hypothalamus releases a substance called gonadotropin-releasing hormone, which signals the pituitary to secrete follicle-stimulating hormone and luteinizing hormone. When a woman's reproductive cycle is functioning normally, the pituitary secretes these two hormones in a coordinated fashion to regulate the growth of the ovarian follicle, which contains the egg, and to induce ovulation. The follicles produce estrogen. After ovulation, progesterone is produced by the corpus luteum, a group of cells that remain after rupture of the ovarian follicle to prepare the uterine lining for the acceptance of the fertilized egg.[15]

The first half of the menstrual cycle is called the follicular phase, during which the ovarian follicle produces increasing amounts of estrogen. At midcycle, luteinizing hormone surges; follicle-stimulating hormone also increases, but to a lesser degree. The ovary also steps up its production of progesterone. Ovulation, triggered by the rapid rise in estrogen, occurs after the surge of luteinizing hormone. The second half of the menstrual cycle, called the luteal phase, begins after ovulation, and the corpus luteum forms at this time. If no pregnancy occurs, it degenerates and menstruation begins.[16]

Beginning in the 1920s with the discovery of estrogen, scientists took the first steps toward deciphering the complex nature of women's reproductive cycle and the relationship of menstruation to ovulation. After that discovery, new findings followed at a rapid pace. Chroniclers of these discoveries have tended to present the "hormone quest," as one popular history called it, as a scientific adventure story: a saga of bold men (and virtually no women), underfunded but imaginative, who created an entirely new understanding of the ways in which our bodies function, who conquered disease, and who made possible both the control of fertility and the modern treatment of infertility.[17] Such a view is misleading. The discovery of estrogen inaugurated an ambitious research program that involved not only scientists, clinicians, and technicians but also foundations and pharmaceutical companies. The "hormone quest" was in fact a collective enterprise, for which scientists secured considerable financial support, and in which they often had definite ends in view. Although there were a few iconoclasts among them, institutional support was hardly lacking, and much of it came in the early days from the Rockefeller Foundation, which funded the Committee for Research in Problems of Sex.[18]

Founded in 1921 under the auspices of the Bureau of Social Hygiene, a Rockefeller-supported organization, the committee's initial intent was to develop a plan "for systematic research on sex problems, designed to provide a better scientific foundation for an understanding of sex in man." Its first act was to secure the sponsorship of the National Research Council, and therefore to align itself with the natural rather than the social sciences.[19] During its first year or so of operation, the committee floundered, unclear about its direction, incorporating sociology and anthropology into its vision of natural science, and providing money for projects as disparate as the estrus cycle of the guinea pig and the sex lives of university students. Within a very few years, however, according to Sophie Aberle and George Corner, authors of the official history of the committee, endocrine research provided the group with a mission, and money for endocrine projects poured into various university laboratories. Sociology and anthropology were forgotten, and experimental biology came to the fore.[20]

In 1915 George Corner had discovered the function of the corpus luteum, a discovery that within fifteen years would lead to the isolation of progesterone. In 1923 Edgar Allen and Edward Doisy isolated estrogen, and after that, noted Aberle and Corner, "to a very great extent, the Committee's program was determined by these discoveries." The moving force in these early years was embryologist Frank Lillie, who had done pathbreaking work in 1917 on the ways in which hormones determine sex differentiation in mammals. By 1923 or so, Lillie gained agreement from the committee on a list of six research priorities, most of which were in the area of experimental biology.[21] From that time until it began to support Alfred Kinsey's studies of human sexuality in the 1940s, the Committee for Research in Problems of Sex earmarked a major proportion of its resources for research aimed at the isolation and synthesis of the hormones influencing reproduction. After his initial discoveries in 1923, Edgar Allen received yearly grants for his work on ovarian hormones. Indeed, during the committee's first four-year grant cycle, ovarian hormones and the female cycle were its principal priority.[22]

Overall, the Rockefeller Foundation, in part directly through the committee and in part by acting favorably on the committee's recommendations regarding underwriting larger projects, funded much of the basic research on the hormones affecting the reproductive cycle from the 1920s through the 1940s. As historian James Reed has noted, "the committee virtually paid for the development of endocrinology in the United States during the twenty-year period when the female sex hormones were identified and clinicians began to use hormone extracts to treat disease."[23] In all, the committee directed the expenditure of more than $2.5 million in the first twenty-five years of its existence. Aberle and Corner were particularly proud of the committee's role in hormonal research, but they concluded their history of its first twenty-five years by reminding both funders and the scientists who depended on them of the power and the responsibility inherent in the command of such sums of money: "A devoted group of scientific leaders, given financial means and operating wisely at a strategic time, may exert world-wide influence on a course of research . . . and sway the activities of whole segments of the scientific profession. This is a sobering thought for those who give money and those who direct its expenditure for intellectual purposes."[24]

It would be an exaggeration to conclude that either the committee or the Rockefeller Foundation directed the entire program of research into the biology of reproduction, but they nevertheless exerted a powerful influence. In addition, pharmaceutical companies, which were not slow to see the clinical possibilities of the hormones once they were synthesized, began to support research directed toward that end.[25] Synthesizing, however, proved at least as difficult as discovery. From the 1923 isolation of the "ovarian hormone" (named oestrin in 1926), it took until 1930 to create it in a pure crystalline form and another half-decade until the first synthetic estrogen, stilbestrol (later known as diethylstilbestrol, the infamous DES), became available.[26]

The isolation and synthesis of estrogen was, of course, a crucial step toward understanding the female reproductive cycle and ultimately treating its disorders. But scientists had long suspected that there was an additional ovarian hormone, one that proved more elusive than the first. In 1929, George Corner solved most of the mystery, producing the first "corpus luteum extract," which he wished to call progestin. By 1932, several teams working separately had obtained it in an "almost pure" crystalline form, even though its structure remained undetermined. Four research teams who had been working independently managed to isolate it by 1934, and an international conference was called to give it its name, which became progesterone.[27]

In 1940, the American chemist Russell Marker, who had previously synthesized estrogen from plant steroids, concluded that other hormones, including progesterone, could be synthesized cheaply and in large quantity from similar sources. Sapogenins, a plentiful source of which reposed in the roots of wild Mexican yams, provided the answer. By 1943, he was making large quantities of progesterone in a home-built laboratory in Mexico City and had founded a company, Syntex, to produce the product. By the early 1940s, therefore, both estrogen and progesterone were available in synthetic form. These products, together with the recent discovery that the female menstrual cycle could be tracked by means of vaginal smears, held out the possibility that fertility (and infertility) in women could be both understood and controlled.[28]

The male hormones were not entirely neglected during this period, although American scientists seemed to lag behind the Europeans. One reason may have been lack of adequate financial support. The Rockefeller Foundation provided some funding, but its principal interest was birth control, and work on the male reproductive process had so far not produced promising results in terms of prospects for contraception. As a result, the Rockefeller interest was limited. Another reason may have been the unsavory association between research on male hormones and the now-discredited rejuvenation theories of Brown-Sequard or the less reputable Poehl. Or perhaps the Europeans simply outran the Americans. Extracts of male hormones from bull's testicles were first reported in 1927, and Frank Lillie at the University of Chicago clearly expected that his colleague, biochemist F. C. Koch, would be the first to succeed "in the purification of the male hormone." But Dutch researcher Ernst Laqueur was the first to do so, isolating testosterone in crystalline form and giving it its name in 1935.[29]

From the Scientists to the Clinicians

The research scientists who isolated these hormones, along with those who chronicled their achievements in later years, have given us an image of scientific progress that was orderly, precise, and clearly demarcated by specific dates and the names of individual researchers who deserved the credit for each successful experiment. But if one moves outside the laboratory, which is, after all, a controlled environment with captive subjects, to the practice of a busy clinician, where order and method were often overthrown by the needs of patients for the physician to take care of their particular problems, the scene was entirely different. Physicians faced with patients urgently insisting that their infertility be "cured" were less likely than research scientists to await a precise demonstration, confirmed by chemical isolation, of the ways in which hormones functioned, before attempting their use. If research scientists wanted to see chemical structures, clinicians wanted to see pregnant women. And they were more likely to draw conclusions based on their own experience, mediated perhaps by some cursory reading, than they were to await a definitive scientific proclamation. For example, several years before George Corner isolated progesterone, the clinical authority Charles Gardner Child accurately described the ways in which he surmised such a hormone would function.[30] Although hormones did not begin to become available in standardized forms until the 1930s, that does not mean that clinicians patiently waited for definitive laboratory results before attempting to take matters into their own hands.

Hormonal discoveries seemed to have considerable promise for some of the heretofore untreatable sterility cases in both men and women. By the end of the 1920s clinicians, therefore, sought both to understand how hormones operated within the reproductive system and to put them to practical use. Skeptical historians might protest at this point that there should have been a *diminishing* demand for infertility treatment around this time, since the high level of childlessness in that era appears to have been a result of choice rather than chance. Nancy Cott, for example, has argued that the high overall rate of childlessness for the decade of the twenties—18 percent of married women never produced a child—demonstrated "in a unique way . . . the positive volitional element in modern motherhood." But there are other dimensions to what at first glance seems like fairly straightforward data. Economic historian Claudia Goldin, for example, does not associate the higher rates of childlessness with prosperity but rather with economic depression. Using twenty-five-year cohorts to analyze her data, Goldin has found that about 28 percent of ever-married women of color and about 20 percent of their white counterparts born in 1905 bore no children. Goldin ascribes this childlessness rate, first, to the virtual closing of immigration in 1924, and then to the American economic decline, which in several regions and economic sectors began several years before the great crash of 1929.[31]

Susan Householder Van Horn's study of twentieth-century fertility patterns supports at least the second part of Goldin's analysis. Economic decline, she argues, fueled the deep fertility drop of the late twenties and thirties. Evidence drawn from data on both preferred and actual family size suggests that "most women would have chosen higher fertility if their economic circumstances had permitted it." Indeed, "for the small group with extremely high income," high birthrates persisted, according to Van Horn, suggesting that "many married couples modified their fertility behavior because they felt the constraints of inadequate resources." If Goldin and Van Horn are correct, then, higher levels of voluntary childlessness had less to do with avoidance of emotional responsibilities of parenthood than with economic anxieties, and one cannot therefore conclude that a significant erosion in pronatalist sentiment had occurred.[32]

Physicians in the 1920s and 1930s, however, saw the matter differently. Conceding that much of the increased childlessness in American society was indeed voluntary, they began to argue that this made medical treatment for the involuntarily childless all the more important. In fact, the greater proportion of couples who decided against parenthood, when added to the generally accepted figure of 10 to 13 percent of women who were involuntarily childless, gave heightened visibility to the dramatically lowered birthrate during the Great Depression and to the demands of those who wanted children.[33] Physicians as a result used the increase in voluntary childlessness to argue for the greater urgency of treating the involuntarily childless. That they found a receptive audience is evident from the fact that the depression years seemed to bring a renewed interest in infertility treatment on the part of practitioners, after a period of quiescence in the early 1920s.

In the aftermath of World War I, up-to-date treatment for infertility was available at only a few hospitals in urban centers, thereby limiting access to such services to urban dwellers or those who could afford a stay away from home. Even though practitioners' guides and journal articles enabled physicians far from large urban centers to keep up with current literature, in fact, considering that many gynecologists in the late nineteenth century had considered sterility one of the specialty's greatest challenges, medical interest seems to have ebbed considerably. Perhaps the doctors were discouraged. After all, high hopes had led to disappointments; only in rare cases did surgical treatments for sterility result in pregnancy. In the late 1910s and early 1920s, even in the practices of the most highly regarded infertility experts, pregnancy rates hovered at best at around 16 percent, and physicians never tried to provide figures on how many of those pregnancies resulted in live births.[34]

A dramatic change occurred with the discovery of the hormones and with the development of new, nonsurgical methods of determining the patency of the fallopian tubes (that is, whether they were open). Practitioners felt a new surge of confidence, and the public was deluged with new information. By the 1930s, couples troubled by infertility could find information in popular periodicals, books written by physicians in nontechnical language, and films. According to journalist Gladys Denny Shultz, by 1940 medical advances had made "offspring possible for . . . childless couples in all but absolutely frontier settlements."[35] The decade of the 1930s therefore was an era of high expectations, with popular articles claiming that half of the infertile couples could conceive through the new therapeutic techniques.

Gynecologists encouraged infertile couples to have hope, although their own studies produced more modest pregnancy rates of less than a quarter of their patients. Samuel Meaker, a nationally known expert who practiced in Boston, was a diagnostic and therapeutic innovator. His success rates were among the highest reported. Out of a sample of 64 patients, 48 were treated; of those, 16 delivered living babies, a success rate of 25 percent overall, and 33 percent of the treated patients. After developing a more extensive treatment plan in the 1930s, he treated 36 patients who produced 15 living babies. But these were the best statistics. Samuel Siegler, querying 200 gynecologists in the early 1940s, found that pregnancy rates were around 28 percent; he did not discuss the proportion of these pregnancies that ended in live births. By the 1940s, in fact, the experts, stung by their inability to deliver on the promises of the thirties, began to temper their rosy projections.[36]

In addition to the hormonal discoveries discussed above, perhaps the most important diagnostic advance was I. C. Rubin's announcement in 1921 that he had developed a nonsurgical test to determine the patency of the fallopian tubes. Until then, the only way a physician could discover whether the fallopian tubes were blocked was through major surgery. Now, using a relatively simple apparatus that could be set up in an office, a doctor could insufflate the tubes with carbon dioxide. If the tubes were patent, then the gas would pass through them easily and enter the abdominal cavity. The patient would know the gas had passed by feeling a pain in the shoulder region; the clinician would judge patency by how much pressure was needed to force the gas through the tube. By the end of the decade, both the Rubin test and a similar procedure known as a hysterosalpingogram, in which a patient underwent insufflation with an oil-based solution while the physician watched the progress of the procedure under x-ray guidance, had become common diagnostic procedures.[37]

Tubal blockage was, and remains today, a significant cause of infertility. During the 1920s and 1930s, clinicians argued that the major culprit was gonorrhea, although they also noted that infections from an earlier birth, appendicitis, and other pelvic infections could have the same result. Some physicians attributed as much as 70 percent of tubal inflammation to the gonococcus, and as much as 25 to 50 percent of all cases of sterility. There were a few dissenters. In 1924, infertility experts Edward Reynolds and Donald Macomber argued that the role of gonorrhea had been vastly overstated, and that at least among men of the "intelligent classes," husbands "rarely expose their wives to contact with acute gonorrhea." But theirs was a minority view. In spite of the Progressive Era and World War I campaigns against venereal disease, many gynecologists insisted, men of all social classes still consorted too often with prostitutes. Such a thoughtless man thereby "doomed" his bride "to a childless life for the rest of her days."[38] Although Rubin and other clinicians used tubal insufflation to treat tubal blockages as well as to diagnose them, it was of no use in cases of severe damage. Insufflation could dislodge tiny bits of debris, thereby opening a tube with a small blockage, but surgery remained the only recourse if the tubes were truly occluded. Because successful operations were extremely rare, in the 1920s practitioners seldom advocated surgery.[39]

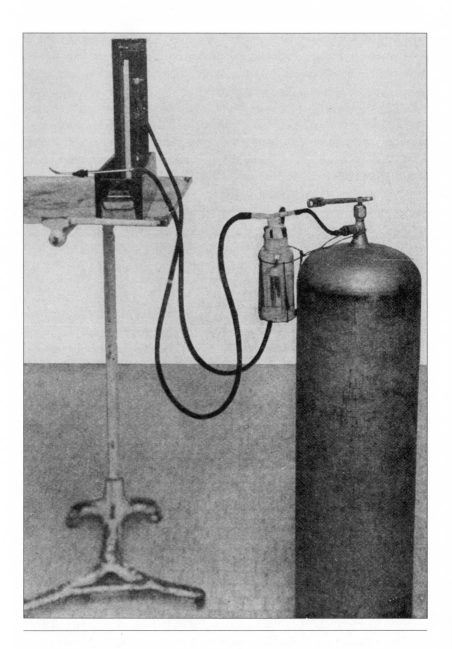

Equipment used in the 1920s for insufflation of the fallopian tubes to determine their patency, a test developed by I. C. Rubin in 1921. Until then, the only way to know if the tubes were open was to perform major surgery.
Courtesy of the College of Physicians of Philadelphia

Tubal insufflation, therefore, provided a relatively less invasive method of diagnosing a long-recognized condition, but it did not appreciably increase the rates of successful treatment. New discoveries unveiling the properties of hormones, however, at least appeared to promise advances in both diagnosis and treatment. As a result, by the end of the 1920s physicians started to prescribe thyroid, ovarian, and testicular extracts for couples having difficulty conceiving. From the time of Galen, practitioners had noted that that women "too fat or too thin" often experienced difficulty conceiving, and prescribed dietary regimens. By the 1920s, physicians seeing a woman at either extreme would suspect a probable thyroid disorder and would prescribe one or another of the commercially available extracts. In addition, the recently discovered vitamins brought new life to dietary therapy; when animal studies demonstrated that rats deprived of vitamin E lost their ability to procreate, clinicians hastened to encourage their patients to fill their plates with foods rich in that substance. However, diet took a back seat to extracts manufactured from desiccated animal organs by drug companies in Europe and the United States long before scientists were able to create pure crystalline forms of many of the hormones. In addition to the thyroid preparations, physicians could prescribe the ovarian extract ovolglandol, or a preparation of the frontal pituitary lobe called prolan.[40]

A vogue—one is tempted to call it a craze—for glandular preparations swept the medical community at all levels by the late 1920s. It is hard for an observer a half-century removed to tell the difference between the moderates and the wholehearted enthusiasts. One self-described moderate, the international authority Theodore van de Velde, spoke out forcefully against overprescription of hormones. But he considered it prudent, in the case of any suspected but not demonstrated hormonal imbalance, to prescribe the medication thelyglan, which combined "ovarian, thyroid, and pituitary hormone, [plus] calcium and the vegetable extract yohimbin." (Yohimbin had a long history of use as an aphrodisiac. This mixture touched all bases!) All these preparations, we must remember, had become available before any of the hormones that govern the reproductive process had even been synthesized. By the end of the twenties, therefore, before the synthesis of the hormones that would revolutionize infertility treatment, clinicians attempted to make practical use of the information filtering out from the research laboratories.[41]

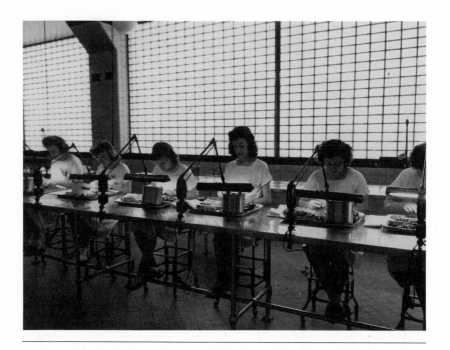

Workers at the pharmaceutical company Parke, Davis in 1943, where animal glandular preparations were manufactured. These women are separating the anterior from the posterior lobe of the pituitary glands. Such preparations were used in infertility treatment from the 1920s onward.
Courtesy of the Library of Congress

Setting Standards

Such new diagnostic procedures and therapies—the latter unproven but fashionable—called practitioners' attention to new opportunities for treating infertility successfully. Perhaps of at least equal significance in the long term, however, was the strategic decision by birth control advocate Robert Latou Dickinson to attempt to connect in his colleagues' minds the treatment of infertility and the advocacy of contraception. Just as scientific research was beginning to provide new diagnostic and therapeutic options for infertile couples, Dickinson's Committee on Maternal Health, with funding from the Rockefellers as well as a number of women philanthropists, attempted to promote research on and treatment of infertility as a part of its agenda.

John D. Rockefeller and many of his fellow advocates of birth control in the 1920s and 1930s, it must be remembered, viewed contraception as a way to enforce smaller families on the poor; indeed, many of birth control's staunchest supporters were eugenicists who also advocated forced sterilization. Looked at in this way, one might argue that any marriage of birth control and infertility treatment would have to be a way of trying to coax the middle classes to have more children and the poor to have fewer. The full story is more complicated than that, although there is no doubt that eugenicists did make those connections and that such may have been the intention of the Rockefeller Foundation when it put up the money for reproductive research.

Birth control was still controversial during the depression, and the medical community remained divided on the ethics of contraception until well into the 1930s. Dickinson tried and failed to elicit the full support of John Rock, for example, a practicing Catholic who was an infertility specialist in Boston. (Several decades later, Rock became the leading clinician in the development of oral contraceptives.) And the American Medical Association refused to endorse birth control until 1937, even though its Section on Obstetrics, Gynecology, and Abdominal Surgery had done so as early as 1925. However, during this period Dickinson and his allies within the Committee on Maternal Health successfully exploited practitioners' interest in learning about infertility as an entering wedge into changing their colleagues' negative views on contraception.[42]

Dickinson, an obstetrician-gynecologist from Brooklyn, had retired from practice in 1920 and resolved to devote the rest of his life to the promotion of happy marriages through good sexual adjustment. Contraception, he was convinced, was an essential element of such happiness for the affluent as well as the indigent. An astute committee politician with the ability to work cooperatively even with colleagues who disagreed with him, Dickinson founded the Committee on Maternal Health in 1923, supported by funding from the Rockefeller Foundation through its Bureau of Social Hygiene and by donations from a number of wealthy and philanthropic women. John D. Rockefeller Jr.'s main interest, of course, was contraception, which placed him at variance with many physicians. Dickinson recognized that to win over the medical profession as a whole, he needed to promise a broader program, to "bracket," in his words, "contraception . . . with sterility."[43] Dickinson's idea to incorporate infertility treatment in his vision of the planned family was not entirely Machiavellian. He had maintained a substantial infertility practice before his retirement and had been one of the early pioneers in donor insemination. It was a combination of expediency and conviction that led him to use infertility as a wedge into the profession to promote the legitimacy of birth control.

Just as the hormonal research begun in the 1920s shaped the ways in which scientists constructed an explanation of fertility, the clinical research either conducted by the Committee on Maternal Health directly, or supported by its funding, was instrumental in developing standardized modalities of infertility treatment. From the design of a widely used form on which physicians would record a couple's medical history to the classification of the steps in a diagnostic evaluation, the committee's hand was visible.[44] The period from about the mid-1920s to the mid-1930s marked the turning point during which the lineaments of modern infertility treatment became clear. This is not to say either that such standardization reached into every city or small town or that Dickinson planned or even anticipated all of the results. However, by creating an organization that functioned as a clearinghouse both for basic research and clinical studies, he was able to pilot his committee in such a way that it not simply stayed abreast of new developments but to a great extent also shaped them.

Two far-reaching examples of the ways in which Dickinson's primary interest in birth control spurred advances in the understanding of infertility are his encouragement of systematic data gathering in infertility practices and clinics and his support and encouragement of research on male fertility. The committee supported the pioneering research of Gerald L. Moench on the structure of sperm in humans, which for the first time allowed physicians to determine what "normal" male fertility was in terms of sperm quantity, motility, and morphology.[45] It was Dickinson who proposed that the Committee on Maternal Health fund a new study of sterility. Initially, he anticipated that new clinical research would form the basis for the study. In the end, however, he concluded that what was really needed was an assessment of current developments and a guide for practitioners to the most advanced new therapies. After at least one false start, the committee turned to Samuel Meaker, of the medical school at Boston University, who had an excellent reputation, a thriving infertility practice, and no scruples against birth control. The last was central to one of the purposes of the study as Dickinson envisioned it—to lay to rest a time-honored view that contraceptive practices brought on sterility.[46]

The resulting work, entitled *Human Sterility* and published in 1934, was perhaps the most significant publication for practitioners that had yet appeared in the twentieth century. Although not based on original clinical research, this book both codified the current state of knowledge about reproduction and broke new ground in several areas. First, Meaker gave reproductive endocrinology a central place in his typology of the etiologies of infertility, suggesting that endocrinological disturbances occurred in more than half of infertile couples. Second, he gave new prominence to Gerald Moench's research on sperm motility and morphology, although he refused to consign a man to a fatherless future unless untreatable azoospermia was present. Third, he popularized among practitioners the idea that infertility usually resulted not from a single cause but from a number of predisposing factors. These three general conclusions led him to argue that successful treatment of most infertility required a team of specialists rather than a single practitioner, and he pressed in this work for the creation of group infertility practices consisting of a gynecologist, a urologist, an endocrinologist, and a pathologist.[47]

Human Sterility set a new standard of practice for the diagnosis and treatment of infertility in both men and women. Even before its publication, Meaker had been considered a national authority on the subject by gynecologists and the public. An influential work by a prominent figure, *Human Sterility* offers historians a snapshot of the ways in which elite physicians approached infertility treatment in the mid-1930s. In addition to his new contributions, however, Meaker's work suggested that some things had not changed. J. Marion Sims would have been delighted to find that his successors still considered an anteflected cervix worthy of treatment. But those of Sims's contemporaries who had eschewed the knife, prescribing instead dietary and similar therapies to improve the general health, would have experienced more ambivalent feelings. Meaker endorsed their viewpoint, but labeled it a new discovery, calling the realization that poor health affected fertility "one of the great modern advances" in practitioners' understanding of the condition. Other ideas came full circle. While late-nineteenth-century physicians had denigrated the centuries-old belief that lack of orgasm inhibited fertility, Meaker and his colleagues resurrected it in the diagnosis of "chronic passive congestion" in women, a condition, they claimed, that resulted from sexual arousal without orgasmic satisfaction and that led to temporary and sometimes permanent closing of the fallopian tubes.[48]

Meaker's book included the first systematic attempt to uncover the extent to which Americans experienced infertility; but, as he soon realized, and just as researchers before and after him discovered, this is a figure that eludes precision. Meaker argued, in contrast to the race suicide alarmists of the teens and twenties, that infertility rates had remained fairly constant since the late nineteenth century, and perhaps longer. After all, he noted, those who saw a rising tide of sterility had relied on genealogical studies to confirm their views. Meaker, however, cautioned practitioners to remember that "those who were sterile . . . are the very ones most unlikely to come to the notice of the genealogist." His own estimate of the prevalence of infertility was between 10 and 13 percent of married couples.[49]

Meaker attributed the growing public interest in infertility treatment not to a rise in the condition itself but to advances in medical science. Endocrinology, in particular, had created an "unprecedented wave of interest . . . [within] the medical profession both in this country and abroad," and demands for treatment followed.[50] Rightfully so, he suggested. *Human Sterility,* written during a time when discovery seemed to follow discovery and practitioners believed that scientists would soon both elucidate the remaining mysteries of reproduction and point the way to treating their disorders, exudes an air of optimism. Even though severe tubal damage remained intractable, with surgery the only treatment and success rates low, less serious tubal occlusions, he argued, often responded to insufflation. But his greatest hopes rested on endocrine therapy, particularly in thyroid and pituitary extracts. The new "oestrus producing hormones," he noted, were still in an experimental phase but could be used if other treatments failed to work. In men, he believed, thyroid and pituitary hormones could reverse low sperm counts, while dietary changes, moderation in alcohol and tobacco use, and increased exercise also promoted increased fertility. Only a very small proportion of men, he believed, among them those whose azoospermia resulted from a case of adolescent mumps, were irremediably sterile.[51]

In the literature of infertility, *Human Sterility* signaled the beginning of a new era. Most significant of all for practitioners was Meaker's assessment that "the usual clinical problem is . . . not that of one definitely sterile partner mated with one who is unqualifiedly fertile, but rather that of two individuals of whom both exhibit some degree of infertility."[52] This analysis led, at least among the gynecologists who practiced in big-city hospitals, to a transformation of infertility treatment. By the late 1930s, most major cities could boast of one or more private group infertility practices, as well as infertility clinics for indigent patients at major hospitals. Numerous diagnostic tests, followed by complex treatment plans, replaced the ad hoc therapy of the twenties.

"What Is Wrong with Me?"

In 1922, twenty-year-old Mrs. F. S., married just over a year and living in Cincinnati, wrote an anxious letter to the Children's Bureau. Shortly after her marriage, she had become pregnant. Young and frightened, her mother dead and no trusted woman friend nearby to reassure her about her severe morning sickness, apparently afraid to see a physician, she took the advice of a neighbor and had an abortion. Now more settled, the young wife was plagued by fears that her abortion would prevent a future pregnancy. "My only goal in life is to become a mother," she wrote. Ethel Watters responded for the Bureau with perhaps more optimism than current medical views would have encouraged. "I am very sorry that you should have so unfortunate an experience," she responded sympathetically, "but nature is usually very kind and she does not always punish by depriving women [who have had a single abortion] of children. . . . It would be wise for you to go to some good physician and have a careful examination made."[53]

Mrs. F. S.'s potential for childbearing would have depended on the skill of the person who performed her abortion. A botched procedure could result in pelvic inflammatory disease and permanently occluded fallopian tubes. According to the most advanced medical opinion in the 1920s and 1930s, infections following abortions ranked just after gonorrhea in responsibility for such inflammations. There is no way of knowing whether Mrs. F. S. succeeded in becoming pregnant; what this exchange, and others like it, demonstrate is that women were beginning to acknowledge more openly their hopes and anxieties about their childlessness.[54]

Many of the letters to the Children's Bureau in this period came from rural areas where access to medical care remained limited. From a small town in Indiana, Mrs. E. M. wrote that "I . . . has always wanted children in my home of my own, and hasn't any." Having "taken all kinds of medican" (probably proprietary products such as Lydia Pinkham's tonic), she asked the women at the Children's Bureau "what I should do that would be a help to me." From women who relied on over-the-counter tonics to those who sought medical help, these letters from the involuntarily childless reveal both hope and sadness. They also show that women did not always accept their childlessness passively but actively attempted to find ways of bearing children, or if that were impossible, adopting them.[55]

In the early 1920s, women in infertile marriages may have turned to the Children's Bureau because they had few other sources of specific information. But by the end of the decade, mass circulation magazines geared to various audiences discussed infertility and offered advice. From *Hygieia* (a health magazine published by the American Medical Association for a general readership) to *Readers Digest,* from *Parents* to *Pictorial Weekly,* general interest periodicals took up the issue. In part, such interest reflected the growing body of scientific knowledge about reproductive issues; but perhaps more important was the ever-growing willingness of Americans to air issues that previous generations would have found entirely out of place in a public forum. The circumlocutions still required of mass circulation magazines during the Progressive Era crusade against venereal disease now gave way to frank statements about "the seminal discharge," "vaginal secretions," and "the frequency of marital relations." Whether such publicity was the cause or the effect of increased interest in infertility is difficult to pinpoint, but the fact remains that the 1930s, the high point of *voluntary childlessness* in the United States, also witnessed an extensive interest in, and transformation of, medical treatment for involuntary childlessness.[56]

By all accounts, both popular and medical, it was not usually couples, but wives, who sought medical help when pregnancy failed to occur. They entered the doctor's office asking, as did "Evelyn Salisbury," Maxine Davis's infertile everywoman, "What is wrong with me?" Women, however, did more than simply internalize the responsibility for the couple's infertility. Many a wife, apparently abetted by the family doctor, protected her husband from any suspicion that he might be responsible for the couple's plight. According to New York gynecologist Asta Wittner, a couple's regular physician would rarely inform a man that he was infertile, no matter how low his sperm count, out of "fears that an inferiority complex might develop in his patient if told he is at fault." Wives, Wittner complained, would rather undergo extensive treatment themselves than risk asking their husbands to come in for an examination. Nearly every infertility expert, whether male or female, confirmed the reluctance of most men to believe themselves responsible. Or, as writer Maxine Davis put it tartly, "The husband . . . doesn't think for an instant that the fault might lie with him."[57]

As Meaker's study had made clear, by the 1930s fertility specialists knew full well that men bore a share of the responsibility for a couple's infertility. Nevertheless, although elite practitioners embraced the new techniques of semen analysis, they disagreed among themselves over the percentage of abnormal or weakly motile sperm necessary to render a man incapable of impregnation. Furthermore, the literature clearly suggests that male specialists—who dominated the field—held different attitudes about male infertility from those of their female colleagues. In the interwar years, most of these men remained as sensitive to the possibility of "an inferiority complex" in the husband as had the general practitioners scorned by Asta Wittner.

For a bracing dose of blunt talk to men, one must look to women practitioners. Where Samuel Meaker, the most cited infertility expert of the 1930s, tiptoed gently, women gynecologists often strode forcefully. Although Meaker noted that men bore some responsibility for infertility in from "40 to 50 percent of all cases," he hastened to add that "the aggregate responsibility of wives . . . appears to be greater." It is possible, of course, that Meaker's gentler handling of men came from expedience rather than conviction. After all, if a doctor were unable to persuade a man to come into the office, he or she would never have a chance to determine his fertility. Most husbands, all physicians agreed, submitted to examinations reluctantly, if at all. As Meaker concluded, a man "will go to any lengths of obstinacy rather than run the risk of losing domestic prestige." Another infertility expert warned his colleagues that the mere suggestion to a man that he might be infertile could render him impotent. Husbands, he insisted, "must . . . be handled with great care and tact."[58]

Several prominent women physicians expressed impatience with such delicacy because it too often led to unnecessary treatment of the wife. As Sophia Kleegman remarked in 1939, "Even today the study of the husband is frequently superficial and inadequate, or else entirely overlooked. Sterility is still considered a gynecological problem, and it is the woman who comes to the gynecologist for relief." Sophia Kleegman, born in 1901, was one of a few women gynecologists in the twentieth century who made their reputations as infertility experts. The first woman appointed to New York University College of Medicine, in 1929, she treated infertility in both private and clinic practices up through the 1960s. Her mistrust of both general practitioners and urologists led her to study semen analysis directly under Gerald Moench, so that she herself could determine as accurately as possible the degree of fertility of the husbands of her patients. After all, she noted, "In no field of therapy has the human body been so frequently assaulted as has that of the barren woman. . . . No surgery on the woman should be done . . . unless the husband's sperms . . . are within fertile limits."[59]

Whether bluntly or tactfully, however, by the 1930s the up-to-date gynecologist would have asked a woman to bring her husband in for an examination. Still, many wives continued to protest. Women would "willingly submit," as one doctor noted, to repeated treatment, including

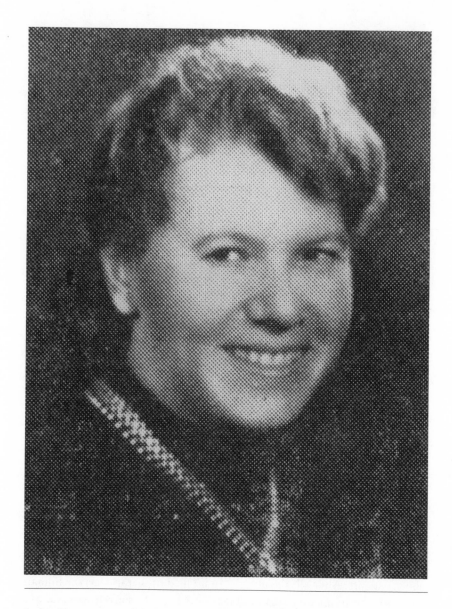

Sophia Kleegman, one of the few women among the pioneers in the treatment of infertility, practiced in New York City and was a member of the faculty of the New York University College of Medicine.
From *Women's Medical Journal* (1948); Courtesy of the College of Physicians of Philadelphia

surgery, rather than bring their husbands in for diagnosis. For this reason some infertility specialists declined to treat a woman whose husband refused to cooperate. But not all specialists were willing to send a woman away just because of her husband's recalcitrance. Furthermore, not all infertile couples consulted a specialist. The woman who went to the family physician may not have been given the same ultimatum. Indeed, specialists' constant reiteration that it was necessary to examine the husband suggests otherwise.[60]

Couples who consulted an infertility expert in depression-era America found themselves facing a time-consuming and often expensive course of diagnosis and treatment. One writer noted with admiration that an eminent (but unnamed) specialist treated his patients with severe financial problems for a flat fee of $75, but such limits on fees were rare. The price of infertility treatment, both financial and otherwise, could be quite steep. A single office visit to a specialist could cost fifteen dollars, and hormonal therapy in the days before the availability of synthetic preparations could run into hundreds of dollars. Samuel Meaker and his team of doctors required their patients to devote an entire week to the initial diagnostic workup, going from office to office, making love at precisely prescribed intervals, and having their bodily fluids—blood, urine, semen—tested and retested. Many of Meaker's patients came from outside the Boston area, so to the expense of the physicians' bills and laboratory tests added hotel charges and perhaps lost wages.[61]

Most infertility specialists did not require a couple to set aside an entire week for diagnostic purposes, but they did establish a similar pattern of physical examination followed by laboratory tests. Both partners had their medical history taken, next undergoing a general physical that included urine and blood analyses. The wife's gynecological examination followed, then evaluation of the husband's semen for quantity, motility, and morphology. Unless the husband was azoospermic, a postcoital examination was next, to determine whether sufficient numbers of sperm reached the cervical canal with adequate motility. The Rubin test or a hysterosalpingogram—and very often both—followed to determine tubal patency. By the end of the 1930s, a few clinicians had begun to perform endometrial biopsies (which allowed the physician to determine, by examining tissue from the endometrium, whether ovulation had occurred). Those patients in whom endocrine disorders were suspected also underwent additional tests to attempt to determine the exact nature of the deficiency.[62]

The infertility evaluation described by Meaker, of course, was an ideal perhaps attained only by specialists with access to the full panoply of laboratory services and complete dedication to the process on the part of both husband and wife; in general outline, however, it served as a goal toward which doctors strove. The potential economic benefits may not have concerned the famous practitioner with the too-large practice. But for many physicians, couples anxious for offspring—when they were able to bear the financial burden of the diagnosis and treatment—provided a welcome new source of income during difficult economic times.

According to Meaker, an infertility workup and subsequent treatment required dedication and tenacity on the part of the infertile couple. Such requirements, he claimed, militated against the treatment of the poor. Charity patients, he asserted, lacked the patience to complete the diagnostic program. They demanded, he sniffed, an answer after the initial visit; his private patients, in contrast, "eagerly welcome[d] an opportunity of having the most thorough possible investigation." It was for this reason, he argued, that free infertility clinics were "unsatisfactory." That he may have had other reasons, however, is suggested by his remark that "superior people," by whom he meant the affluent and well-educated, were not having enough children.[63]

Others disagreed. Sophia Kleegman and Asta Wittner, for example, followed the same diagnostic procedure for both private and clinic patients. Indeed, the 1930s witnessed the growth of a number of free or low-cost infertility clinics, some of which had been started a decade or so previously. Additionally, a number of general gynecological clinics also provided infertility treatment. From the hospital at Philadelphia's Woman's Medical College to the Woman's Hospital in New York to Brookline's Free Hospital for Women, a number of voluntary hospitals offered such services.[64]

Elite physicians, of course, had for several decades (and in the case of the Woman's Hospital in New York, for three-quarters of a century) treated indigent patients as a way to hone their skills, build their reputations, train young physicians, and provide a body of case material for papers to be given before medical societies and for articles to be published in the appropriate journals. With such goals in mind, the gynecologists treating infertility might be seen as doing nothing different from their colleagues who researched other medical problems by experimenting on people. However, a physician seeking boldly to increase the fertility of the poor could not be unaware that many other physicians believed full well that there were already too many poor children. Without some sympathy for the patients' desire to conceive, a practitioner would have to be cynical indeed to treat infertility among low-income and indigent patients.

Perhaps some were. But at the Free Hospital for Women, in Brookline, Massachusetts, just over the border from Boston, patient records suggest that clinic and private patients underwent the same tests and received the same treatments. From hormones by mouth and injection, to surgery for pelvic adhesions or blocked fallopian tubes, to donor insemination, the therapies were the same for the wives of WPA workers and elevator operators as they were for the wives of bankers and engineers. Both groups, however, underwent experimental as well as time-tested therapies. John Rock, the director of the Fertility and Endocrine Clinic at the Free Hospital, was a professor at Harvard Medical School, and the facility served as a research arm of that institution. Women who came to the Free Hospital, whether as private or clinic patients, were both patient and research subject, and that was true at other research institutions as well. The extent to which women understood their dual role is unclear.[65]

Regarding treatment, the general consensus among physicians was that various endocrine factors contributed to infertility in somewhat more than half their patients, men and women alike. Given the excitement over hormonal discoveries and the fact that drug companies competed intensively over the compounding, synthesizing, and marketing of new preparations, it should come as no surprise that these new therapies caught the medical fancy. Readily admitting that they had no clear understanding of the reasons why some women experienced problems with ovulation, as a result of recent scientific discoveries they did have the techniques—vaginal smears and the charting of basal body temperature—to predict ovulation more accurately.

In addition, since the hormones secreted by the pituitary, thyroid, and ovary were known to affect ovulation, practitioners did have at least some scientific basis for believing that various hormonal preparations might be beneficial. The tendency to experiment with unproven endocrine therapies therefore continued unabated throughout the 1930s. Even those physicians who complained that their colleagues used hormones haphazardly generally followed their own trial-and-error method. Samuel Meaker, a self-described conservative on the issue of hormonal therapies, often, in spite of his colleagues' skepticism, prescribed megadoses of a "preparation of the whole anterior lobe" of the pituitary gland when he was unable to determine exactly what caused a woman's failure to ovulate.[66]

Although Meaker put his faith in pituitary extracts, if the published literature is any indication the most overused hormonal preparation was thyroid extract. True metabolic disorders existed, of course, but they were very difficult to diagnose. Any man or woman who was either obese or extremely thin, therefore, seemed a likely thyroid case. When physicians found themselves unable to locate a specific cause for a couple's inability to conceive, the wife—and sometimes the husband—received thyroid therapy, either as a first step or after all else failed. Although wives were most likely to be given hormones, physicians believed that men with relatively low sperm counts could increase sperm production with the help of thyroid or sometimes pituitary extracts.[67]

Most women and a good number of men therefore could expect some form of hormonal treatments. Women might also find themselves subject to repeated tubal insufflations. According to I. C. Rubin, tubal factors contributed to infertility in 47 percent of women unable to conceive. Others confirmed his figures or placed the proportion even higher. Furthermore, Rubin and others believed, insufflation alone might remove tubal blockages. Among his own patients with completely nonpatent tubes, he reported that 6 percent conceived after insufflation. Among those with partial obstructions, 12 percent conceived, as did 25 percent of women diagnosed with tubal spasms.[68]

In 1938, New York gynecologist Frances Seymour reported that in a series of 300 cases she obtained an astonishing 77 percent pregnancy rate with tubal insufflations. Seymour, however, performed the procedure only on women whose tubes demonstrated some degree of patency already; and she repeated the procedure over a period of up to nine months. As a result, there was no way to judge whether it was the insufflation or something else that enabled the women to get pregnant. As infertility authority Samuel Siegler noted about the Rubin test a few years later, "It is impossible . . . to assay the true value of tubal insufflation as a therapeutic agent. . . . *Many extraneous factors enter into statistical data,* but in general it may be said . . . that conception in not a few cases may be directly attributable to this procedure."[69] In the abstract, infertility specialists expressed reservations about the efficacy of surgery to open blocked fallopian tubes. But since the usefulness of the Rubin test as a therapeutic measure remained in doubt, most gynecologists, when confronted with an infertile woman whose tubal blockage appeared to be her only obstacle to conception, agreed to perform surgery.[70]

More women than men were treated, in part because although experts agreed that men bore some degree of responsibility, they disagreed over how much. Sophia Kleegman, for example, found that men were the "sole cause" in about one-third of her cases. Samuel Meaker, in contrast, in spite of his contention that male factors contributed to infertility in somewhere between 40 to 50 percent of cases, believed that men were absolutely responsible "only in rare instances." Male physicians in general, like Meaker, seemed reluctant to pronounce a man sterile unless he had complete azoospermia. For anything less than absolute sterility, they expressed optimism about the efficacy of treatment.[71]

The most common advice to men was to change their eating habits, cut down on smoking, get more exercise, work less and relax more, avoid excessive exposure to substances such as x-rays and carbon monoxide, and limit their sexual indulgence. (Too frequent intercourse, doctors argued, lowered a man's sperm count.) In addition, practitioners often prescribed thyroid medication for men. For what one physician referred to as "genital underdevelopment" (probably cryptorchidism, which is an undescended testicle), some doctors injected an extract made from bull's testicles.[72]

By the end of the decade, a number of doctors treated both cryptorchidism and abnormalities of the sperm with a newly developed gonadotropic hormone. "Tom Salisbury," who figured in one of the popular stories about infertility in this period, had chronic tonsillitis and was underweight. His doctor prescribed (unspecified) hormone injections and a tonsillectomy. In addition, he reduced his hours at work, gave up coffee, and gained weight. We do not know the resultant effect on his sperm count, but if these measures had no effect, little else was available.[73] At least he did not have azoospermia; that condition remained untreatable (and still is) unless caused by a blockage in the vas deferens that would respond to surgery. In reality, unless his low sperm count actually resulted from correctable dietary deficiencies, a true thyroid disorder, or a constitutional infection that responded well to treatment (such as an infected tooth that could be pulled, or an abscess), all the extract of bull's testicles in the world would not have helped. If his sperm count remained low and his wife, Evelyn, were fertile, the couple's two recourses would have been artificial insemination using donor sperm, or adoption.

"Ghost Fathers"

On April 17, 1934, Lillian Lauricella, a Long Island housewife who had been childless for eight years, gave birth to twin girls. For years, in spite of undergoing an unspecified "series of treatments" for her supposed sterility, she had failed to conceive. Finally, her husband, Salvatore, a

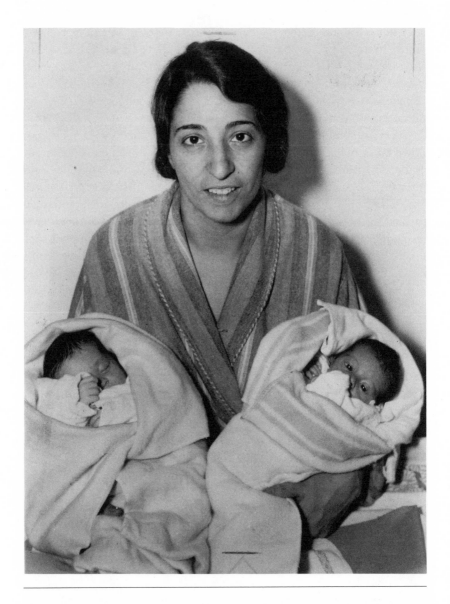

Mrs. Lillian Lauricella and her twin daughters, conceived through donor insemination and born in April 1934. The event was widely covered in the news media and was evidence of a growing interest in artificial insemination.
Courtesy of the Library of Congress

garage worker in Manhattan, bemoaned his childless state to one of his customers, infertility specialist Frances Seymour. She agreed to look into their problem—which, as it turned out, was that Mr. Lauricella's semen contained no sperm. The Lauricellas had come to the right place: Frances Seymour was a vocal and prominent advocate of artificial insemination using donor semen. After receiving several inseminations, Lillian Lauricella conceived her twins.[74]

It was during this period that artificial insemination came to public attention. Numerous articles appeared in the popular press, and physicians debated the question among themselves. In some ways, it may seem strange that in an era of breathtaking new scientific discoveries regarding the biology of reproduction, a relatively old reproductive technology captured so much attention. But in fact, without the hormonal discoveries of the previous two decades that had elucidated the menstrual cycle, artificial insemination—which had been practiced at least occasionally since the end of the eighteenth century—would not have been very practical. Still, most physicians found the technique morally palatable only in cases where infertility resulted from "faulty reception of the spermatozoa" by the wife, and the semen came from the husband.[75]

Even then, a number of moral authorities as well as doctors continued to oppose all artificial impregnation, even with husbands' semen. The Catholic Church condemned the practice (and still does) as unnatural. Some physicians, including a few who might consider such therapy as a last resort found it "at best . . . distasteful" and, at worst, fraught with the danger of infection, no matter how great the "aseptic precautions." Physicians' unwillingness to perform artificial insemination using the husband's semen resulted at least in part from the procedure itself. Many doctors either could not bear to ask men to masturbate (or, in the medical parlance of the day, to provide a "friction specimen") or they were bluntly turned down. As a result, doctors often were handed a condom specimen; in fact, doctors found that some husbands even refused to use a condom. In such a case, at least a few physicians agreed to visit the patient's home, wait while the couple had intercourse, then, just as J. Marion Sims had done eighty years before, draw out the semen from the vagina with a syringe and "inject" it into the cervical canal. But if many doctors were repulsed by the idea, others argued, at least when the insemination involved the husband's semen, that the end justified the means. As Edward Griffith remarked, "If the motive for our action is right and positive there can be no objection to the use of any scientific discovery which may enable us to reach our end. And what is more worth striving for than the creation of healthy living children?"[76]

Some physicians extended Griffith's argument into the realm of donor insemination, but the main spur to donor insemination seems to have come not from the medical profession but from the involuntarily childless themselves. Several months before the birth of the Lauricella twins, the popular science magazine *Scientific American* commissioned a survey of physicians on the question. John Harvey Caldwell interviewed 200 doctors from New York, Chicago, Milwaukee, Cleveland, Philadelphia, Newark, and Washington, D.C. Of the 200, although 15 refused to discuss the issue, and another 129 reported that they discouraged the practice, the remaining 56, presumably the most receptive to the idea, claimed to have received nearly three hundred requests to have the procedure done, all of them because the husband was sterile. Of these fifty-six, twenty-two ultimately decided against performing the inseminations, most of them fearing either legal complications or a change of heart on the part of the husbands. (In some cases, wives wanted to conceal the inseminations from their husbands entirely.)[77]

Several gynecologists who expressed disapproval of the practice claimed that "the public was not ready to sanction it." Yet it was "the public," at least in the form of childless wives with sterile husbands, who seemed most ready to accept the idea. In fact, the New York City Community Church—led by activist minister John Haynes Holmes, with more than two thousand congregants—provided a service to match up those seeking donor insemination with physicians willing to provide it. Why the interest in this not so new, albeit newly practical, technique? For the press, of course, it was partly a matter of sensational copy: *Newsweek* referred to babies born of "Ghost Fathers," while the *New York Times* called the babies themselves "synthetic infants." But there was more to it than that. In the first place, much male sterility was proving itself intractable, physicians' hopeful pronouncements notwithstanding. It took until the 1940s for clinicians to accept the pronouncement of the distinguished group of research scientists who authored *Sex and the Internal Secretions*, who had remarked in profound understatement in 1932, "the treatment of the male for infertility is less satisfactory than that of the female."[78]

Some physicians objected not so much to using donor insemination but to allowing couples—or, in some cases, unmarried women— to resolve the issue for themselves rather than leaving the decision up to their physician. The doctor "himself," a number of male physicians argued, should be responsible for determining that the couple seeking donor insemination had a stable marriage, that the husband was truly willing to rear a child not biologically related to him, and that more good than harm to the marriage would be the likely result. Some practitioners were willing to go even further. Robert L. Dickinson suggested that physicians could be justified in deceiving the husband (for his own good, of course). If a man had such a fragile ego that knowledge of his sterility would cause psychological damage, in Dickinson's view the wife and physician might agree to a subterfuge—the doctor telling the husband that his fertility had somehow been restored and inseminating the wife without his knowledge. But others showed much less eagerness to play the role of the Creator, as evidenced by Sophia Kleegman's unadorned statement that she performed inseminations "at the request of the couple." Among the physicians advocating donor insemination, Frances Seymour provoked the most apoplectic response from Dickinson and his colleagues, who wished to keep the procedure within the tight control of a few specialists. One of their greatest objections to her practice was that she appeared willing to accommodate her patients, as long as they seemed healthy and eager for children.[79]

Seymour was certainly not averse to publicity, even if she had not sought it in the case of the Lauricellas. She had no qualms about making the procedure as available as possible and did not insist that her patients be married. She later claimed that she had inseminated "many" unmarried career women. Insisting that any woman who wanted children should be able to have them, Seymour viewed donor insemination for women without husbands as "a decent and moral method of acquiring the children nature intended her to bear." In 1941, in the *Journal of the American Medical Association,* she and her husband, Alfred Koerner, reported the results of a survey of physicians that demonstrated the growing success of artificial insemination. Their claim that ten thousand babies had been born as a result of artificial insemination—nearly one-third of them by using donor semen—although challenged at the time, received indirect confirmation within a decade.[80]

During the 1930s, increasing numbers of childless women apparently sought out the procedure in spite of warnings about the ambiguous legal status of the child, fears that the husband might reject the offspring of his wife and a donor, or anxiety that the wife would find being pregnant with a child not biologically her husband's repugnant. Seymour, crusader that she was, downplayed any potential harm to the marriage. The mother, she claimed, would "admire the broadmindedness of her husband" in approving such a course, while the husband, "anxious for an heir, is happy that his wife will resort to this unusual step to make up for his deficiencies." But in fact, the warnings were not without foundation. Although Seymour argued that the child conceived through donor insemination would in law be considered the legitimate child of the husband, the Legal Bureau of the American Medical Association disagreed, advising that the father of record should ensure his paternity by formal adoption. In the 1940s, two divorce cases involved artificial insemination, but neither created a legal precedent, and the legal status of children conceived in this manner remained murky.[81]

In some respects, donor insemination remained a clandestine activity. It is impossible to know definitely the extent to which couples resorted to donor insemination in the prewar years. A number of practitioners, including Dickinson, challenged Seymour and Koerner's figures as outrageously high. But a few years later Dickinson himself estimated the number of babies born as a result of artificial insemination at twice the number they had. Such large figures are puzzling. If male physicians accurately assessed the sensitivity of men on the grounds of their sterility, one would expect that no more than a small number of them would find it possible to agree to a solution to their childlessness that would remind them daily of their inability to be a biological father. Dickinson's suggestion of collusion between the doctor and the wife seems entirely credible.

In the midst of all these speculations, however, one thing seems clear: That with the exception of Seymour, who was anathema to the gynecological elite, it was not physicians but women and men outside the medical profession who brought donor insemination out into the open, and perhaps made it more available. Prominent gynecologists, faced with a demand, brought their professional authority to bear in order to attempt to control access, and most elite practitioners closed ranks to attempt to exclude physicians, such as Seymour and Koerner, whom they saw as making such a procedure accessible to "questionable" couples, not to mention women without husbands.[82]

The AMA-sanctioned *Hygieia,* after the *Journal of the American Medical Association* had published the Seymour-Koerner survey, continued to deemphasize the procedure. Noting that donor insemination was "a possible solution" for "hopelessly sterile" men "in a small proportion of cases," the magazine went on to claim that "remarkably few" incidences of successful insemination "are reported in the medical literature." The author was being disingenuous. The obfuscation of the issue in the *Hygieia* article may have represented the wishes of elite practitioners, but it could not have been accurate.[83]

Legal and moral qualms notwithstanding, artificial insemination became even more acceptable in the popular press during the war years. *Newsweek,* in reporting on the plans of Frances Seymour and Alfred Koerner to supply the decimated countries of Eastern Europe with the semen of "the most superior expatriated donors" in order to build postwar populations, called the idea "daring—but . . . scientific." And a 1945 article on donor insemination in *Woman's Home Companion* faced the issue without moral pronouncements and without acceding to practitioners' beliefs that they alone should have the final say on who could procreate in this fashion. Instead, author Marie Beynon Ray placed the responsibility on the wife. Should a wife choose this way out of an infertility problem, it was her responsibility to anticipate "how the advent of a baby who is truly hers but in no way her husband's will affect him. . . . Will her husband, with a reminder of his inadequacy constantly before him, become jealous and resentful? Might the child . . . create a rift?" Surprisingly, neither this nor any other article on the subject ever speculated on how the children born of artificial insemination might view their unorthodox conception, probably because everyone assumed that the child would never be told. Nevertheless, Ray's view was positive, as she invoked expert reassurance that when "husband and wife are not only willing but eager" to have a child this way, "the doctors who give the treatment state that they have had highly satisfactory reports from their patients and their husbands."[84]

Not every physician performed donor insemination, not every couple would have made such a choice, and many who might have simply had no access to it. Expense could deter some couples. In the early 1930s, Seymour's donors were paid $150, the same fee that a blood donor earned. By the end of the decade, she claimed to rely on volunteers. By the early 1940s, medical students apparently served as regular donors, and the cost per sample had come down considerably. But there were other costs besides the sample. Usually a woman required several inseminations before conceiving, as well as a series of laboratory tests to determine her time of ovulation. An article in *Harper's Magazine* noted that most people who tried donor insemination were unable to afford to continue it long enough to achieve a pregnancy. Still others had moral or ethical objections, or heeded the edict of the Catholic Church, which took an increasingly firm stand against artificial insemination by the 1940s.[85]

The Adoption Alternative

Infertile couples for whom donor insemination was not an option, as well as those in which the wives were infertile, often looked to adoption as a solution to their childlessness. One couple who did so was the comedy team of Gracie Allen and George Burns, who had been married since 1926. After several years of travel on the vaudeville circuit, they achieved spectacular popularity as a radio act in the early 1930s. Their success, according to a 1953 interview with Allen in the *Woman's Home Companion,* provided the stability the couple wanted in order to start a family. After his wife's death, Burns told the story of their inability to have children, but he did not say whether she sought medical treatment when she failed to become pregnant. However, in the early 1920s she had undergone an emergency appendectomy and may have had a pelvic infection as a result. As Burns later recalled, they had both come from large families and were saddened by their inability to conceive. Within a few years they adopted two children from the Cradle, a Catholic foundling home in Evanston, Illinois. They were not alone. Among show business personalities, Burns remembered a half-century later, "Adopting babies was a popular thing to do . . . in the 1930s."[86]

The Cradle was founded in 1923 by Florence Walrath, who had become involved in adoption work a decade earlier by locating a baby for her sister. It courted publicity and provided children to a number of celebrities. Harpo Marx, George Burns recalled, adopted a child from the Cradle. So did Jimmy Walker, the flamboyant former mayor of New York, and his second wife, Betty Compton. Walker, who had no children during his first marriage, married Compton in 1933, when she was twenty-eight and he fifty-one. After adopting a girl in 1936 and a boy in 1937, they divorced in 1941. Most likely Jimmy Walker, who by his own account had sown several acres of wild oats throughout his life, was the sterile partner. Betty, who remarried in 1942, bore a child two years later.[87]

Despite the intense media interest that surrounded celebrity adoptions, in the general literature on infertility the role of adoption as a solution to infertility was in the process of transformation. Beginning in this period, it became increasingly common for articles to claim that pregnancy often followed adoption. Although studies conducted several decades later would demonstrate convincingly that adoptive infertile couples were no more likely to conceive than those who did not adopt, beginning in the 1930s and continuing into the 1950s journalists and physicians alike claimed that the relationship was "scientific fact." One article in *Hygieia* insisted not only that there was a relationship between adoption and subsequent fertility but also that such phenomena demonstrated how important psychological factors were in creating infertility.[88]

It is difficult to know how many couples turned to adoption in hopes of promoting their fertility; it seems more likely that they adopted after having given up all hope for biological children. According to a study of couples who had adopted children between 1931 and 1940, approximately 85 percent adopted because of infertility. Among these, about half had sought medical advice; according to the team of researchers conducting the study, this group divided about equally between those who had avidly pursued medical treatment and those who had pursued it cursorily before deciding to adopt. The remainder, which comprised nearly half of all the couples who had said they adopted because of infertility, had never consulted a physician. Rather, they simply accepted their inability to conceive after trying for a number of years and moved on directly to adoption.[89]

By the 1930s, both private charities and public social service agencies provided children for adoption. Like infertility treatment, adoption often entailed both anxiety and expense. Legal fees, for example, could be particularly burdensome during the depression years, thus limiting the chances of the less affluent to adopt. Among the families in the study noted above, about two-thirds of the adoptive couples were solidly in the middle class. A Pennsylvania study conducted in the 1930s also shows that the more affluent were more likely to adopt. Out of 323 adoptions completed in the state in 1931 and 1932, only 9 percent of adopting families had incomes of less than $25 a week.[90]

There are no definitive statistics on the extent of legal adoption in the United States before World War II, but the Child Welfare League estimated the number to be about sixteen thousand annually. People could also turn to private adoption—what has sometimes been called the "gray market"—and a flourishing "black market" in babies existed as well. "It was not at all uncommon," notes historian Rickie Solinger, "for an abortionist to take on baby selling as a lucrative sideline."[91] There were also more informal, adoptionlike practices, which appear to have been quite prevalent but are uncountable. Couples considering adoption during the 1930s had to worry both about expense and about whether they could even get a baby. Newspapers were reporting that "the baby market is booming," as couples "country-wide scramble . . . to adopt a child."[92]

By the early 1940s, infertility had ceased to be a subject whispered about behind closed doors and had become a staple of popular journalism. Women's magazines heralded a new era of successes in infertility treatments. Physicians trumpeted their new endocrinological therapies and their streamlined treatment methods. Voluntary hospitals provided services for those unable to pay. And if infertility treatments failed, fertile women with sterile husbands could try donor insemination, and others could attempt to adopt. Lillian Lauricella posed with her donor insemination babies for a New York newspaper, Burns and Allen with their adopted children in fan magazines. Optimism about future progress prevailed.

Perhaps it was this optimism that led one clinician to believe that it would be possible to tackle one of the most intractable problems in infertility—blocked fallopian tubes. Although John Rock was arguably one of the most skilled and successful practitioners of the surgery known as tuboplasty—the reconstruction of damaged fallopian tubes—his success rates remained very low.[93] In the late 1930s he began to wonder whether it might not be possible to bypass the fallopian tubes altogether, and in 1938 he and his assistant Miriam Menkin began a series of experiments to fertilize a human egg in vitro. Their experiments would ultimately shake the foundations of contemporary reproductive medicine and raise profound ethical and moral questions about the nature and direction of reproductive technology. The quest for technological innovation, combined with the urgency for procreation that fueled the postwar baby boom, formed the basis for the postwar developments in infertility treatment.

"Such Great Strides"

Reproductive Technology in
Postwar America, 1945–1965

It is a distressing fact that at least one out of every ten married couples in this country wants children but is unable to have them. And yet such great strides have been made in the study of infertility in recent years that today, with treatment, nearly a third of these cases can achieve parenthood.

Grace Naismith, "Helping the Childless," Today's Health, February 1954

In the summer of 1944, John Rock and Miriam Menkin of Harvard University and Brookline's Free Hospital for Women astonished readers of *Science* by reporting the fertilization of four human eggs in vitro. No one had ever achieved such a feat before. Although some scientists would later raise questions about the experiment, their contemporaries acknowledged this as a major achievement; soon journalists began to predict that in the not-too-distant future, in vitro fertilization would allow women whose fallopian tubes were blocked or absent to bear children.[1] Their forecasts were premature. Babies born through in vitro fertilization were more than three decades away. But these first glimmerings of the possibility of creating human life outside the body signaled a sea change in the ways in which scientists, clinicians, and the public defined infertility and envisioned possible means of overcoming it.

Rock and Menkin's announcement appeared at a time when science and scientists reigned, and few Americans doubted that technological advances promoted the public good. Medical science and clinical practice basked in such a favorable climate. Funds poured in for basic and clinical research, as the national government joined pharmaceutical houses and foundations in underwriting research. Optimism prevailed in all fields of medicine. Scientists and clinicians interested in infertility research and treatment, who had recently banded together to form the American Society for the Study of Sterility, in 1950 founded the journal *Fertility and Sterility* for the exchange of information on new discoveries and developments. Established infertility centers expanded, and new ones opened up all over the country. Infertile couples, convinced that scientists either had already or soon would find a way to make them parents, filled the waiting rooms.

John Rock, who directed the Fertility and Endocrine Clinic at the Harvard-affiliated Free Hospital for Women and later founded the Rock Reproductive Center, embodied the postwar era's new directions in research and treatment. Although Rock's later fame resulted from his work on the development of the birth control pill, his life's work had been in infertility. From his and Menkin's pioneering attempts at in vitro fertilization in the 1930s and 1940s to clinical research on new fertility drugs in the 1960s, Rock was one of a handful of nationally recognized figures who stood at the head of a new elite corps of infertility specialists and who, over the course of two postwar decades, fundamentally altered the ways in which researchers conceptualized, and practitioners treated, the problem of infertility.

John Rock had considered attempting human in vitro fertilization at least as early as 1937, when he wrote anonymously in the *New England Journal of Medicine* that if it were only possible to initiate conception outside the body, "What a boon for the barren woman with closed tubes!" Inspired by the successes of his friend Gregory Pincus, who had not only fertilized rabbit ova in vitro but had also successfully implanted an embryo conceived in vivo—that is, in the body—from one rabbit into the uterus of another, Rock became convinced that in vitro fertilization would work with humans. But if Pincus had provided a scientific precedent, it was

Rock's decade of treating women with blocked fallopian tubes, mostly unsuccessfully, that fueled his determination to succeed.[2]

John Rock was a Harvard-trained M.D. who directed one of the nation's longest-lived infertility clinics, which he had started in 1926, when he was thirty-six years old. He had originally viewed his gynecological training as a way station to psychiatry or neurosurgery. In later years he claimed that he tarried so long in obstetrics and gynecology that he simply grew too old to do anything else. When he began his career, he was in fact somewhat older than the typical neophyte physician—nearly thirty by the time he had completed his residency—and he was eager to get started in his life's work. He had early expressed an interest in infertility, in 1923 reopening the defunct sterility clinic at Massachusetts General Hospital once under the direction of Edward Reynolds. Shortly thereafter he opened his own clinic at the Free Hospital for Women, all the while still continuing to practice obstetrics and general gynecology. By the early 1930s, however, his interest centered almost entirely on infertility.[3]

Rock was a practicing Catholic who at the beginning of his career expressed a firm belief that without children a couple could hardly be a family. He later modified that rigid view, but despite his later fame as the father of the birth control pill and his crusade against overpopulation, he always believed that every measure possible should be employed to assist infertile couples to conceive. An involuntarily childless marriage was for him one of nature's saddest stories. Rock and his wife had five children themselves, and by all accounts he was a devoted husband and loving father. He appears to have been a beloved doctor as well, his patients in both his private and his clinic practice expressing a personal gratitude for his care and attention that went beyond appreciation for his medical services.[4]

When Rock began his career in the mid-1920s, he held fairly conventional ideas about infertility, but by the 1930s he began to question a number of his profession's long-held beliefs concerning its treatment. Possessed of an open and curious mind, he pioneered in the clinical use of a number of new techniques, including the tracking of ovulation by dating the lining of the endometrium. He seemed ready to investigate nearly every therapeutic innovation that might hold out the promise of some success. He experimented with hormonal therapies, treating both female endocrine disorders and male infertility with thyroid extracts and performing clinical trials of other hormonal preparations such as equine gonadotropins, which were designed to stimulate the pituitary.[5]

But if Rock believed at the time that he could help couples with an en-

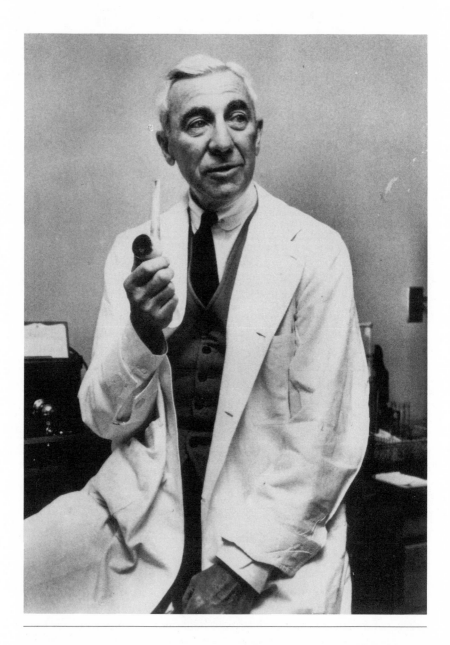

John Rock's career in reproductive medicine spanned much of the twentieth century. He and his assistant Miriam Menkin in 1944 reported the first successful in vitro fertilization of human ova.
Courtesy of the Countway Library of Medicine, Harvard University

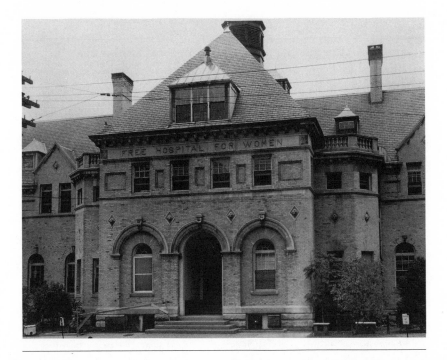

The Free Hospital for Women, where John Rock directed the Fertility and Endocrine Clinic until his retirement from Harvard University in 1955.
Courtesy of the Countway Library of Medicine, Harvard University

docrine disorder, he was less optimistic about the nearly 20 percent of his patients with blocked fallopian tubes. Caused by infections including gonorrhea, complications from abdominal surgery and appendicitis, and endometriosis, tubal occlusions could only be remedied surgically. Rock was perhaps one of the most skilled operators in the delicate surgery of tubal reconstruction, but even his success rate was only around 7 percent. And if disease had made it necessary to remove the tubes entirely, most practitioners agreed that there was no hope for pregnancy.[6]

A little-known gynecologist in Bethlehem, Pennsylvania, however, believed otherwise. In 1909, William Estes had developed a procedure similar to one devised earlier by Robert Tuttle Morris. Estes implanted the ovary, or a portion of it, in the uterine wall at the point where the tubes and uterus normally connected. In 1924, Estes' son claimed four pregnancies out of a series of ninety-five cases that occurred during both his and his father's career. But no one seemed able to replicate their success, and the procedure appears to have been rarely used by the time Rock began to consider the possibility of bypassing the tubes entirely by means of in vitro fertilization.[7]

When Rock decided in 1938 to attempt in vitro fertilization, he hired Miriam Menkin as his research assistant, thereby beginning an association that would last for the rest of both of their careers. Menkin had been a technician for Gregory Pincus at the time he was engaged in his in vitro experiments with rabbits. Originally she had planned to be a doctor herself, but she abandoned her goal in order to work as a technician to put her husband through medical school. Talented and hardworking, Menkin was a member of that large, and almost entirely female, technical support army that staffed twentieth-century scientific laboratories. She was in some ways luckier than most, however, because in John Rock she found an employer who publicly and frequently acknowledged her contributions and considered her a collaborator in his research. When she went to work at the Free Hospital for Women, she threw herself wholeheartedly into the experiment that she came to call "egg chasing."[8]

Their methodology evolved over a period of years.[9] Rock obtained the ova from women undergoing elective gynecological surgery who had consented to participate in the project. The women agreed to keep temperature charts for several months to determine their dates of ovulation. When the experiments first began, Rock used only those matured eggs that were present in the tubes following ovulation, since that was what Pincus had done in the rabbits. This decision raised two problems. First, only women undergoing complete hysterectomies could be asked to participate in the experiment, and second, Rock had to time the operations very precisely to coincide with ovulation. The first resulted in a relatively small group of women available to donate their organs, and the second proved extremely difficult to predict. Even the most regular menstrual cycle, the researchers discovered, exhibited occasional irregularities. Eventually, Rock performed the surgeries earlier in the cycle and cultured the less mature ova until they seemed ripe for fertilization.

After Rock or another physician performed the surgery, one of the nurses rushed the excised organs to Menkin in the laboratory. It was Menkin's job to extract the ova, culture them, and then attempt the fertilization, using semen left over from donor inseminations. Between 1938 and 1944 Rock and his fellow surgeons had obtained 800 ova, and Menkin had attempted to fertilize 138 of them.[10] After six years of unremitting failure, between February and April 1944, Menkin managed to fertilize four ova from three women. Why this success after so many years? According to Menkin, accident and exhaustion both played a part. Until the first successful attempt in February, she had washed each sperm suspension three times with Locke's solution before initiating contact with the egg. This time, worn out from having been kept awake by her teething baby for two nights, she washed it only once, and then used a more concentrated suspension. She made another change as well. Having previously allowed the sperm and egg no more than a twenty-minute contact period, because that was what had worked with the rabbit sperm, this time "I was so exhausted . . . that I couldn't get up, so I just sat there, watching this remarkable sight, . . . which never fails to fascinate me [—]the human egg, with a mass of spermatozoa on its surface. . . . so great is the force of their combined efforts that the egg is made to rotate around and around." Transfixed, she sat for an hour.[11]

This first success was not, however, an absolute triumph. In all the excitement, but fortunately not before a sketch had been made, she somehow lost the newly fertilized ovum. Although she endured a great deal of teasing about her "miscarriage in vitro," she had at least corrected her technique. Unsure which of the new factors altered the results, Menkin incorporated all three changes into her procedure and was successful in two more experiments, using three ova from two women. These fertilized ova were carefully photographed before being fixed for preservation.[12]

To her lasting regret, Menkin was forced to abandon the project at that critical point. Her husband, who appears to have had a difficult temperament and a penchant for losing or quitting jobs, lost his position in Boston. Rock tried to find him another opportunity but was unable to do so. So Menkin followed her husband to Duke University, which had hired him and also offered her a position as a technician. Duke's medical faculty, however, was appalled at her research interest; behind her back, one of the doctors called it "rape in vitro." Eventually she persuaded one of the pathologists to allow her to use autopsy material for fertilization purposes. But her sojourn at Duke was short. Just as she believed she had convinced some doctors to help, her husband moved on to Philadelphia, where she was only marginally more successful at getting support. Her successors back at the Free Hospital, who apparently lacked her technical proficiency, were having difficulties of a different kind. In 1949, Rock wrote her, "This pm Dr. Finkel lost a beautiful 3 cell in vitro fertilized egg, fortunately after photography. A 2 cell one was lost only a few months ago just before photography. We need you badly."[13]

Rock and Menkin's report of their results in *Science* caused a popular as well as a scientific stir. On the day the article appeared, journalists began to converge on Rock. His comment that pregnancy via in vitro fertilization was "not beyond the realm of imagination, and it seems to offer about the only hope for women whose tubes have been destroyed," made national news.[14] Almost immediately letters began to pour in to Rock and Menkin from women whose fallopian tubes were blocked or absent. With the appearance of each new article, another batch of letters arrived. Most of them came from relatively young women whose fallopian tubes had been surgically removed. While a number of the writers mentioned appendectomies and a few had suffered from ectopic pregnancies, many had no idea why doctors had removed their tubes. A woman from California wrote that when she was 29 her doctor "said her tubes were dried up so he removed them" during an appendectomy; she hoped for "a modern surgical miracle" that would allow her to have another child. Mrs. H., of Richmond, Virginia, who had lost both tubes and one ovary and had "often thought of something in an experimental way," wrote to ask specific questions about the procedure of human IVF. A twenty-three-year-old bride from Shamokin, Pennsylvania, explained that at the age of nineteen she had surgery during which her doctor removed her right ovary and both tubes for adhesions. She hoped that Rock could provide the child she wanted. In a touching postscript she concluded, "Please answer."[15]

Rock answered most of the letters himself, with kindness and sympathy. To women in their late twenties or thirties, he tried to put an end to futile expectations, but for those in their very early twenties—betraying his own hopes that these experiments would lead quickly to clinical application—he expressed some optimism. To one he wrote his regrets that "our research work has not progressed to the point where it is of any clinical value. Fortunately you are young yet so don't give up hope."[16]

More than one woman embraced the idea of an egg donor. Mrs. J. R. wrote from a small town in Illinois offering "to let myself be used as an experiment." She did not say why doctors had removed her fallopian tubes, but since she still had her uterus and one ovary she hoped that Rock could do something for her. Her life, she said, "was so empty and useless as it is without any children." Finally she suggested, "if nothing else use another woman's ovum and my husband's spermatozoa and place it in my uterus." In a sympathetic but discouraging reply, Rock promised that "if by a miracle I learn of something in the near future that can be done for you, I will let you know." And to a similarly unhappy childless woman, he expressed the hope that in vitro fertilization "may some time in the future be able to help people like you . . . , but there is still a tremendous amount of laboratory work to be done before the work can be applied on patients."[17]

After Rock and Menkin published a full account of their experiments in the *American Journal of Obstetrics and Gynecology* in 1948, another spate of popular articles appeared, the most sensational of which was published in *Look* in 1950. Entitled "Babies by Proxy," the article juxtaposed Rock and Menkin's experiments with attempts by cattle breeders to develop a method of IVF and implantation in order to allow purebred cattle to provide the genetic material while "scrub cattle" actually underwent the pregnancy. Human beings, author J. D. Ratcliff suggested, would soon follow the cattle. For women with blocked fallopian tubes, one possibility would entail "an egg taken from a woman's ovary . . . fertilized and incubated outside the body, then implanted in the same woman's womb." And for a woman without a uterus or whose uterus was diseased, "motherhood would still be possible with egg-transfer breeding." In the only note of caution in the entire essay, Ratcliff wondered whether it would be difficult to find women willing to bear babies for others; but then again, "many women today sell their milk to nourish infants who cannot be fed by their mothers. . . . Tomorrow, they may offer their bodies as incubators for the babies of women who are denied motherhood."[18]

The *Look* article, later condensed in *Coronet,* brought Rock a torrent of letters from women who now believed that in vitro fertilization was near at hand. One young woman, engaged to a man she loved very much, was devastated when surgery for pelvic inflammatory disease robbed her not only of her tubes and an ovary but of her fiancé as well. He "wanted children very much," she wrote. "We have never married because of this." Another had thought she was undergoing "a minor operation" while her soldier husband was overseas, to enable her to become pregnant when he returned. Instead, she found herself without her fallopian tubes. "I have never," she wrote, "felt that this operation was absolutely necessary." Her husband, as well, was "deeply grieved" about their childlessness.[19]

One of the most touching letters came from a twenty-four-year-old woman from Geneva, New York. Like many of Rock's correspondents, she had lost both tubes and one ovary to surgery when she was twenty-two and thought of Rock as her last hope. Calling the *Look* article "the most importance [sic] article of my life," she recalled how she "read this article over and over so that I wouldn't make a mistake when I write to you." She and her husband, she said, would be willing to take any risks involved; parenthood "means just that much to us." Like others, she ended her letter with the urgent postscript, "Please answer this letter." Rock did answer, just as he had the others, expressing both his sympathy for her situation and his outrage over the way in which the magazine had irresponsibly raised false hopes.[20]

Perhaps Rock was as frustrated by his own inability to offer these women a solution to their plight as he was by the magazine's misleading story, because soon after receiving all these letters he began to consider whether he could revive and improve upon the Estes operation. From Scandinavia, one physician reported in 1951 that out of twenty-three ovarian implantations, four pregnancies had ensued. Although he did not indicate whether any live births had resulted, these were by far the highest rates of conception yet recorded.[21]

That same year Rock received a letter from Mrs. R. T., a young woman from a tiny hamlet in Kentucky, who said that immediately after the birth of her first child, her doctor without her knowledge sterilized her by completely removing her fallopian tubes. Her baby died when he was just over a year old. Devastated, she then learned of her sterility. Writing with great formality in an uncertain hand, she asked Rock for his help. Sympathetically and with barely suppressed rage over her sterilization, Rock asked for more details. He needed to know if there had been a legitimate medical reason for her sterilization, he said, because he was considering making a series of surgical attempts to allow "the eggs when they come out of the ovary [to] pass into the womb, even though there are no tubes present." But before he would think about operating on her, he reiterated, he needed to know more. At this point, she told him the full story. "I knew when I wrote you before," she responded, "and maybe I should have told you then I have heart trouble." Having gotten more detailed information, Rock was convinced that her health, in spite of her protestations that she was "a lot better I do my housework my washing and ironing and have a garden and hoe in it," was in fact much too poor for her to risk pregnancy.[22]

For unknown reasons, Rock appears to have abandoned the notion of reviving ovarian implantation after this. He did consult with a plastics company about the idea of creating artificial fallopian tubes, but here too the obstacles seemed insurmountable. With his hopes for in vitro fertilization put off indefinitely and no other possibilities for bypassing the tubes near at hand, Rock once again devoted himself to improving his surgical techniques for repairing blocked and damaged tubes. For the women without them, there was indeed no hope.[23]

Their early hopes notwithstanding, Rock and Menkin were unable to progress beyond these initial stages of in vitro fertilization. Menkin returned to the Free Hospital, but the research failed to advance. The two persisted with some work on IVF into the early 1950s; eventually, however, they discontinued it entirely, both because of their own lack of progress and because others—especially Landrum Shettles of Columbia–Presbyterian Hospital in New York, who believed that he had replicated the Rock-Menkin achievement in 1951—began to concentrate intensively on the problem. Rock had in fact been more interested in the practical application of IVF, and it had begun to look to him as if it might take decades instead of years to succeed. Fundamentally a clinician rather than a scientist, he refocused his attention on more immediately promising fields.[24]

Changes in Medical Practice

The research funds that began to pour into medical training within a decade or so after World War II "radically changed academic medicine," as Paul Starr has noted. Federal funds complemented the support already provided by private foundations and pharmaceutical companies, producing opportunities for highly specialized practitioners and young physicians who competed for residencies and staff positions with eminent authorities.[25] Infertility specialists associated with thriving medical centers shared in this expansion. Established clinical facilities augmented their research and treatment capacities, and new centers were founded in response to the growing perception that a specialized medical problem required a specialized physician.

Some infertility experts had long contended that an infertile couple should not put their problem in the hands of a general practitioner who might fail to examine the husband before initiating invasive treatment of wives, perform procedures that worsened a condition, or at the other extreme simply not take the couple seriously. Now their voices were joined by journalistic exposés of shoddy practitioners who at the very least misdiagnosed their patients and at the worst did them actual harm. "Sheer lack of experience and knowledge," insisted one reporter, led physicians to perform unnecessary surgeries, treat nonexistent thyroid conditions, or declare fertile men sterile. Impelled by large fees and visions of an army of "child-hungry" patients, a "swarm of general practitioners . . . have been edging into fertility work," and the only way a couple could be sure of adequate and honest treatment was to see a specialist connected to an infertility center with a medical school affiliation.[26]

Studies of patients treated outside these centers seemed to bear out such contentions. In the early 1950s, for example, staffers at Duke University's infertility clinic completed a study of the records of five hundred women who had been referred to their clinic. They compared the histories of women with identical diagnoses who had or who had not undergone surgery before coming to Duke. Their conclusion: the women who had undergone no treatment before their arrival at Duke had greater success in subsequently becoming pregnant. In 1956 Anna Southam and C. Lee Buxton, two New York infertility specialists, conducted a study of infertility patients with ovulatory dysfunctions that suggested that a woman who received no treatment was more likely to conceive than one who had been treated. Some specialists went even further, arguing that not only general practitioners but also general gynecologists ought not to take on an infertility case. At the "risk of offending some and antagonizing others," an article in the *New England Journal of Medicine* quoted one unnamed infertility specialist who stated "emphatically . . . [that] the family doctor and many eminent specialists need to admit their inadequacy in infertility study, and to acquaint themselves with the proper places to send these patients."[27]

In fact, increasing numbers of couples traveled long distances to see eminent specialists not just at Duke University but at the Woman's Hospital and others in New York, Yale University Hospital in New Haven, and centers around the country. The American Society for the Study of Sterility (today the American Society for Reproductive Medicine) provided names of its members on request, and Planned Parenthood, which until the 1940s had been the Birth Control League, began to provide infertility services across the country at low cost. Between 1952 and 1955 alone, the number of infertility clinics jumped from 66 to 119. Since most of the centers were in urban areas, it might be thought that outside such places couples were more likely to trust their family doctor. Many of them undoubtedly did, but the hundreds of letters that John Rock received from small towns and rural areas all over the country seeking referrals suggest that faith in specialists was not limited to the urbanite. Given the extent to which young women were subjected to excessive and unnecessary surgical procedures, it does not seem that their distrust was invariably misplaced.[28]

A number of major figures in practice during the postwar expansion of infertility treatment had been working in the field for years, some of them for decades, including Rock. The Fertility and Endocrine Clinic—or F&E, as its staff always called it—was originally called the Sterility Clinic. Rock changed its name, Menkin later recalled, because the term "fertility" lent a higher note of optimism. In the 1940s and early 1950s, with the growth of Rock's reputation, the F&E became one of the most important infertility research and treatment centers in the country. Its patient base had increased from around two hundred in the late 1930s to about two thousand by the end of the 1940s. In the early 1950s, the clinic was adding about 200 new patients a year.

In the early years, Rock's clinic had little in the way of financial resources and received its funding largely from the hospital, augmented by some donations. Rock's own income derived mostly from his private practice; although infertility was his primary interest, for most of his career he was never able to make a full-time living from it. Until 1938 he continued to practice obstetrics and afterward general gynecology.[29] After the war, he was able to devote himself nearly full time to problems of infertility and later to birth control. Grant funds from the Committee for Research in Problems of Sex and from the Carnegie Foundation, as well as donation of experimental drugs by pharmaceutical houses, underwrote research and clinical trials. The expansion and specialization of the medical profession provided Rock with more fellows, residents, assistants, and researchers. By the 1950s, physicians from the United States, Europe, and Asia were coming to observe at the clinic, and Rock served as a mentor to a number of young doctors who would form the next generation of infertility experts, including Celso-Ramon Garcia and Luigi Mastroianni.[30]

But if new sources of funding allowed Rock to enlarge his training and treatment facilities, it was the growing patient base that enabled the expansion to continue. Something of a boom in infertility treatment emerged alongside the baby boom in postwar America. During the 1950s, an almost religious faith in the progress of medicine and an intense pronatalist sentiment that accompanied the surge in childbearing combined to make infertile couples less likely simply to accept their childless state. Seeing a specialist might even be seen as a duty.

Childless Couples in a Pronatalist Era

Young married couples in the postwar generation expected marriage to bring them good-sized families and to bring them quickly. When Janet

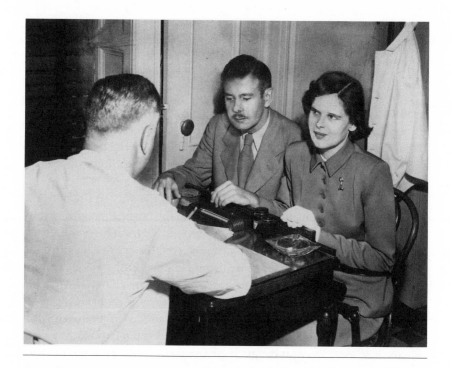

Illustration for an article on infertility in the *New York World* in 1950. The caption reads, "In almost every case, the cause of infertility can be determined . . . if the couple will confront the doctor intelligently."
Courtesy of the Library of Congress

and Herman Schwartz married in 1946, they assumed that parenthood would soon follow. Every month, Janet Schwartz recalled, "I waited for the 'dreaded' period and every month it happened." Because she was, in her own words, "very inexperienced," she simply had no idea what to do. This situation went on for a year. Mrs. Schwartz first found out, from an article on infertility in *Redbook*, that treatment was available at a nearby clinic in Brooklyn, New York. Soon, once a week for several months, she and her husband went together to the clinic. Mr. Schwartz's sperm count was normal. ("And so," his wife remembered, "his ego was intact.") After ruling out other possibilities, the physicians concluded that a uterine fibroid, which they removed, was the likely cause of her infertility. Mrs. Schwartz promptly conceived and safely carried to term. She eventually became pregnant three more times and bore two more children.[31]

Some surge in births after the war was expected. The birthrate had already begun to edge up during the war; women over thirty-five, reassured as wartime prosperity calmed depression-era anxieties, began or completed their families. Although the younger men were off to war, births to older couples increased. Then, after the war and continuing for more than twenty years, Americans reversed a century-old pattern of declining family size. Historians have provided various explanations for the subsequent baby boom. Susan Householder Van Horn has noted that there is always at least a brief surge in the birthrate after wars, a reaffirmation of life after a period of destruction. In Europe as well as in the United States, birthrates rose in the aftermath of war. What is harder to explain is the baby boom's continuation. Unprecedented prosperity surely was a factor. Bankbooks bulged with wartime savings, and the federal government was subsidizing low-interest mortgages.[32]

But there were other determinants at work as well. It may be a truism to bring up the pervasive propaganda campaign to return women to the home to rekindle the fires of domesticity after World War II, as well as the eagerness with which many women complied; but as the birthrate rose, traditionalists breathed a collective sigh of relief. Historian Elaine Tyler May has elevated that reaction to the status of a belief system, arguing that during the postwar years there emerged "a fully articulated baby boom ideology that . . . fit [Americans'] belief in abundance, progress, and productivity." Robert Griswold's study of fatherhood confirms May's views, suggesting that early marriage and parenthood enabled men to keep at bay a number of anxieties and fears, both personal and civic, that confronted them after the war. According to Griswold, "Understanding why young men marched to the altar at a younger age than their own parents and grandparents, and why they seemed so eager to assume the responsibilities of fatherhood involves issues of male identity and cultural anxieties in the postwar era. . . . In short, the willingness to shoulder the responsibilities of fatherhood and breadwinning was the hallmark of mature manhood in the 1950s."[33]

The baby boom cut across class and racial lines; nevertheless, fertility behavior was changing most dramatically among educated white Protestant and Jewish women. True, working-class white women and Catholics of all social classes had a higher overall birth rate than these women during the 1950s, as they had for decades, but their fertility patterns actually remained rather consistent with the past. Fertility patterns of African Americans were more complicated. Although black women had a higher rate of childlessness than whites in the 1950s, as they had for decades, nevertheless at the baby boom's peak in 1957 the overall birthrate among black Americans was 100 percent higher than it had been in 1940.[34]

Young married couples moved quickly into parenthood. In the mid-1950s, the average white woman was just under twenty-two when she gave birth to her first child; among African Americans, the average age was just over twenty. The average age for their mothers would have been about twenty-four and twenty-one, respectively. Couples planned large families; Americans considered four children to be the most desirable number to have, and they wanted to have them soon after marriage. Birth control—except among Catholics, some orthodox Jews, Mormons, and a few nonmainstream Protestant denominations—had become widely accepted, largely as a means to space births, rather than a way of providing women with sexual freedom outside marriage. The Birth Control League had metamorphosed into Planned Parenthood, its image transformed. Even though the baby boom peaked in 1957, the cultural imperative for large, planned families did not abate until the mid-1960s, when young people began to marry later and once again have fewer children.[35]

Until that shift, young men and women were expected to seek early marriage and, within two years at most, parenthood. Not to do so was to seem "different," somehow odd. Women who expressed ambivalence about childbearing were labeled neurotic. Even those who simply wanted to postpone motherhood could face extreme pressures from family and friends. A twenty-year-old woman, married just under two years, wrote *Redbook* in 1963 that her family and friends all were dismayed that she and her husband had as yet had no children. Judy Seabaugh had no intention of remaining childless forever, she said, but everywhere she turned she heard accusations of selfishness, warnings that if she put off getting pregnant much longer she would be "too old to enjoy" her children. From her family, she faced blunt questions about how long she intended to wait. Another woman, married in 1942, who when she found herself unable to conceive considered herself "lucky," still wondered in 1994 if she were the only woman in the country who had not minded being infertile. Surely not, but the happily infertile kept their mouths shut.[36]

Couples having difficulty conceiving found that all around them were messages of both alarm and hope. Media accounts declared that on the one hand, involuntary childlessness was on the rise, afflicting perhaps as many as 15 to 17 percent of all American couples, but on the other hand scientific advances had made possible cure rates for up to 50 percent of those affected. Neither of these claims was accurate. The 1950s had an actual childlessness rate among married couples of less than 10 percent, the lowest proportion of childless Americans for nearly a century. These figures do not take into account the difficulties of couples with secondary infertility—what was sometimes called "one-child sterility"—but they do include the voluntarily as well as involuntarily childless. In fact, the proportion of infertile couples probably was about where it had been in the 1870s.[37]

If the rates themselves do not appear to have changed, both public attention to infertility and demands for treatment among infertile couples had increased. Whether perusing *Redbook* or *Good Housekeeping,* leafing through *Look* or *Ebony,* or reading one of the general interest health magazines such as *Hygieia* or *Today's Health,* Americans would find that medicine was on the verge of conquering infertility. Most magazines did not make the outrageous leap of faith that *Look* did in 1950 when it suggested that in vitro fertilization would soon be available, but all expressed optimism and enthusiasm. Cures, they declared, were on the rise. Almost every article, whether written in 1947 or 1957, began by saying that until "recently" (whenever recently was), physicians were baffled by infertility, but *now* they had increased cure rates to anywhere from one-third to two-fifths of the couples they treated. If more couples would come in for treatment, these stories suggested, success rates could be so much higher. Indeed, "relatively few couples are hopelessly sterile," *Good Housekeeping* assured its readers in 1953. In the immediate postwar era, physician Joseph Wassersug wrote in the American Medical Association's *Hygieia* that "many groups of expert workers" in the infertility field were able to cure "fifty percent or even greater" numbers of their patients.[38]

Whatever the statistical realities, young couples in the 1950s with fertility problems were eager to find solutions. When authorities suggested that perhaps a couple should seek medical help after six months of trying to conceive, young women declined to wait even that long and showed up at doctors' offices three months after marriage. Short fiction in popular magazines as well as increasing numbers of articles stimulated more interest. Magazines aimed at black Americans as well as those directed to a mostly white audience focused on the issue. *Tan Confessions,* which was directed at working- and middle-class African Americans, published several fictional accounts of infertility, in one of which the infertile partner was the husband. The publisher of one of the popular books on infertility, Sam Gordon Berkow's *Childless,* advertised the book in *Ebony,* which also published a number of articles on infertility clinics, artificial insemination, and adoption. Interest was widespread. If the letters that reached John Rock every time his work was reported in the popular press are any indication, the popular magazines did not overestimate Americans' desire to know more about how to become parents.[39]

Such active interest could cut in several directions for infertile couples. Their desire for parenthood was treated with respect, and they were able to make more informed choices about various treatment facilities and kinds of therapies. However, the importance placed on parenthood could bring enormous pressure both on those ambivalent or uninterested in parenthood and on those unable to conceive. Two-thirds or more of the involuntarily childless, in fact, would find themselves unable to conceive no matter how extensive their treatment. The survey conducted by Samuel Siegler in the early 1940s had indicated that practitioners were achieving a pregnancy rate of about 28 percent. There was little change over the course of the decade. In the late 1940s, even the best specialized infertility practices claimed pregnancy rates of about 25 percent; by the end of the 1950s, the proportion had risen to about one-third. Some clinicians reported higher numbers, but as one practitioner cautioned, doctors might be claiming pregnancies unrelated to treatment. One English physician complained in 1952 that her analysis of infertility cases demonstrated that the statistics had not improved in over a decade, regardless of "so-called therapeutic advances." Most treatment centers reported only their pregnancies, not their birthrates. In fact, one five-year survey of a thousand infertility patients who sought help at the Mayo Clinic, published in 1953, found that physicians were able to diagnose the condition causing the problem in only 60 percent of the cases. The author did not even attempt to give pregnancy rates, either because the clinic did not follow up the patients adequately or because the numbers were not very encouraging.[40]

In the immediate postwar period, Rock himself reported a 15 percent pregnancy rate among his clinic patients and a 25 percent rate in his private practice. By the mid-1950s, just before his retirement from Harvard and subsequent founding of his own nonprofit reproductive center, his success rates for private patients reached about 30 percent, and for the clinic population ranged between 21 and 30 percent. Rock's infertility clinic was one of the oldest in the country, and by looking at the increase in its patient base one can judge the dimensions of the postwar upsurge in both demand for, and supply of, infertility treatment. In the late 1930s and early 1940s, the F&E treated a total of just over 200 patients. Between 1942 and 1946, Rock estimated that the number grew to 500. During the next five years, however, more than 2,000 patients—792 clinic and 1,540 private—strained the resources of the practice.[41]

The evidence suggests that postwar infertility clinics, including Rock's, were nearly as jammed as labor and delivery rooms. Long periods spent in a crowded waiting room were followed by an appearance in what must have seemed like an equally full examining room. Residents and visiting physicians often sat in on both examinations and consultations. As a clinic became more famous, so did the numbers of medical observers. Some women put up with the inconvenience because they had no money and hence no choice, while others were drawn by the renown of the clinic director. Even in the private practices of most well-known infertility specialists, although there was no crush of neophyte and visiting doctors in the examining room, the wait both to schedule an appointment and to see the doctor could be almost as onerous. In fact, one knowledgeable journalist advised his readers—whether monied or not—to grit their teeth and bear the clinic experience in order to get the most up-to-date treatment.[42]

Rock's patient population continued to grow in the early 1950s. In both clinical and private practice, Rock and his assistants had traditionally treated women with a variety of reproductive complaints, not only infertility. Until 1951, about half of the approximately two hundred new patients each year came principally for infertility treatment and the other half for various endocrine disorders, such as failure to menstruate, extremely painful menstruation, or profuse bleeding. From then on, from 70 to 80 percent of the new patients were coming specifically for treatment of infertility, and the numbers steadily rose, to a peak of 224 new infertility patients reached in 1955.[43]

The evidence also suggests that Rock's practice enlarged from the largely working-class clientele that had traditionally formed the bulk of the clinic population. Now it was augmented both by the desperately infertile of all social classes who came to Rock after months or years of unsuccessful treatment and by young couples just starting out, including the wives of medical and graduate students, who were perhaps impecunious, but only temporarily. By the early 1950s, Rock's international reputation, enhanced by the residents and fellows from around the world who returned to their homelands and sent back a stream of letters sharing views, asking advice, and making referrals, brought patients from as far away as Pakistan and several African nations. Correspondence with infertile women and men from hamlets in Appalachia to small towns in Texas and California extended not only his understanding of ways in which couples coped with infertility but his influence as well.[44]

Despite the diversity in Rock's patient population, one thing remained constant: the difficulty in persuading husbands to come in for treatment. Although Rock, like his colleagues, tried every means of involving husbands in the diagnostic and treatment process, he complained often about men's unwillingness to cooperate. A separate clinic for men, begun in 1949 under the direction of Fletcher Colby, seemed to ease the situation somewhat; although no figures exist on the total number of men treated, the extant patient records suggest that treatments for male infertility in Rock's practice increased in the 1950s.[45]

In the clinic, Rock and his assistants treated patients for a small fee or none at all; private office patients either paid the full cost or were billed on a sliding scale. Rock's fees for treatment ranged widely. Some women apparently paid nothing, while a small number paid the prevailing fees. Most fees fell somewhere in between. In 1951, for example, a first visit could run for a paying patient anywhere from $15 to $29, with most patients paying $20. Second and subsequent medical checkups appeared to run around $10 for most. Laboratory tests cost extra: Among the routine steps in an infertility workup, a woman could expect to pay around $10 for a postcoital test, $5 for a vaginal smear, $15 for an endometrial biopsy, and $15 for a Rubin test. These seem to have been the standard fees for the tests for those in a position to pay. Records of individual patients suggest that some women were not billed for the tests. To attend the afternoon clinic sessions and have the basic workup could run as little as $25. If an operation were required, the hospital assumed the cost for those unable to pay. In a few cases, Blue Cross benefits were apparently available. At the Rock Reproductive Center, which Rock established after his mandatory retirement at the age of 65 from Harvard and his directorship of the F&E, all patients paid on a sliding scale based on their income level.[46]

As early as the end of the 1940s, as visits by physicians from around the country and the world increased, and the interest of medical students brought more of them to observe his clinic, Rock had complained that he and his staff were increasingly unable to give the patients the attention they deserved. The reasons were both financial—before the boom years of the 1950s, he usually seemed to have had only one or two staff physicians and a single fellow—and historical. Medical students and interns naturally expected to learn by doing, or at least by closely observing. Medical schools relied on their clinic patients to provide the "learning material." So, when a clinic patient walked into a consulting room, she was likely to sit across the table from anywhere from three to six men—until the mid-1950s there appear to have been no women physicians at the clinic—during a consultation, and the examining room was likely to be equally crowded. There is a telling photograph from an undated news clipping, too poor to reproduce here, which shows a young woman sitting across the desk from six business-suited men. The caption reads, "Dr. Mulligan putting a patient at her ease," but the photograph shows anything but ease.[47]

By the early 1950s, as demand for infertility services soared, some patients began openly protesting the conditions at the clinic; others left. More than half of the new patients, Rock noted in 1953, did not stay around long enough for their evaluation to be completed. They were, he told his hospital board, dissatisfied "with clinic routine." By 1954, the clinic was better funded. With more staff and better facilities, Rock determined to provide clinic patients with as close to the same environment as his private patients received. He banned teaching from examining and consultation rooms, relying instead on full patient records that were presented in seminar fashion after the clinic closed. Apparently, the changes worked. Visits were up the next year, and patients were less likely to drift away. When William Mulligan took over the clinic after Rock retired and opened his own center, he continued to try to "accord the patients care which closely approximated that only obtainable on a private patient basis," with interviews and examinations conducted "in relative privacy" and instruction carried out in the patients' absence.[48]

In altering the clinic routine, Rock was attempting to do for patient relations what he had always done with treatment. His therapies, he noted in his report for 1955, "were applied indiscriminately to private and clinic patients."[49] Infertile patients who could afford the cost of treatment were perfectly willing to pay to serve as experimental subjects. In examining the records of Rock's clinic and private practice, it is impossible to separate out which were the clinic and which were the private patients by the therapies they received. The big difference was that the private patients received more consistent—and more individualized—attention.

In Rock's practice as elsewhere, four kinds of conditions plagued most of the couples who had difficulty conceiving: ovulatory abnormalities; blocked fallopian tubes; a variety of what physicians call cervical factors, including infections and poor mucous quality; and male sperm deficiencies. According to an estimate in the *New England Journal of Medicine*, endocrine dysfunctions, particularly ovulatory disorders, affected about 15 percent of infertility patients, tubal abnormalities about one-third of the women, and a "cervical factor" appeared in 40 percent. Some degree

CAUSES OF INFERTILITY

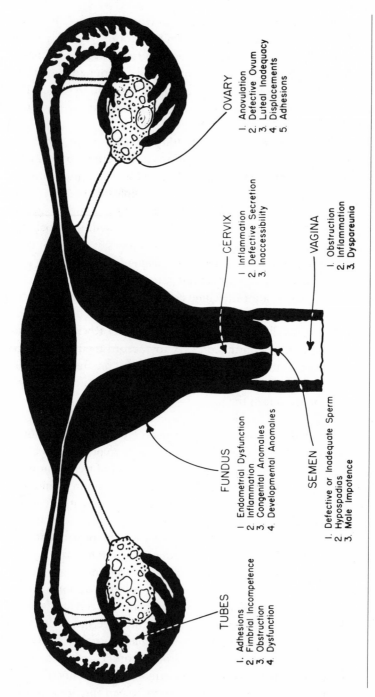

OVARY
1. Anovulation
2. Defective Ovum
3. Luteal Inadequacy
4. Displacements
5. Adhesions

CERVIX
1. Inflammation
2. Defective Secretion
3. Inaccessibility

VAGINA
1. Obstruction
2. Inflammation
3. Dyspareunia

FUNDUS
1. Endometrial Dysfunction
2. Inflammation
3. Congenital Anomalies
4. Developmental Anomalies

SEMEN
1. Defective or Inadequate Sperm
2. Hypospadias
3. Male Impotence

TUBES
1. Adhesions
2. Fimbrial Incompetence
3. Obstruction
4. Dysfunction

This chart depicts the causes of infertility as leading specialists in the immediate postwar period defined them. Courtesy of the Countway Library of Medicine, Harvard University of male responsibility existed in anywhere from 30 to 50 percent of couples.[50]

Ovulatory problems had become easier to diagnose. Rock, along with two of his colleagues, had been among the pioneers in analyzing endometrial biopsies, which enabled them to know whether ovulation had taken place. The therapeutic value of such knowledge in the short run, however, was limited, since ovulatory dysfunctions remained difficult to treat. Some women did not ovulate at all, or only irregularly. By the middle of the 1950s, Rock, in common with many of his colleagues, had become convinced that the animal gonadotropins that had enjoyed such a vogue in the 1930s and 1940s simply did not work, and he appears to have ceased relying on them. But in spite of the skepticism of a number of his colleagues, he prescribed estrogen and progesterone, alone or in combination, both for ovulatory disorders and in cases of unexplained infertility. Other ovarian dysfunctions could result from Stein-Leventhal syndrome (also called polycystic ovarian disease) or other cystic conditions, including those caused by endometriosis. Rock treated ovarian cysts surgically in cases of infertility, but the patients rarely conceived. In one series of fifty-six ovarian resections between 1946 and 1958, only four of the women became pregnant.[51]

Tubal occlusions continued to be a nearly intractable problem. Although one surgeon claimed to have achieved a pregnancy rate of 53 percent among his operations to repair damaged tubes, his numbers evoked considerable skepticism. The published literature by the early 1950s more commonly cited pregnancy rates ranging from about 4 to 13 percent. Some doctors, however, included cases in which only one tube was occluded, claiming success even though the other tube had never posed an obstacle to conception. Others included ectopic pregnancies in their success rates. And even more did not indicate the extent or location of the tubal obstruction in reporting their cases.[52] A number of clinicians argued that tubal insufflation, or the Rubin test, was useful as a therapy. Some gynecologists reported that insufflation alone allowed patients to become pregnant in as many as 18 percent of carefully selected cases. (A "carefully selected" case, in this instance, was one in which the blockage was not total.) Surgery remained the only alternative if neither insufflation nor its radiological partner the hysterosalpingogram restored patency, but according to one authority, "the trial-and-error method is still rampant." Others cautioned surgeons to remind their patients that at best, they could expect a 5 percent chance of conceiving after surgery.[53]

At midcentury most infertility specialists took a cautious approach to all forms of surgery, which with some exceptions had taken a back seat to medical therapies since the 1920s, when endocrinology burst on the infertility scene. More surgery was done on women than men, but even on women, among the most advanced infertility specialists, surgery was never an immediate resort. Rock's expressed views on the usefulness of surgery were somewhat more optimistic than those of some of his colleagues; nevertheless, he reiterated that only after a careful study "of all factors of fertility . . . and assiduous attention toward perfecting them— short of surgery—will a conscientious gynecologist" begin to consider resorting to the operating room.[54]

His actions, while they did not wholly belie his words, nevertheless did demonstrate that he had more faith in surgery than did many of his colleagues, especially those who had come into infertility work from endocrinology. Rock had, after all, trained as a surgeon. Even though surgical treatment of infertility had gone out of fashion in the 1930s and 1940s he never gave up on a belief in its efficacy. He also continued to perform diagnostic laparotomies, in spite of new diagnostic advances that would appear to have made them less necessary. The culdoscope (an instrument that allowed the visualization of the internal reproductive organs through a small, puncture-like incision in the vaginal wall) now made it possible to diagnose intrapelvic disease without resorting to surgery. Rock used the culdoscope, but when it failed, he did not hesitate to operate. He also continued to refine his techniques of tubal surgery, pioneering in the use of new plastics to retain patency after surgery. "For good results in fimbrioplasty," he recommended that the "conventionally everted ends should be covered with a polyethylene hood, which unfortunately requires a second operation for removal about six weeks later."[55]

Tubal surgery was a tempting proposition for both patient and practitioner, simply because it did sometimes work. As one gynecologist remarked, "there is always the patient in a 'hopeless case' who has children." The decision on whether or not to operate, insisted Harvard gynecologist Fred A. Simmons, should be left to the woman. Some women, unfortunately, were unable to give up the idea of motherhood until they had been operated on repeatedly, and surgeons continued to agree because they believed they could beat the odds. But even Rock had an overall success rate in the 1950s of less than 10 percent, and in general successes stood at about half that. Still, it was hard for Rock to deny surgery to someone like the young Mrs. S., eighteen years old when she came to the clinic in 1953 for her infertility. Both of her fallopian tubes were occluded. Her first surgery was unsuccessful, and she returned again

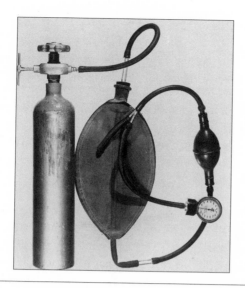

The equipment used for conducting a tubal insufflation, or Rubin test, had changed very little since the development of the test in 1921, as this image from the post–World War II period shows.
Courtesy of the Countway Library of Medicine, Harvard University

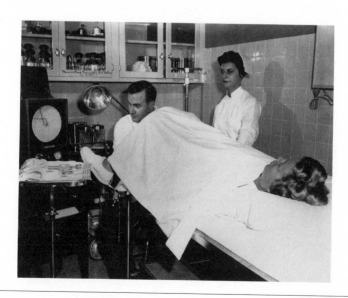

Doctor performing a tubal insufflation in 1956 as a nurse looks on.
Courtesy of the Library of Congress

in 1955. Her youth made the doctors wish to try again. Once again they failed. Another woman who did not give up for eight years also underwent two unsuccessful surgeries. Of the forty-eight women in this series of cases, only four got pregnant.[56]

But if Rock did employ surgery sometimes when there seemed little chance of its working, at least he never succumbed to the newly fashionable idea that a considerable amount of female infertility—some estimates placed it as high as 75 percent—resulted from psychological rather than physiological disorders. Although like most infertility experts he believed that sufficient data existed to suggest a relationship between the ovulation process and emotional stress, he was not prepared to accept the more extreme ideas finding their way into the pages of medical journals. According to one typical account, "A deep-seated conflict between husband and wife, a wish to thwart his desires, [and] unconscious rejection of motherhood" could cause infertility. These views appeared in general interest publications and all too often in the respected journal *Fertility and Sterility;* women could therefore expect to face these attitudes in the doctor's office as well as in the pages of their favorite magazines. Chicago gynecologist W. S. Kroger insisted that some women did not conceive not only because of hostility to their husbands but also because they refused to give up their careers. "We have all seen," he claimed, "a long desired pregnancy follow the renunciation of a career."[57]

No other believers in what was often called psychogenic infertility suggested, as did practitioners Earle Marsh and Albert Vollmer, that women solve their home and career conflicts by continuing their careers. Although Marsh and Vollmer agreed with Kroger that "frequently, sterility is a somatic representation of a conflict in the unconscious," their resolution in one case was to convince the patient that her career desires were perfectly reasonable. Stop feeling so guilty, they told her. If she wanted to spend more time at home, she should work part time and hire more household help rather than give up her job, which was what she thought she should do (having herself read all the advice to that end). Such counsel helped her relax enough, or so they said, to conceive. "As her attitude toward herself changed," they claimed, "her pelvic physiology underwent change," and she subsequently bore two children.[58]

But many prominent practitioners simply dismissed the whole idea that any such relationship existed between "pelvic physiology" and "a conflict in the unconscious." One gynecologist complained about "the plethora of undocumented psychiatric papers currently crowding the clinical data from the pages devoted to problems of reproduction." It hardly matters, he said, whether a woman " 'has a mother complex and really does not want a child'; perhaps she does not, but often her husband has no spermatozoa at all, or too few." Or as another concluded, "In essence, everyone is subject to psychosomatic influences," whether fertile or not.[59] It is impossible to know how many women were treated by physicians who blamed their infertility on a lack of femininity, but such an idea was prevalent enough to cause considerable anxiety. John Rock and his colleagues, however, do not appear to have succumbed to these ideas. Even though the F&E referred patients for psychological counseling, its staff appeared to do so mostly in cases of troubled marriages or situations in which continued infertility resulted in severe stress and anxiety.

Many of the most physiologically inclined practitioners dismissed the notion of emotional hostility as a cause of infertility, but they did have faith in another form of hostility—the "hostile mucous." J. Marion Sims had first promoted the view that cervical secretions could destroy sperm. In the 1950s, a century later, the idea came once again into prominence. Some practitioners prescribed estrogen therapy, others antibiotics. Rock, who had pioneered in some of the new antibiotic treatments of cervical abnormalities, admitted that he had become skeptical of their efficacy. In spite of successes in animal experiments, he said, "we have had but indifferent results with intensive antibiotic treatment, although, like some other over-optimistic frustrates, we have been guilty of ill-considered reports to the contrary." Although antibiotics worked some of the time, he said, as did conization (removal of the core of the cervix), Rock concluded that "a cervical barrier is for us a hard one to crack," resistant even to uterine insemination.[60]

By far the most difficult situation to treat, whether in the 1950s or today, is "unexplained infertility," that troubling a healthy couple, with no discernible impediment to fertility, who do not conceive. It was in such cases that clinicians in the 1920s had prescribed treatments like "thelyglan," a mixture of animal extracts with an aphrodisiac thrown in for good measure. In the 1930s and 1940s, practitioners had often prescribed thyroid extracts, even when a woman had a normally functioning thyroid gland. In the 1950s, Rock had come to rely on progesterone. In these cases and others, he told a group of doctors, "when I am darkly defeated in the presence of a really hypoplastic uterus, as also when I am led to theorize that perhaps the normal trophoblast fails to find easy access to a sparse vascular network, I give, sometimes with an estrogen, such large doses of progesterone as to inhibit ovulation . . . for three or four months, hoping thus to stir the uterus and its lining into more helpful function."

By the mid-1950s, John Rock had acquired "newer progesterone-like steroids," which he claimed were producing "somewhat encouraging" results.[61]

In Rock's practice and elsewhere, infertility treatment for women in the first decade or so of the postwar era relied on a combination of new and old diagnostic techniques and therapeutic agents. The culdoscope, developed by Albert Decker in 1942, was the principal new diagnostic instrument, taking its place alongside the Rubin test and the hysterosalpingogram as a means of diagnosing disease in the pelvis without resorting to laparotomy. Used together, they reduced the need for major diagnostic surgery but did not entirely replace it. In treatment, some recent therapies had fallen by the wayside. Thyroid treatments, except for women with evident thyroid malfunctions, had been largely debunked, although some clinicians were still likely to prescribe them when all else failed. John Rock may have found animal gonadotropins unsatisfactory, but they had not disappeared from all clinical practice.

Prominent new treatments included various estrogenic preparations, used both to promote ovulation and to prevent miscarriages (the use of diethylstilbestrol in pregnancy would turn out to have disastrous consequences), and progesterone. Rock was testing the newly developed progesterone derivatives that would soon be called progestins, but they were very much at an experimental stage. Many gynecologists still treated ovulatory failure with surgical resection. And although insufflation or a hysterosalpingogram might remove a slight obstruction in the fallopian tube, only surgery could repair an occluded one. New refinements in surgical techniques in tubal surgery had yet to result in significantly higher pregnancy rates.

The "Male Factor"

Wives continued to be the ones most likely to seek treatment for infertility, but by the 1950s men were coming in for a considerable share of attention. Motivated in part by a pervasive but undocumented sense that male infertility was on the rise and in part by an equally unverified idea that greater success in treatment was possible, researcher and clinician alike turned their attention to this problem. The idea that male infertility had increased derived from observation of wartime experiences. Soldiers faced exposure to radiation and hazardous chemicals and were subjected to high scrotal temperatures, which practitioners suggested might have af-

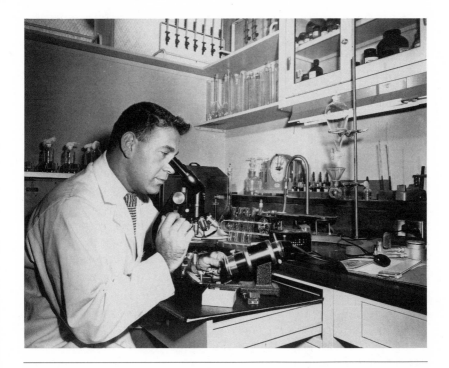

Performing a semen analysis, 1956. By the 1950s, after decades of urging by infertility specialists, semen analysis had finally become a routine part of a diagnostic workup for infertility.
Courtesy of the Library of Congress

fected their sperm production. In addition, new treatments appeared to promise a better outcome for the infertile male. Although these therapies would turn out not to merit the optimism with which they were greeted, for a while it appeared that cures were at hand. A 1949 article in *Better Homes and Gardens* entitled "What Every Husband Should Know about Sterility" suggested that most male infertility could be corrected either by endocrine therapy or by surgery.[62]

Clinicians, however, faced three major difficulties in the 1950s in treating male sterility. First was simply getting men into the examining room. Since the late-nineteenth-century practitioner William Goodell first begged his colleagues "in the name of humanity as well as science" not to operate on women before they had examined their husbands, physicians who specialized in infertility treatment deplored the fact that women often underwent treatment when their husbands were infertile. But the fact was that women were the ones who sought treatment, that most practitioners in the field came from gynecology, and that husbands proved elusive creatures when it came to having their genitals probed or their semen examined. One young wife, after her first visit, alone, to an infertility clinic, admitted that her husband simply refused to be examined himself, although he said he wanted children. "I can't force him," she said. "Rather than risk breaking up our marriage, I'll go without a family." Others told the same story.[63] To get a man to cooperate, physicians appealed to his love for his wife, reminding him that tests for male infertility required much less invasive procedures, that sometimes a semen sample was all that was required. Of course, should that semen sample reveal a low sperm count or other abnormality, further tests ensued. A few men took the initiative, although when a husband rather than his wife called one infertility clinic in the mid-fifties, the staff took that as a signal that the wife might not really want to be a mother.[64]

Second, there was profound disagreement among experts as to what actually constituted male infertility. Everyone agreed that a man with a seminal emission of more than 2.5 cubic centimeters, a sperm count of at least a hundred million sperms per cubic centimeter, with a high proportion of the sperm active and normally shaped, was fertile. And they agreed that a man with no sperms at all was sterile. But in between, disputes abounded. When the American Society for the Study of Sterility had attempted to standardize diagnosis by providing guidelines in the late 1940s that set the fertility standard at sixty million sperms with 60 percent active and 75 percent normally shaped, such definitions met resistance. Some clinicians believed that infertility started at eighty million sperms, others argued for forty, and a few insisted that a man with only twenty million sperms per cubic centimeter, as long as most of them were normal and active, was fertile.[65]

Third, therapeutic disputes abounded. For years, physicians agreed that azoospermia was untreatable, except in rare cases in which sperms were produced but their passage had been blocked. Oligospermia (inadequate sperm count) was a different matter, and many did believe it could be treated. The usual therapies were those advocated in the 1930s: regular rest and exercise; abstention from alcohol, tobacco, and caffeine; a healthy and varied diet; avoidance of "sexual excess"; reduction of stress; decrease in exposure to lead, automobile emissions, and x-rays; and thyroid therapy. When New York physician Abner I. Weisman decided to determine the efficacy of a treatment that combined these measures, however, he found himself stymied. Out of six hundred men that Weisman treated and followed up for two years, only three pregnancies resulted.[66] Soon, physicians would be giving men one benign new recommendation—to switch from jockey to boxer shorts—while also subjecting them at the same time to new experimental therapies using testosterone and gonadotropic extracts from animal sources.[67]

The new testosterone therapies received widespread publicity. Testicular implants gained favor with some practitioners. Others preferred injections of megadoses of testosterone over a period of months. Clinicians believed that testosterone therapy, although absolutely suppressing sperm production at first, would produce a "rebound" effect that could raise sperm counts much beyond pretreatment levels. Urologist Morris Heckel reported surprising success in one series of cases with the latter method, and during the early to mid-1950s testosterone became the rage. Even after the abysmal results of further studies failed to confirm Heckel's results, a few researchers continued to hope that a variation in dosage or technique might turn the tide, in part because the therapy had succeeded in animal experiments.[68]

By the middle of the decade John Rock, discouraged with the results of almost all therapies for men, derided some of his own attempts to increase sperm counts. He had, he told a group of fellow physicians at an informal lecture, tried everything. He had encouraged men to eat large amounts of lettuce, since it was "high in the necessary vitamin E, and rabbits are so prolific." He had put men on diets, since lean dogs in one study were found to be more fertile than fat ones. In a more serious vein, he went on to criticize most of the therapies for male infertility. He had given vitamins and testosterone, in small and large doses, as well as gonadotropins from various sources; he injected thyroid extracts. He also had tried the new steroids, "only to be shocked . . . to find azoöspermia after a few weeks—and worse than that, deplorable loss of all libido and finally of potency. Fortunately, . . . the results were reversible." So far, he said, no matter what treatments appeared to work on animals, they failed when applied to humans. In spite of generations of research on the semen of bulls and boars, stallions and rams, clinicians still knew "pitifully little . . . that is of practical value" in treating men. The most they could hope for, he said, was that "by testicular biopsy, the source, and occasionally a probable cause, . . . of defects may be found, and sometimes a prognosis from our lamentably few and faulty therapeutic methods may be guessed at." In the end, he said, the best thing to do was advise a regimen of hygiene, diet, and "adjusted coital frequency."[69]

Because it seemed so difficult to increase sperm counts, some practitioners, including Rock, turned to new techniques of artificial insemination that were intended to boost the fertilizing power of the limited number available. Using the husband's semen, they centrifuged it, sometimes suspended it in solution, and tried various methods of placement. They finally settled on the method developed in the 1940s by James Whitelaw, which used a cap placed on the external os. In the mid-1950s, Rock and his associates had a success rate of about 8 percent. (Not all of these inseminations were for male infertility, however. Insemination with the husband's sperm also served to bypass a problem cervix.) By the 1960s, Rock's success rate had doubled to about 16 percent. In many cases, husband insemination was the only hope, short of donor insemination, for pregnancy in some cases of inadequate sperm count. "Until means of increasing spermatogenesis are available," Rock noted, "we must make use of what we have."[70]

Given the disappointments with the various nonsurgical therapies for male infertility, some practitioners returned to surgical techniques. As early as the era of World War I, the Dutch researcher Theodore van de Velde and a little later the American Donald Macomber had suggested that varicocele—what the nonmedical person might think of as a varicose vein in the male reproductive organ—was a factor in male infertility. More recently, British infertility experts, who put more faith in surgery than their American counterparts, had reported that surgical treatment of varicoceles sometimes resulted in higher sperm counts. Fred A. Simmons, who urged his colleagues to reconsider their reluctance to perform surgery on men, treated seven men this way in the 1950s and was encouraged by the fact that five pregnancies resulted.[71]

During the latter half of the 1950s, as their faith in each new hormone preparation faltered, infertility specialists appeared to "rediscover" surgery for both men and women. Greater meticulousness and the wider use of antibiotics rather than new advances appeared to account for the very slight rise in pregnancy rates after tubal surgery. Operations on men increased as well, as American specialists adopted some of the ideas of their British counterparts about the role of varicoceles in promoting male infertility. Practitioners seemed to experience greater successes in increasing male sperm counts by surgery than they had by the plethora of hormonal treatments that had been tried and discarded.[72]

Insemination and Adoption

This success, however, was only partial. Sperm inadequacy remained an exceedingly difficult condition to treat in the postwar era. Donor insemination, as long as the wife herself had no fertility problem, found increasing favor among the medical establishment. By the 1950s infertility experts, especially members of the American Society for the Study of Sterility, overwhelmingly endorsed its use in cases of male infertility. Although some physicians still insisted that they and only they had the right to decide which couples should be "accepted" for donor insemination, many infertility specialists now claimed that only a couple could make such a decision. "The attitude of the physician should be permissive and objective," declared Sophia Kleegman in 1954. The couple, as a unit and as separate individuals, she said, possessed "the freedom of decision" and the "responsibility [of] choice."[73]

Because of the private, almost clandestine, way in which donor insemination was still conducted, it is impossible to estimate its impact or to know the characteristics of the couples who sought it. It does appear that demand cut across lines of class and race. Some practitioners claimed that they refused to provide donor inseminations to Catholic patients, suggesting that some level of demand, in spite of church proscription, did exist. Attitudes among African Americans are equally difficult to measure. New York infertility specialist Abner Weisman, whose patient population included a number of African Americans, said in 1950 that in his entire career he had performed only fifteen such procedures for black couples. In 1950, journalist Allan Morrison suggested in *Ebony* that although blacks appeared less likely than whites to take advantage of donor insemination, demand had begun to grow. The fact that the procedure was expensive as well as time consuming, with pregnancy usually taking three to six months of inseminations, served as a deterrent to the less affluent and leisured. Infertility clinics associated with Planned Parenthood made referrals, but most did not perform inseminations themselves; as a result, many low-income couples still had to seek out a private physician and negotiate payments.[74]

Since the 1930s, donor insemination had routinely appeared in news reports and women's magazines, almost always in the context of whether or not physicians and the public would accept it. By 1960, it was clear that many couples and their physicians had rendered a verdict. About fifty thousand children, estimated Milton Golin in the *Medico-Legal Digest,* had already been born of donor insemination. In making the decision to take this route to parenthood, however, doctors and patients were thrust into a legal limbo and an ethical quagmire. Orthodox rabbis as well as the Catholic and Anglican churches opposed its use outright. Mainstream American Protestant denominations, including the Episcopalians, were more equivocal, although in the 1950s none delivered a wholehearted endorsement. Legal guidelines were equivocal. Between 1945 and 1965, there were only five court cases, all divorces, that involved donor insemination. Their rulings created no precedents, but they might have given advocates of the procedure pause. In one case, in spite of the husband's consent, the wife was declared an adulteress. In two others the courts declared the child illegitimate but nevertheless required the husband to pay child support on the grounds that his consent to the procedure implied a promise of support. In not a single state in these years was there a law regulating *or prohibiting* donor insemination. Couples truly were on their own. They had to rely on the doctor to find them a healthy, fertile donor and to keep their confidence. And they had to rely on each other to keep their secret.[75]

To be sure, the moral and ethical questions about donor insemination did not disappear; however, among physicians who treated infertility it was increasingly viewed as a reasonable solution to a sorrowful situation. Although his church condemned it, John Rock had long ago consulted his conscience and found it clear. Patients from his clinic and private practices had received donor insemination since the early 1940s at least. At the Rock Reproductive Center in the late 1950s, he continued to refine insemination techniques and improve the birthrates. In reality, donor insemination allowed couples to evade the infertility of a male partner rather than providing a cure. But physicians who endorsed it and infertile couples alike considered it a medical treatment. Indeed, since the practice involved a series of medical procedures and took place in a doctor's office, such an image was not farfetched. Perhaps somewhat more implausible was the way in which some of the psychoanalytically inclined "experts" insisted that adoption could be viewed as a therapeutic measure.[76]

During the 1950s, there were about 75,000 to 100,000 adoptions in the United States annually. Although national figures do not exist on the proportion of adoptive couples who had experienced infertility problems, the evidence suggests that probably as many as 85 percent chose adoption when they failed to conceive.[77] At least since the 1930s, both popular and medical articles on infertility suggested that more often than not, adopting a child led to pregnancy. In the postwar era, this belief was most often held by those who considered that infertility had psychological causes, from tension and nervousness, or, as the psychoanalytically inclined would have it, unresolved feelings about femininity. Therefore, these actual and armchair psychologists reasoned, adoption, by bringing about parenthood, would alleviate whatever problems it was that the woman suffered.

Psychiatrist William Menninger was so convinced that conception very frequently followed adoption that he insisted that "the occurrence of pregnancy following the adoption or decision to adopt a child are frequent enough to belie the explanation of coincidence for even the most organically minded doctors."[78] Another psychiatrist informed his colleagues of his treatment of an infertile couple who, after five hundred hours of psychoanalysis, "brought out evidence in each member of conflicts dealing with repudiation of femininity and masculinity." Believing that these conflicts would make it impossible to conceive, the couple decided to adopt. Soon afterward the wife became pregnant. The psychiatrist was overjoyed at his cure, but as two of his critics pointed out, the wife had a history of endometriosis, for which she was surgically treated about a year before she finally became pregnant.[79]

The belief that adoption promoted fertility, which had become so pervasive among psychologists, psychiatrists, a number of physicians, and the general public, was powerful because everyone, it seemed, knew of a situation in which it had occurred. Take the case of Sarah Rosen, for example. When her physician husband returned from military service in 1945, she was twenty-three and eager to start a family. After a year of trying, she and her husband saw an infertility specialist. Dr. Rosen, as it happened, had a low sperm count, which he and the specialist both concluded had resulted from the conditions of his wartime service, during which he was exposed to very high temperatures for long periods. Deciding to adopt, the doctor and his wife were easily approved by the adoption agency. Six years later, Dr. Rosen's sperm count having rebounded on its own (his physician, using considerably more restraint than many of his colleagues, had never suggested treatment), his wife conceived. It is stories like that of the Rosens that continue to give credence to the idea that adoption promotes fertility.[80]

But for every such case, couples had stories that demonstrated the opposite. Mary Dixon and her husband, Peter, married in 1941, consulted a gynecologist when they failed to conceive after two years of trying. Mr. Dixon's sperm count, according to the gynecologist, was normal. Mrs. Dixon never received a specific diagnosis, but since physicians knew that pregnancy occasionally followed dilatation and curettage (D&C), Mrs.

Dixon underwent one. She and her husband then spent two years trying to time intercourse to coincide with ovulation. Finding it nerve-wracking and unproductive to tie their sex lives to a calendar, at the urging of her mother—who was very anxious for a grandchild—Mrs. Dixon saw another physician, one of John Rock's associates, in fact. Since he "really didn't suggest anything more than we were doing, . . . I didn't go back."[81]

As the baby boom accelerated, the Dixons felt even more isolated by their childlessness. Not having children, Mrs. Dixon had continued her career, but most of her friends were having children, giving up their jobs, and gearing their social lives around family activities. The Dixons were not excluded from social events, but all the other couples brought their children. "After a while," she said, "[we] almost felt like declining the invitations." They also found themselves under "pressure" from family and friends. In 1947 they adopted their only child, after which, all their friends told them, she would surely get pregnant. She did not.[82]

A few skeptical gynecologists began to question the soundness of the purported link between adoption and pregnancy. John Rock and Frederick Hanson had begun to investigate the subject systematically after World War II. In their first study of two hundred adoptive couples, conducted in 1949, they found that 8 percent subsequently conceived. Citing data from the medical literature that demonstrated a 10 percent rate of "spontaneous cures" that occurred among infertile couples in general, Hanson and Rock concluded that their study could not establish a definitive connection between adoption and subsequent fertility. When they later made a more extensive study of adoptive parents, which employed a control group of nonadoptive infertile couples, the results were clearer: Among the *nonadopting* infertile couples there was a pregnancy rate of 14 percent, while only 5.7 percent of those who had adopted later conceived.[83]

The Advent of Fertility Drugs

If in the face of such evidence clinicians could still consider adoption a form of therapy, skeptics might well wonder whether the confidence many of them expressed, not to mention the faith their patients placed in them, was at all warranted. In fact, practitioners in between the mid-1930s and the mid-1950s had added few effective new therapies to their repertory of treatments for infertility, although they had made technological improvements in such procedures as tubal surgery and artificial insemination.

Such improvements may have been responsible for the rise of overall success rates for infertility treatment from about a quarter to a third of patients. It is also possible, however, that the fact that many women were
seeking treatment within six months of attempting conception may have
played a role. Achieving pregnancy without intervention often takes a
year, and can take longer. It seems likely that at least some of the rise in
pregnancies may not have been the result of treatment at all.

Women could receive a myriad of treatments and still not conceive.
Their husbands could be injected with hormones, told to wear boxer
shorts and avoid environmental toxins, eat a healthy diet, and rest. A
couple could try artificial insemination with the husband's sperm. Perhaps
two-thirds of them, however, would still not conceive. Next to severely
occluded fallopian tubes, ovulatory disorders had proved perhaps the
most intractable. Those who had once been convinced that extracts from
sheep's pituitaries could be made purer and more effective, simply because
they seemed *almost* to work, had been disappointed. What had worked
on rats failed when used on women. Anovulatory women also received
progesterone therapy, but that too worked only under fairly limited conditions. Some women with ovulatory dysfunctions recovered sponta-
neously, but many did not.

Young Grace Fuschetto was a case in point. Married in 1958 at the age
of eighteen, like many young women of her generation Grace planned to
have children immediately. As another woman married at about the same
time remarked, having children seemed to be the main reason to get married.[84] The Fuschettos immediately bought a three-bedroom house and
decorated one bedroom in pink and one in blue, in anticipation of the ad-
ditions to their family. After three months, Grace asked her family physician what was wrong. He told her to have patience. Nine months later she
was back, still not pregnant. She began to avoid her friends, the sight of
whose pregnancies distressed her. Her family kept hinting that she should
try harder, and her husband felt helpless to ease her sadness. The couple
never considered adoption because of objections from his family. For
seven years Mrs. Fuschetto underwent various forms of treatment. In
1965, her doctors put her on an experimental drug being used in clinical
trials, and she conceived.[85] Grace Fuschetto had joined the ranks of a
growing number of women who were able to have babies for the first time.

The drug was Pergonal, a human gonadotropin hormone, and it provided the breakthrough for which clinicians and patients alike had hoped.
In the late 1950s two researchers working separately, one in Sweden and
one in Italy, succeeded in extracting and purifying this hormone, which

initiates the ovulation process. Carl Gemzell, in Sweden, took the pituitaries of women who had died during their reproductive years and developed a technique to create an injectable form of the hormone. Of fifty women he treated between 1957 and 1963, twenty became pregnant, half of them with twins. Ten of the women carried their pregnancies to term.[86] Soon, physicians outside of Sweden were attempting to replicate Gemzell's success. In the United States, C. Lee Buxton at Yale was the first to report that he had done so, and in fact had improved upon Gemzell's technique by following up the human pituitary extract with an injection of chorionic gonadotropin. By 1963 Buxton and his group had treated eleven patients, and although they were very disappointed to report only two pregnancies, they remained optimistic.[87]

Whereas Gemzell's technique required a supply of human pituitaries taken at autopsy, Pietro Domini in Rome found a way to utilize a renewable source, the urine of postmenopausal women. Domini developed a technique to isolate and purify the hormone, as well as a stable source of donors—retired nuns living in Italy and Spain. Soon researchers around the world were testing his drug, which was named Pergonal. In the United States, the first trials were under the direction of Eugenia Rosemberg, in Worcester, Massachusetts. Although John Rock apparently did not test Pergonal, a fellow Boston physician, Janet MacArthur, at Massachusetts General, was among those who did. California infertility specialist Edward Tyler and others began to report pregnancies in the first half of the 1960s. The major side effect of Pergonal was the risk of multiple births, a risk that remains to this day.[88]

While a number of clinicians were testing Pergonal, others were pinning their hopes on a new synthetic preparation—clomiphene citrate, which most Americans recognize by its brand name, Clomid. A group of researchers in Georgia first discovered clomiphene citrate's ovulation-inducing properties in the late 1950s. Beginning in 1960, both the Rock Reproductive Center and the Free Hospital for Women tested Clomid as an infertility remedy, and by 1964 the Brookline clinicians reported a 35 percent pregnancy rate among seventy women who were treated with the drug. The cumulative results of trials in several centers on a total of seventeen hundred women yielded a pregnancy rate of about 20 percent. Although the results were encouraging, doubt about the precise way in which Clomid worked remained. "To date," noted Elliot Rivo in 1965, "the mechanism of action of this drug is still not known."[89]

Before Clomid and Pergonal, women failing to ovulate would have been given, generally to no effect, extracts of animal pituitaries, or had their ovaries resected surgically. (If a woman had true Stein-Leventhal syndrome, surgery might have worked. But Stein-Leventhal syndrome, it appears, had become dramatically overdiagnosed in the 1950s.) Or she would have been told that nothing could be done, which might have been more effective. According to Anna Southam and C. Lee Buxton in a study conducted before the development of Pergonal and Clomid, this last was unquestionably the most effective therapy of the three, since the untreated succeeded in becoming pregnant, they found, more often than the treated in cases of ovulatory failure. With Clomid and Pergonal, for the first time in decades, infertility medicine had made a therapeutic leap, although in 1965 the impact was just beginning to be felt.[90]

During the two decades following World War II, infertile couples in unprecedented numbers sought medical advice for their predicament. Practitioners in turn experimented with a variety of surgical and hormonal therapies. John Rock himself had participated in nearly every therapeutic advance, and a number of therapeutic misadventures, not only of this era but of nearly the entire twentieth century. By the early 1960s, he had helped to usher in a new era in reproductive medicine, with its twin symbols of the birth control pill and technologically assisted reproduction.

The era of the postwar baby boom came to an end around 1965, when the oldest baby boom babies themselves began to reach their reproductive age. Since 1960, fertility had been declining, but until about mid-decade the fundamental fertility pattern set in the late 1940s continued to prevail. After 1965 birth rates would begin to plunge, and larger numbers of couples would choose to be childless. At the same time, dramatic advances would occur in the ability to treat infertility effectively. The next chapter explores the complexities, and the ironies, of therapeutic progress in infertility during a decade of antinatalism.

seven

"The End of the Beginning"?

From Infertility Treatment to Assisted Reproduction, 1965–1981

We're at the end of the beginning—not at the beginning of the end.

Robert Edwards, one of the researchers responsible for the first IVF baby, on the occasion of Louise Brown's birth, 1978

When Linda Anderson sought medical help for an infertility problem in 1967, she recalled her doctor jokingly suggesting that she would be better off childless. Susan Lennon remembered that in the late 1960s and early 1970s, when she and her husband were trying unsuccessfully to conceive, "there was no support for couples with infertility problems." Rachel Wolf, who underwent infertility treatment for three years in the 1970s, said that her inability to conceive made her feel "like a freak." Instead of sympathetic support from her family, she got unwanted interference. Eventually the Wolfs adopted two children; still, after more than fifteen years, "the hurt and bitterness . . . remain with me way back in my mind whenever I see a new mother with a baby." Kathleen O'Donnell, whose doctors were never able to pinpoint the reasons why she and her husband failed to conceive in the 1980s, was a Yale graduate with a thriving professional life who nevertheless found herself "astonished to see that a major part of my self-concept revolved around my ability to reproduce."[1]

These women's experiences, which span the years from the late 1960s to the 1980s, illustrate some new dimensions of the experience of infertility. Attitudes toward the infertile, it appears, were changing, as antinatalist sentiments challenged the pronatalist consensus that had held sway among the postwar generation. Instead of sympathy, in the 1970s couples feeling anguish over their inability to have a baby might be reminded that pregnancy was unattractive or that the world was overpopulated anyway. Such opinions did not, of course, diminish their desires. Nor did the impact of a feminist movement that enabled some women to attend Ivy League colleges and succeed in careers inevitably create a generation of women antithetical to motherhood, despite fears held by advocates of the "traditional" family.

Women and their husbands who faced infertility in the post–baby boom era may have had the same parental longings as the generation that came of age in the 1950s, but the context of their experience differed demographically, culturally, and medically. Demographically, 1965 marked the inception of a new fertility pattern in the United States, one based on later marriages and smaller families. The birthrate slid, then plummeted in the 1970s; even the later rise in birthrates in the 1980s remained considerably lower than the postwar explosion of births. Culturally, the late 1960s witnessed the rise of a youth movement that combined antiwar sentiment with new ideas about what it meant to love, to have sex, and to take on "adult" responsibilities. A new feminist movement defied conventional ideas about gender roles. The challenges to authority and the received wisdom implicit in these movements had direct ramifications for those who experienced infertility, but they also affected those who treated it. Physicians, accustomed to be seen as authority figures, were surprised to find themselves on the defensive, wondering how it had come to be that Dr. Welby had turned into Dr. Frankenstein.

In the middle of the 1960s, as demographers have pointed out, a new pattern of fertility appeared. The oldest members of the baby boom generation were about to turn twenty, an age at which many of their mothers were pregnant with their first child. The new generation, numbering some 63.5 million, was the largest in this nation's history. These young men and women did not intend to replicate their parents' lives. They would marry later than their parents had, and they would have smaller families. The birthrate, standing at 23.7 in 1960, slipped to the depression-era rate of 18.4 in 1970, and to 15.9 in 1980. Nevertheless, in spite of their dilatory slouch to the altar, more than 90 percent of the baby boom daughters did eventually marry, and the overwhelming majority have produced offspring, even if they often waited until their thirties to have their first child. Of the cohort of women born between 1948 and 1952, only 16 percent—including both married and single women—remained childless, a figure far below the historical high of childlessness set for women born in the 1880s.[2]

To say that more than nine-tenths of the baby boom daughters married and that more than 80 percent would bear children—even if we assume that those born later will end up with a higher overall childlessness rate than their older sisters—is not to deny that fundamental changes were taking place, which historians, economists, and demographers have interpreted in various ways. One might even argue that it was the postwar youth who exhibited aberrant behavior in marrying so young and having such large families and that the small families of the late 1960s and 1970s were a continuation of the older pattern.

Such a contention has some merit. After all, the baby boom had been fueled by a prosperity that, although it did not touch every sector of the society, was the most broadly based to date. Skilled blue-collar workers had benefited substantially from an economic growth rate centered in the housing, automobile, and defense industries. The prosperity was as long-lasting as it was broad. From 1947 through 1965, industrial productivity rose at an average annual rate of 3.3 percent a year. But then, just as the children of postwar America were becoming adults, the economy changed. For a number of reasons—the cost of the escalating war in Vietnam, rising inflation, and international competition—the new generation's realities did not meet expectations. By 1970, industrial productivity rates had slipped to 1.5 per cent; during the second half of the decade, growth was a mere .2 per cent annually. Skilled blue-collar jobs became a scarce commodity, as steel mills and other plants closed their doors.[3]

All this was at a time when enormous numbers of young people sought entry into the economy. The largest generation of young adults in American history, many of whose anticipations of their own economic worth had been shaped by postwar abundance, entered a very different economic world from that of their parents. Victor Fuchs had argued as long ago as 1956 that "the direction and change of income," rather than "the absolute level of income," serve as the best predictors of a nation's fertility rate. He later concluded that in the 1970s the failure of the economy "to meet the rising tide of expectations undoubtedly contributed to the increase in the age of marriage and the low fertility rate of that decade." This notion of a change in income relative to expectations, rather than an absolute decline in prosperity, helps to explain why, although fertility rates declined across the entire spectrum of young Americans, the sharpest downward trend emerged among the most highly educated. "After 1960," Susan Householder Van Horn has noted, "economic factors and fertility behavior resumed the strong inverse relationship characteristic of the early decades of the twentieth century."[4]

Recession and inflation were not the only aftereffects of America's post World War II economic high. The divisive war in Vietnam highlighted the costs of cold war prosperity; the sexual revolution, the explosion of a counterculture among the country's more privileged and affluent youth, and the rise of feminism all pointed to a growing unwillingness of the children of postwar affluence to make the same choices as their parents had. Of course, not all young Americans deplored the war in Vietnam, went to Woodstock, or stayed in college until an age at which their parents had owned a house and had already produced two or three children. Nevertheless, Vietnam veterans, unlike the young men who served in World War II, did not invariably rush home to marriage and early parenthood. The young men who opposed the war, with the exception of that small number who had "deferment children" in the conflict's early years, remained single or childless while they stayed in college as long as possible to avoid the draft. Among college women, the feminist movement had by the early 1970s encouraged a reexamination of the wholehearted commitment to childbearing and childrearing that had characterized their mothers' generation.

These changes were accompanied by a generalized cultural shift away from unquestioning pronatalism. By the late 1960s and early 1970s, some environmentalists had begun to attack pronatalist values as one of the causative agents in the deterioration of the world's environment. Although "overpopulation" in the nonindustrialized world had attracted the attention of scientists and demographers since the 1950s, the problem now seemed closer to home. Paul Ehrlich, who would become one of the most powerful voices of American environmentalism, argued that saving the planet required a direct attack on pronatalist views. As historian James Reed has suggested, "The deterioration of the American habitat provided a focus for criticism of the quality of life in a mass society. Social order everywhere suddenly seemed threatened by human fertility."[5]

In 1970, *Look* magazine published an article entitled "Motherhood—
Who Needs It?" with an even more daring subtitle: "A Provocative Report on What May Be History's Biggest Fallacy: The Motherhood Myth."
It would have been inconceivable to imagine such an article appearing a
decade before. Challenging the widely held idea that children made marriages happier, the article suggested that they worsened it. "Often when
the stork flies in, sexuality flies out," *Look* noted. The shattering of the
"motherhood myth," predicted *Look,* would mean that motherhood
would no longer be "compulsory," and therefore, "there will, certainly,
be less of it. . . . It is not a question," the article concluded, "of whether
or not children are sweet and marvelous to have and rear; the question is,
even if that's so, whether or not one wants to pay the price for it. It does-
n't make sense any more to pretend that women need babies, when what
they really need is themselves. If God were still speaking to us in a voice
we could hear, even He would probably say, 'Be fruitful. Don't multiply.'"
By the middle of the decade, survey research conducted by the University
of Michigan's Institute for Social Research suggested that having children
decreased marital happiness, and syndicated advice columnist Ann Landers was stunned by the reaction to her request for her readers' views on
parenthood in which 70 percent of her respondents said that if they could
make their choices again, they would have remained childless.[6]

Some observers claimed that antinatalism resulted from an overwhelming sense of futility about the future prospects of human survival.
Psychiatrist Nathan Ackerman believed that the young had succumbed to
a "a doomsday attitude." Perhaps. But as one young husband told
Newsweek reporter Martin Kasindorf, "I don't know any happy young
parents." According to his wife, "What turned me off about children was
moving in young married circles and seeing what a drag it is."[7] The National Association of NonParents (NON), founded in 1972, provided an
institutional base for antinatalism. NON's organizers committed themselves to advocating childlessness "as a way of creating 'social space.'
That means 'a combination of time, money, and energy' that can be used
to conserve planetary resources, beat the high cost of living and free husbands and wives for political activism and the pursuit of free life-styles."
For an organization that started out with only two hundred members and
reached its peak in 1976 with two thousand members before it faltered
and ultimately collapsed in the early 1980s, NON received an extraordinary amount of publicity. In the 1970s *Time* and *Newsweek* covered its
events and meetings, and its membership lists provided the case-study material and interview subjects for the numerous popular and scholarly ar-

ticles on voluntary childlessness in the 1970s. That such a relatively small organization could garner so much national publicity (a great deal of it uncritical) suggests that in spite of the insistence of NON cofounders Ellen and William Peck that "pronatalist pressure [was] everywhere," in fact at least some of the pressure appears to have been coming from the opposite direction.[8]

Aggressive antinatalism among the "childfree," a growing belief in the existence of a worldwide population crisis, and the heady confidence among young women that birth control pills would enable them to delay childbearing as long as they desired made voluntary childlessness a "respectable" choice for larger numbers of young Americans. On the whole, such changes marked a step forward for tolerance. The pronatalist consensus had been both dogmatic and oppressive, castigating those who chose not to procreate as selfish neurotics and unreasonably extolling the joys of parenthood. Now, the strong challenge to the consensus helped to empower the voluntarily childless.[9]

It had a different impact, however, on the infertile. About three million couples acknowledged an infertility problem in 1965, or about 11 percent of all married couples. About a half-million of these were childless, or afflicted with primary infertility; the other 2.5 million couples had at least one child but were unable to conceive again. Such couples often came to believe that both the medical profession and society in general had become indifferent to their pain. In the 1950s and early 1960s, a couple having difficulty conceiving could at least be confident that their friends and family would be hoping for the same outcome as they did, since having children was considered almost essential for a happy marriage. By the 1970s, such a couple might be told they were lucky, and be deprived not only of a much-desired pregnancy but also of compassionate understanding.[10]

Even popular articles devoted to infertility problems in the 1970s bore the stamp of the new consciousness, as writers struggled to justify their desire to provide couples with information on how to *have* babies when allegedly the real social need was for population control. One typical article in *McCall's* began by reminding readers that "the exploding population" was the world's primary health crisis; only after underscoring everyone's responsibility to control family size did the author suggest the acceptability of assisting the infertile to conceive. "We are now living in a contraceptive culture," claimed the famed sex research team of Masters and Johnson. Only a few articles suggested that in such a culture the infertile might feel as disenfranchised as had the voluntarily childless in the previous generation. "In this era of birth control, the Pill and the Population Explosion, [the infertile are] too often forgotten or simply dismissed as unimportant," one writer in *Good Housekeeping* perceptively noted. The focus on birth control affected physicians as well, claimed Albert Decker, the infertility specialist who had invented the culdoscope; more and more, doctors had come "to believe that they have no real obligation to cope with infertility." Another physician similarly urged his colleagues to consider the needs of the infertile. "These couples should not be denied the right to have children simply because others have too many."[11]

Infertile couples expressed disappointment that not only did their problems seem of little concern to society but also their friends showed little understanding. One woman complained that a friend of hers, "who has three children herself," upon hearing about the woman's sadness over an infertility problem, "told me that the world was overpopulated anyway." A childless husband whose wife suffered from an ovulatory disorder that failed to respond to treatment seethed when a friend of his, the father of four, remarked that "he wished he had our problem." Indeed, if the infertile women who wrote us of their experiences are at all representative, those suffering from an infertility problem in the late 1960s through the late 1970s seemed more isolated and less supported than had most of those who faced the same problem in the baby boom years. As chapters of the infertility support group RESOLVE, founded in Massachusetts in 1973, began to proliferate toward the end of the decade, that situation changed for some couples. For others, however, RESOLVE did not provide an antidote.[12]

If it would be unfair to stereotype the voluntarily childless as either career-obsessed feminists or irresponsible young hedonists, it would be equally unfair to stereotype those who attempted to conquer their infertility as desperate housewives who believed that motherhood alone legitimized their existence, or as overbearing men determined to leave behind some genetic evidence of their existence. There was no necessary antipathy between feminism and motherhood, regardless of the media images. Susan Viguers, author of a poignant memoir of her experience with infertility and adoption in the 1970s, was certainly a modern woman—a writer and university professor married to a playwright and editor. Children had always been a part of her plan for life; in a very contemporary twist to an old story, she and her husband-to-be even began trying to conceive about a year before they married. Many of her friends had children, and Viguers contended that her infertility, which resulted from an ovulatory problem, made her feel more than "empty" and "defeminized"; it "came to symbolize being uncreative in general."[13]

One thing had not changed: women still more often initiated treatment for infertility, and in many cases, even if it turned out that the husband had the infertility problem, women nevertheless took on the principal responsibility for it. Some women apparently went so far as to lie by claiming a defect in themselves, rather than let their husbands know their sperm counts were too low. At least some doctors apparently encouraged them to do so. As one psychologist claimed, a husband's knowledge of his sterility would certainly "strike at the heart of his self-esteem" and might "even make [him] impotent." Very few infertile men have left their own accounts of their feelings. In fact, of all the personal accounts, memoirs, and articles that we have seen on the subject up through this period, only one man wrote of his own experience for publication. Discovering that he was azoospermic, this young man felt "stab[bed] to the core. . . . At first, I was so wrecked emotionally that I couldn't think of anything except the fact that fate, cruel destiny or God (I didn't give a damn which) had singled *me* out, had deprived *me* of what . . . I wanted most in life: children." Eventually, this man and his wife chose to have a child by donor insemination, a choice that thousands of couples made annually. This essay, however, was unique.[14]

Among the respondents to our own small survey, only two husbands were responsible for the couple's infertility. Both husbands had low sperm counts, both experienced rebounds without medical treatment, and both couples succeeded in having children. A few of the couples surveyed experienced "unexplained" infertility, but in most instances blocked fallopian tubes or an ovulatory disorder caused the difficulty. Several of these women found their husbands curiously remote, as if their wives' intense desire for children were not entirely comprehensible. A number of men, even among those who actively wanted to be parents, appear not to have given the matter much thought until their wives brought it to their attention. Susan Viguers's husband, Ken Arnold, was a case in point. Married previously to a woman who had expressed the wish to remain childless, he had been on the verge of having a vasectomy when the marriage dissolved. Although he supported his second wife's desire for a child and acknowledged his own wish to be a father, he still had difficulty comprehending her anguish. "In spite of my best efforts," he admitted, "I couldn't identify with her ups and downs. I didn't quite understand the sensation she had of being tied to an unknown, uncooperative body."[15]

Because women in the 1970s were delaying childbearing later than their mothers and grandmothers had, the issue of age became important for the first time. Two issues dominated the discussion: whether older couples could adjust to the demands of parenthood, and whether or not their babies would be healthy. Couples themselves appeared to be deciding the first question in the affirmative. In 1974, for example, the National Bureau of Health Statistics reported a 12.5 percent increase in the number of women over the age of thirty who, during the past twelve months, had had their first children. On the second, the development of amniocentesis, coupled with the option of legal abortion, allowed a woman whose fetus exhibited abnormalities to end her pregnancy. Amniocentesis became widely available in the mid-1970s. By 1976 more than 140 medical centers offered the procedure, which enabled physicians to detect chromosomal abnormalities by analyzing amniotic fluid. At that time, its principal use was for the detection of Down's syndrome, which disproportionately appears in the children of mothers over thirty-five. If the problem were discovered, a woman could choose to terminate the pregnancy. The ability to terminate such a pregnancy made the decision to conceive at a later age somewhat easier. In fact, beginning in the 1970s and continuing to the early 1990s, women in their thirties have been the only group to show significant and consistent increases in childbearing.[16]

But if amniocentesis, coupled with the possibility of abortion, allowed some couples to enter pregnancy with a greater degree of choice over the outcome, the very notion of controlling a pregnancy in this manner appalled others. During the 1970s, infertile couples were no longer simply people trying to conceive. They became one symbol of the cultural battle over the meaning of family life that had begun to rage in the United States in that decade and that continues today. The struggle over abortion rights stood at the center of the controversy, but underlying that struggle were larger questions: who had the right to control a pregnancy? What was a family? Was there a morally correct way to achieve pregnancy? Among sexual conservatives, there was a growing sense that some of the new technologies being promoted as aids to the infertile were in fact attacks on the traditional family itself. However, although the challenge to reproductive research originated as part of the antiabortion, antifeminist movement, one wing of the feminist movement developed its own critique of reproductive technology, stating that it was a tool in the hands of a male power structure designed to subordinate women to the ends of a false technological imperative.[17]

The implications of new reproductive technologies—especially in anticipation of the impending success of in vitro fertilization—sparked a fierce debate over the relationship between science and morality. According to a 1969 *Life* magazine article, "Startling advances in the science of reproductive biology" were about to "bring about a sweeping transformation in the style of man's life on earth." The author, the magazine's science editor, Albert Rosenfeld, confirmed the fears of the baby boom generation's parents that a sexual revolution was already taking place, and that new reproductive technologies would only accelerate the changes. The rootlessness and restlessness characteristic of the rebellious young, so different from their rooted and stable elders, would only accelerate. "In vitro" babies, according to the article, conceived in anonymity, "raised by a state nursery, . . . might never know [their] genetic parents, nor . . . have any brothers and sisters." Both fascinated and repelled by such a chilling notion, Rosenfeld asked if society could ever devise "adequate substitutes" for the conventional family. "Could the trans-human of post-civilization survive without love as we have known it in the institutions of marriage and the family? If each of us is 'forever a stranger and alone' here and now, then how much more strange, how much more alone, would one feel in a world where we belong to no one, and no one belongs to us?"[18]

Perhaps more interesting than the article itself, which in many ways simply rehashed the premises of *Brave New World,* was the Harris Poll that accompanied it, in which respondents clearly invested the new reproductive technologies with social and cultural meanings. "We should not mess around with the laws of nature," said one man. "Family life is already deteriorating now. We need stabilizing, not the emancipation of women." Another envisioned "sperm drive[s] every year to replenish the supply. Spermobiles would be around like bloodmobiles. Support your local sperm bank!" The majority of respondents, while they approved of the use of hormone treatments to promote ovulation and of artificial insemination using the husband's sperm, disapproved of any reproductive technology that did not overtly and obviously serve to abet conventional family formation.[19]

Their anxieties were not entirely misplaced. Feminist radical Shulamith Firestone, for example, in her now-classic work, *The Dialectic of Sex,* eagerly anticipated the day when babies would be not only conceived in vitro but nurtured in an artificial placenta. Technology, she chided her Luddite comrades, was only as bad as the uses to which it was put. If it challenged the traditional family, liberated women from pregnancy ("Pregnancy is barbaric," she said) and childbirth, then it was an undoubted good. "Natural childbirth is only one more part of the reactionary hippie-Rousseauean Return-to-Nature, and just as self-conscious," she insisted. "Perhaps a mystification of childbirth . . . may make a woman feel less alone during her ordeal. But the fact remains: childbirth is at best necessary and tolerable. It is not fun." The full implications of in vitro fertilization, carried to its logical conclusion, in vitro birth, Firestone predicted, would mean that "the reproduction of the species by one sex for the benefit of both would be replaced by (at least the option of) artificial reproduction: children would be born to both sexes equally, or independently of either, however one chooses to look at it. . . . The tyranny of the biological family would be broken."[20]

The *Life* article had illustrated that Americans were developing a more critical attitude toward science and technology. The cold war–era consensus that defined nearly all scientific developments as invariably positive and progressive was coming to an end; henceforth, scientific researchers would no longer enjoy immunity from cultural challenges to the moral and ethical validity of their findings and applications. And Shulamith Firestone's defense of reproductive technology notwithstanding, some of the most aggressive challenges to medical science came from the left. As Paul Starr has argued, the 1970s witnessed a new "health rights movement" that "challenged the distribution of power and expertise" between doctor and patient. The feminist attempt to "demedicalize" childbirth was only the most obvious example of a pervasive distrust of the methods as well as the motives of the medical specialists who treated women. Indeed, Starr views the feminist challenge to medicine as a significant part of "a broader revival of a therapeutic counterculture with political overtones," in which "the content of medical practice was imbued with political meaning."[21] Infertile couples were caught in a crossfire, beset both by changes in social attitudes and by an increasing divergence of views among scientists and physicians themselves. Confidence was giving way to skepticism, as questions arose within and outside the medical community over the efficacy of existing therapies and the desirability of pursuing more controversial areas of reproductive technology.

Conflicts arose early in the decade over the safety and effectiveness of the new fertility drugs. Safety questions were raised by the disclosure in 1971 that a synthetic estrogen compound, diethylstilbestrol (DES), used widely in the 1950s to prevent miscarriage, had serious long-term effects. Daughters of women who took the drug faced a very high risk of developing what had until then been an extremely rare form of vaginal cancer. In addition, as many as 75 to 85 percent of the daughters were found to have abnormalities of the uterus, and as many as 90 percent developed a cervical disorder called adenosis. The fact that some groups within the medical profession, especially the American Medical Association, attempted initially to downplay the findings simply encouraged greater public mistrust of doctors.[22]

Aids to Ovulation

The shocking revelations about DES may have been one of the factors that slowed the federal government's approval of Pergonal for several years and caused some to question the easy approval of Clomid. Four years earlier, Clomid had had its official debut, after years of testing, with a well-orchestrated advertising campaign that appeared to promise that nearly every woman with an ovarian dysfunction who took the drug would wind up pregnant. One skeptical physician, however, analyzed twenty-eight of the studies on which the manufacturer of the drug based its claims and found that the Clomid trials had included women with a very wide range of ovulatory problems, including numerous women who ovulated on their own, although not consistently. Such a fact was important in assessing the efficacy of Clomid because the research also suggested that 40 percent of women who ovulated irregularly could expect to conceive on their own. Even by including such women, claimed Massachusetts gynecologist Walter W. Williams, only 17.5 percent of the 6,714 women in the twenty-eight studies subsequently bore a living child.[23]

Such criticism notwithstanding, Clomid was effective in inducing ovulation in about 30 percent of those anovulatory women who were producing naturally some level of both estrogen and follicle-stimulating hormone. What these women needed, and what Clomid seemed to induce, was the essential surge of luteinizing hormone that normally occurs at midcycle and triggers ovulation. In spite of the skepticism of some practitioners, therefore, or their own misgivings, many women with ovulatory disorders looked to Clomid as their only hope. By the middle of the 1970s, some 20 percent of anovulatory women who took Clomid became pregnant. The vast majority would never have conceived naturally.[24]

Pergonal, although developed before Clomid, did not earn approval for general distribution until a decade after Clomid. In part, its manufacturers wished to move more slowly, because Pergonal was a more powerful drug with more severe side effects. Unlike Clomid, it was able to induce ovulation even in women whose hypothalamus appeared to be producing no gonadotropins naturally. One grave problem, however, as physicians conducting the clinical trials found, was how to determine an effective dosage. Susceptibility to the drug varied from woman to woman. Too high a dose often resulted in multiple births. The attempt to control these effects had kept Pergonal in clinical trials for a decade when a New Jersey woman gave birth to quintuplets in February of 1970 after having been treated with the drug. It was Margaret Kienast's third Pergonal pregnancy—the first two had resulted in single births—and a team of seventeen physicians attended her delivery.[25]

The national publicity encouraged infertile women to clamor for access to the drug, despite the questions being raised in the press about its safety. Within weeks, fertility clinics all over the country were swamped with inquiries. Edward Tyler, one of the pioneers of Pergonal therapy, had already prescribed it for three hundred or so patients who either were failing to ovulate or whose infertility was unexplained. Nevertheless, he counseled caution. "Pergonal may help [anovulatory women] ovulate," he said, "but it won't necessarily make them pregnant." Eugenia Rosemberg, one of the first physicians to test Pergonal, had treated only thirteen women with the drug, of whom three conceived; two of them carried single pregnancies to term, while the third miscarried. Cutter Laboratories, which would soon be seeking FDA approval for Pergonal, decried what it called "premature publicity" and would only say that the drug appeared "promising." But women refused to be put off. By March of 1970, only one month after the birth of the Kienast quints, the clinics testing Pergonal were telling everyone that they were "booked solid." In Los Angeles, noted Edward Tyler, "we don't have a vial in the house."[26]

Clomid and Pergonal did not work for everyone, but they offered the only hope of pregnancy for anovulatory women. In the late 1970s, Harvard's Robert Kistner estimated that 70 percent of women treated with Clomid for secondary amenorrhea would ovulate, and 40 percent of them would become pregnant. Pergonal often succeeded where Clomid failed. These two drugs, used sometimes separately and sometimes sequentially, must be seen as a major therapeutic advance in infertility treatment. Although there was some controversy over their safety, for the most part practitioners, infertile couples, and the American public viewed such therapies as encouraging manifestations of the new reproductive medicine.[27]

Male Infertility

But if ovulation therapies provided treatment for one of the principal causes of infertility, other problems still lacked solutions. Male infertility, in particular, remained intractable. Some feminists contended that the failure to address male infertility stemmed from the fact that infertility specialists, most of them men, were willing to experiment on women but not on men. It is easy to see why they would think so. After all, women continued to be the ones who sought treatment for an infertility problem, and they usually sought it from a gynecologist.

The reluctance of husbands to submit to examination; the continued association in men's minds between their masculinity and fertility; and the extreme lengths to which some wives and their doctors would go to protect men from the reality of their responsibility all attest to the fact that women bore a disproportionate burden. But to recognize that burden is different from suggesting that infertility researchers ignored male reproductive inadequacies. In fact, specialists since at least the 1930s had attempted a host of solutions to the problem of male oligospermia, but with little success. During the 1950s, in fact, a number of prominent clinical researchers took at least as great an interest in male as in female infertility. And in 1969, after the development of Pergonal and Clomid appeared at last to point the way to a solution to female ovulatory dysfunction, John Rock announced that he intended to concentrate his attention on the next reproductive challenge, "the oligospermic male." By then, however, Rock was eighty years old, realistically stating, "how much more I can do with it I do not know." Neither Rock nor anyone else was able to come up with any new solutions. As Edward Tyler noted in 1971, "the treatment of male infertility is practically nil. Nothing so far has worked."[28]

Men with sperm inadequacy usually received the same advice in the 1970s that they had in the 1950s—lose weight or gain weight, eat healthfully, wear boxer shorts, and treat any "constitutional diseases." In addition, however, by the 1970s two recent techniques now enabled some persistently oligospermic men to produce biological offspring. First, surgical treatment for varicocele, to which American physicians turned in growing numbers from the late 1950s onward, seemed increasingly successful. By the 1970s, the sperm counts of about one-third of patients who underwent the surgery showed considerable improvement.[29] Second, new methods of artificial insemination using the husband's sperm enhanced the chances for pregnancy. Since the 1950s, clinicians had attempted to separate the more active and vigorous sperm from the malformed or slug-

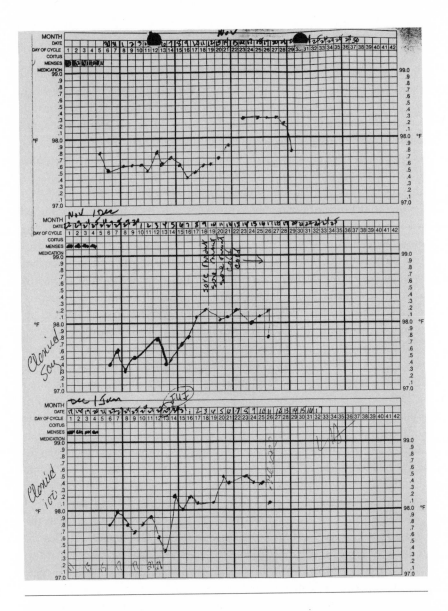

Basal body temperature charts. Beginning in the 1930s, infertility specialists had patients take their temperatures and plot them on a chart. The approximate time of ovulation can be determined by daily measurement of a woman's temperature throughout an entire cycle. After the development of the ovulation-inducing drugs Clomid and Pergonal, these charts helped to determine the result of such therapy.

Used with patient's permission

Follicular development scan. Today, women taking medications such as Clomid and Pergonal are often monitored with ultrasound. Both ovaries are measured for size and the number of follicles—where the ova reside—is recorded in each.
Used with patient's permission

```
                        SEMEN ANALYSIS

Date_____

Patient's Name                        _____ Wife's Name_____

Doctor_                          ___

Sterile Container:   Yes__XX__ No_____

Volume_____3.2_____

Viscosity____1_____

Sperm Concentration____70 million/cc___

% Motile_____50%_____

Progression____2.5_____

Debris_____yes_____

Agglutination_____moderate_____

Morphological Forms (%)___30% abnormal forms___

Progression:  0- non-motile, non-moving

              1- moving in place

              2- sluggish forward motion

              3- progressive forward motion

              4- vigorous forward motion

Viscosity:   0- watery, thin

             1- fluid

             2- viscous, gelatinous

Post-wash

Concentration_____

Volume_____

% Motile_____

Progression_____

% Normal Morphology_____

Agglutination_____
```

Semen analysis chart. This husband was fertile.
Used with patient's permission

gish ones in cases of oligospermia. Cryopreservation of sperm, developed in the 1950s and perfected by the 1970s, enabled them to take this process one step further; it became possible to cull out the most "promising" sperm from several ejaculates and use this augmented sample for insemination. In addition to cryopreservation, clinicians had also developed newer techniques of intrauterine insemination, which would more successfully treat cases in which cervical secretions inhibited the passage of the sperm into the uterus.[30]

By the end of the 1960s, artificial insemination using the husband's sperm no longer seemed immoral to many Americans. A poll taken in 1969 revealed that 62 percent of women and 49 percent of men accepted as ethical and reasonable the use of what was generally called A.I.H. (for artificial insemination, husband). The Catholic Church continued to disapprove of the practice, but most other religious denominations determined that couples themselves ought to make their own decision in this matter. Donor insemination, however, remained controversial. When surveyed about their views on using donor sperm in the case of a husband's sterility, fully two-thirds of the male respondents and 63 percent of the women rejected the idea under any circumstance. By 1978, when *Parents* magazine conducted a similar poll, A.I.H. had become so acceptable that the pollsters did not even ask about it. But Americans remained ambivalent about donor insemination. Although nearly half of the respondents believed that when a husband was sterile a couple should have the opportunity to choose such an option, 78 percent maintained that they would never consider it themselves. Fully 88 percent of respondents who had themselves faced an infertility problem in their marriage claimed that they had never considered donor insemination.[31]

Members of the medical profession as well as the public disagreed over the appropriateness of donor insemination. At one extreme stood practitioners who disapproved of the procedure entirely. Their numbers may have been substantial, given that nearly 20 percent of the members of the American Fertility Society could be numbered in that group. At the other extreme were the wholehearted advocates, including nearly 10 percent of the members of the Society who performed the procedure for single women and lesbian couples as well as for married couples with infertility problems. In between appear to have been the majority of infertility practitioners, who sometimes had reservations about the effect of donor insemination on the marriage and the father's relationship with the child, but who believed that in the end, the couple must make its own decision.[32]

Shrouded in secrecy and distrusted by a majority of Americans, donor insemination also earned the censure of some moralists and theologians. Jesuit scholar Francis Filas, for example, insisted that "the sperm bank is the scientist gone mad and the scientist gone mad plays God. . . . donor insemination . . . will take away human dignity and privacy and put the doctor/scientist in the place of God." Physician Edward Tyler rejoined, "If you wish to use that term, then the doctor 'plays God' in almost anything he does. So far as I'm concerned, [donor insemination] is just another phase of medical practice."[33] The evidence suggests that Tyler would have the last word.

Most couples who chose this route to parenthood in the 1970s, like their counterparts in earlier decades, kept their decision private; as a result, it remained impossible to state definitively how many couples employed it. But compelling indirect evidence exists. For example, during this decade several states passed legislation legitimizing offspring conceived through donor insemination; many more would follow in the 1980s. Court decisions affirming the parenthood of the social rather than the biological father also served to give the procedure greater legitimacy. More and more physicians performed donor inseminations, and sperm banks proliferated. By the end of the decade, estimates of the numbers of children born in the United States through donor insemination ranged from 250,000 to 350,000.[34]

Couples who utilized donor insemination and the overwhelming majority of physicians who performed it agreed that such a choice should remain a secret decision within the marriage. "Without exception," said one group of physicians surveyed about the practice, patients "don't want to recall the experience." According to another prominent practitioner, "Not even the grandparents should know." A few physicians disagreed, suggesting that such secrecy made it impossible to know whether the procedure lived up to expectations: that is, were the couples happy with the result? Infertility specialist Herbert Horne felt troubled enough by the lack of information about the social dimensions of donor insemination that he limited his practice of it to couples in which the husband was azoospermic; the more ambiguous condition of oligospermia, he believed, could cause the husband to have doubts about his paternity. In addition, he suggested that parents consider telling the children about their origins. A group of his colleagues disagreed wholeheartedly, reminding Horne that "the family is not a mere biologic relation" but one of "deep emotional involvement between parents and children regardless of the circumstances of conception." The children, these clinicians concluded, "need not be informed" of the way in which they were conceived.[35]

Proponents of donor insemination made several related arguments in its favor: It enabled a couple to have a child with a biological relationship to one of the parents; it offered more privacy than adoption; it allowed the wife to experience pregnancy and childbirth. In short, it provided some childless couples their best hope of becoming parents. Some couples believed that it would be impossible for them to adopt; others insisted that "they could love a baby from the wife's body more than one they might adopt."[36]

Male infertility continued to defy solution throughout the 1970s, in spite of continued attempts both to diagnose and to treat it. Donor insemination allowed the fertile wife of an infertile husband to conceive, but it did not, of course, cure his infertility. In cases of female or joint infertility, when treatment failed, adoption remained the only way to achieve parenthood. Many couples pursued that option, adopting children from Korea or Latin America when the shortage of infants eligible for adoption in the United States became acute. Those who could afford it paid thousands of dollars to adopt so-called gray market babies in private transactions. But adoption, like donor insemination, evaded infertility; it did not "cure" it. Infertile couples continued to hope for technological miracles. In the 1970s, one seemed imminent.

In Vitro Fertilization

When John Rock and Miriam Menkin announced in 1944 that they had achieved in vitro fertilization, near-universal acclaim followed the news. The two researchers and an enthusiastic public believed that these first steps toward creating human life outside a woman's body advanced human knowledge and brought motherhood one step closer for women with blocked or absent fallopian tubes. Menkin, who witnessed the fertilizations, expressed a sense of awe and privilege. Rock, when questioned some twenty years later about his own attitudes, declared that he had discussed the idea with a Catholic theologian beforehand and proceeded with an absolutely clear conscience. Rock received only a few letters critical of his experiments and little negative press for this work. Indeed, during his long career, only his advocacy of the birth control pill caused controversy and criticism.[37]

The initial public excitement over in vitro fertilization seemed to have worn off by the 1950s, when neither Rock and Menkin nor Landrum Shettles of Columbia–Presbyterian Hospital, who became the most visible researcher in the field in the 1950s, appeared to make any significant progress. For about a decade, as animal experimentation continued and researchers worked with little fanfare, in vitro fertilization made few headlines. The situation changed in 1963, when an Italian researcher announced that he and a small research team had succeeded in culturing an embryo for twenty-nine days. A storm of criticism from the Vatican greeted the announcement. Calling the experiment "sacrilegious," *L'Osservatore Romano,* the official Vatican newspaper, editorialized, "God surrounded the act of creation of a human being with the most supreme assistance of love, nature, and conscience. . . . It would be monstrous to violate these conditions." Dr. Petrucci responded immediately that "he did not believe he had done anything immoral as a Catholic" and vowed to continue the experiments, but in fact he did not; whether he was forbidden to do so or made the choice himself is unclear.[38]

Although Landrum Shettles continued his research in New York, outside the laboratories in vitro fertilization once again faded from public view after this brief flurry of attention. In 1969, however, British embryologist Robert Edwards and his gynecologist collaborator Patrick Steptoe published an account of human in vitro fertilization that left little doubt of their plans to carry their research to the point of pregnancy and birth. Controversy immediately swirled around them. At first, some physicians refused to believe that they had actually succeeded, insisting that until a healthy baby emerged out of such experiments, skepticism should remain the order of the day. But because Steptoe and Edwards had carefully documented on film every step of the procedure, most experts were prepared to acknowledge their achievement.[39]

The controversy owed more to a changing culture than to a changing science. In the late 1940s, Americans were still reveling in their wartime technological feats; advances in science and technology, they believed, could only make their lives even better. Then, too, pronatalism amounted to a national religion, and the public was disposed to view any new development that would enable the infertile to conceive as a social good. By the end of the 1960s, however, mistrust of science, medicine, and technology had become more prevalent. Some Americans, pointing to nuclear weaponry, industrial pollutants, and deterioration of the environment, had become antitechnological. Others, many of them moral conservatives, while they certainly favored enabling the infertile to conceive, feared that in vitro fertilization, like abortion, provided one more piece of evidence of declining morality. As if to reinforce that last idea, some radical feminists hailed in vitro fertilization as one step toward women's ultimate liberation from their biology.

Some opponents of in vitro fertilization in the 1970s clearly viewed it as an attack on the traditional family. Physician and ethicist Leon Kass asserted that in vitro fertilization brought human beings one step closer to destroying the biological nature of the family unit. Once perfected, he presciently noted, in vitro technology could not be limited to assisting infertile married couples to bear their own biological child but would be broadened to include egg and embryo donation, as well as the recruiting of gestational mothers. Kass deplored such uses of reproductive technology as detrimental to "the virtues of family, lineage, and heterosexuality." It would also, he believed, weaken "the taboos against adultery and even incest." Books such as Firestone's *Dialectic of Sex,* which heralded the coming of the new reproductive technologies for the same reason that Kass deplored them, could only contribute fuel to what was quickly becoming a conflagration.[40]

Feminist resistance to the new reproductive technologies would not fully emerge until the 1980s. In the 1970s, most opposition stemmed from conservative and/or antifeminist views. The American Medical Association called for a moratorium on research into human IVF in 1972. Not surprisingly, the specialists who constituted the leadership of the American Fertility Society disagreed. The current president of that organization, in fact, was the distinguished reproductive endocrinologist Georgeanna Jones, of Johns Hopkins University. Like most of her fellow infertility specialists, she welcomed such experimentation.[41] While the American Medical Association urged caution and published the views of Leon Kass on in vitro fertilization, participants in a symposium featured in the *Journal of Reproductive Medicine* took a very different point of view. Although one clinician argued for a longer period of animal research before attempting to achieve a human pregnancy, no one expressed opposition to in vitro fertilization on moral grounds. Ethicist Joseph Fletcher's contribution took direct issue with those who inveighed against the morality of a pregnancy begun in vitro. A longtime advocate of donor insemination, Fletcher could have been expected to weigh in on the side of new reproductive technology.[42]

Of course, one might argue that fertility specialists simply had a vested interest in new techniques. As the baby boom collapsed, without a corresponding decrease in the numbers of ob/gyn specialists, gynecologists and fertility subspecialists alike had an interest in treating infertility as well as in providing the new contraceptive methods, which demanded medical monitoring. But in fact the possibilities of new reproductive technologies could cut in different directions.[43]

When radical feminist Shulamith Firestone espoused a hope for a technological transformation of childbirth, she looked forward not only to in vitro conception but also to in vitro birth. In order for such technology truly to liberate women, she argued, it would have to be part of "a new value system, based on the elimination of male supremacy and the family."[44] Coming from the opposite direction, some proponents of a more conventional value system realized that it was equally possible that the new technologies, by allowing infertile couples to bear children, could strengthen the nuclear family. Catholic moralists faced perhaps the severest dilemma. Forceful advocates for the idea that procreation was at the heart of the marriage relation, and equally strong believers in the biblical notion that human beings were to have dominion over nature, Catholic ethicists also faced several decades of papal injunctions against the separation of the sexual and reproductive acts, regardless of whether the goal was the promotion of reproduction or its prevention. Papal edicts even prohibited artificial insemination using the husband's semen. Nevertheless, American Catholics seemed reluctant to denounce outright all in vitro fertilization, the earlier Vatican condemnation of Daniele Petrucci's research notwithstanding.

Between Petrucci's 1963 censure and 1970, of course, American Catholics had felt the liberating breezes of Vatican II, short-lived as was the reign of its progenitor, Pope John XXIII. In 1971 Father James T. McHugh, at that time director of the family life division of the United States Catholic Conference, told the Catholic newspaper the *Boston Pilot* that in vitro fertilization "should be discussed fully while [animal] research is going on." It was possible, he believed, to "harmonize" the aims of research with the precepts of morality "so that in no way is science posed against theology."[45]

While ethicists debated, journalists sensationalized. In 1970, the Sunday magazine of the *Boston Herald Traveler* offered its readers a "brave new world" account of the 1944 Rock-Menkin experiments that bore absolutely no relation to reality, as readers will recall from Chapter 5. Science fiction had replaced science, as journalist Nicholas Panagakos purported to describe the first in vitro fertilization: "If someone had peeked into the Harvard laboratory of Dr. John Rock a few years ago, he would have seen him staring intently at a . . . human embryo, growing in an artificial womb which Dr. Rock had devised himself. Using deft surgery, [he]

had lifted an egg from a human womb . . . and had introduced spermatozoa obtained from a sperm bank. . . . [In] the artificial womb . . . it had
grown into an embryo. The embryo died at the end of a week, but the important point is that what Dr. Rock almost achieved—the creation of life
outside the human womb—no longer seems impossible of achievement.
Indeed, it may be alarmingly close."[46]

The account was nonsense, but it did accurately convey the new anxiety about reproductive technology. When *Saturday Review* tackled the
same subject, its illustration featured an anxious-looking baby suspended
in a glass beaker. Even when the text of the articles aimed for some degree of balance, the headlines and illustrations invoked alarm. All the
publicity caused researchers to stop granting interviews, but it did not
stop them from continuing to do experiments.[47]

In 1973, Landrum Shettles believed that he had an opportunity to be
the first researcher in the world to succeed in creating a successful in vitro
pregnancy. Doris Del Zio, thirty-three years old and married for the
second time, had blocked fallopian tubes. Although she had had a child
in her first marriage, she could no longer conceive. Two operations
had failed to reestablish patency. Shettles, a member of the staff at
Columbia–Presbyterian Medical Center, had begun to achieve consistent
success in growing embryos to what he considered the implantation
stage of sixty-four cells. He agreed to try to fertilize ova from Mrs. Del
Zio with her husband's sperm. He also decided to do so without informing his department chair, Raymond Van de Wiele, of his intentions. When
Van de Wiele inadvertently discovered the researcher's plan, however, he
destroyed the experiment. He also made it impossible for Shettles to continue to do his experimental work, forcing him within a few months to
leave the hospital.[48]

It was probably not a coincidence that Shettles faced such treatment in
1973, the year of *Roe v. Wade*. The Supreme Court decision granting
women the constitutional right to abortion had unleased a wave of vocal
antiabortion sentiment that also opposed all human embryo research.
Those who believed that life began at the moment of conception found
the idea of in vitro fertilization experiments abhorrent, because of necessity embryos would be sacrificed on the way to achieving a pregnancy. In
vitro fertilization had appeared to offer a technological miracle in
the 1940s. By the 1960s, it had come to seem a morally questionable
endeavor. In the 1970s it became a political minefield, and Landrum
Shettles was one of the first to feel the explosions. In the same year that
Van de Wiele destroyed what Mrs. Del Zio continued to call "my test-

tube baby," several states imposed bans on fetal research. In 1975, the Department of Health, Education, and Welfare suspended any funding of human IVF research until it could convene a National Ethics Advisory Board. Such a board was not created until January of 1978, six months before the birth—in England—of the first IVF baby.[49]

The vocal "Right to Life" movement, flexing its political muscle, had succeeded in shutting down American IVF experimentation at mid-decade. This left the field to scientists in other nations, including Australia, where in 1973 Carl Wood and John Leetong of Queen Victoria Hospital in Melbourne reported that they had implanted a fertilized egg, only to have it survive in the woman's uterus less than two weeks; India, where research was conducted quietly and without fanfare; and England, where Robert Edwards and Patrick Steptoe were growing ever more hopeful that their work would result in the world's first IVF baby.

Robert Edwards was a Cambridge University physiologist in his early forties and Patrick Steptoe a gynecologist a decade older when they began to collaborate on human in vitro fertilization in 1968. Both of them were mavericks who occasionally came into conflict with the British medical establishment. Because the Medical Research Council disapproved of human embryo research, Edwards faced denial of research funds. As for Steptoe, his fellow gynecologists deprecated his interest in treating infertility. According to Naomi Pfeffer, author of a recent history of English reproductive medicine, eminent British gynecologists, unlike their peers in the United States, were by and large uninterested in treating infertility in the years after World War II. Steptoe's pioneering use of the laparoscope, an instrument for which American gynecologists expressed considerable enthusiasm, raised little interest among their counterparts in England. (In the United States, infertility specialists employed laparoscopy as both a diagnostic and a therapeutic alternative to laparotomy. Laparoscopy, performed under general anesthesia, involved a small incision just below the navel, then abdominal distention with the use of carbon dioxide; this allowed for the insertion of the laparoscope and direct pelvic visualization. Although its primary initial use was diagnostic, physicians also were able to perform lysis of adhesions and to cauterize areas of endometriosis if they were not too extensive.) Steptoe's unconventional pursuits apparently cost him an appointment as a consulting gynecologist and obstetrician at a London hospital. As a result, he moved to Oldham, in the north of England. There, according to Pfeffer, "he pursued pet projects, like the laparoscope, which were at odds with those favoured by the gynecological establishment."[50]

Oldham General Hospital, where Steptoe practiced, is located in an industrial city of just over 200,000 people near Manchester. Steptoe and Edwards conducted their experiments at a small private institution nearby, Dr. Kershaw's Cottage Hospital. Steptoe's expertise in laparoscopy was essential to in vitro fertilization, since the extraction of ova from their follicles required delicacy and proficiency. He performed the surgery, while Edwards worked on creating the optimum media in which to bring the sperm and egg together and afterward to nurture the embryo. During the 1970s they refined both their surgical and laboratory techniques, performing at least eighty in vitro fertilizations before they effected a successful implantation. Throughout the decade, as they came closer to their ultimate goal, their evidence of consistent fertilization, in spite of the difficulties in securing a pregnancy, suggested to their fellow researchers that they were likely to be successful within a short period of time.[51]

As Steptoe and Edwards made increasing progress, Americans, effectively barred from work on humans, continued to experiment on mice and rabbits. The British team encountered disapproval from official agencies just as Americans had. Edwards had faced the cancellation of grants as well as the scrutiny of ethics committees. But their situation was different. Steptoe was able to fund much of the research with his own fees from the performance of legal abortions that were not covered by National Health Insurance. (Despite the fact that the National Health Insurance would in theory provide for abortion, long waiting lists apparently sent all those who could afford it to private practitioners.) And the local hospital board supported their work. Whereas, in the United States, universities and hospitals were reluctant to jeopardize funding for other projects by ignoring the federal research moratorium on human IVF, Steptoe and Edwards, fortified with their own funds and with access to patients guaranteed by Steptoe's own hospital board, pressed ahead.[52]

Initially, Steptoe and Edwards used fertility drugs to induce what we now call "superovulation," or the production of a number of ripened follicles per cycle, rather than the single one that nature usually produces. With the woman under general anesthesia, using the laparoscope, Steptoe removed the ova; Edwards then took over, fertilizing the ova with the sperm from the husband and culturing them. At that point, the pair and the prospective parents all hoped, one of the fertilized ova would develop to the blastocyst stage and be suitable for implantation. Until 1975, not a single woman became pregnant; when their first patient did so, she suffered an ectopic pregnancy and required surgery. When no other pregnancies occurred, the two researchers decided to discontinue the use of fertility drugs and returned to single egg retrieval. This method, combined with implantation at an earlier stage, finally succeeded with Lesley Brown, a thirty-one-year-old Bristol homemaker.

Married to truck driver Gilbert John Brown since her late teens, Lesley Brown had wanted to have a child for at least a decade, but her blocked fallopian tubes made pregnancy impossible. Referred to Steptoe in 1976 after a series of failed operations, she saw him as her last hope. The Browns were a working-class couple with little extra money; but England's National Health Insurance covered at least some of her medical costs, including the surgery to remove what was left of her fallopian tubes and the adhesions that blocked Steptoe's view of her ovaries. Once she conceived, it also covered the expensive prenatal monitoring and testing, including the then not-so-routine amniocentesis and ultrasounds. It did not cover her travel expenses. Since the Browns lived in Bristol, some two hundred miles away from Oldham, these costs mounted, and they were not covered either by the nation or the doctors.[53]

Louise Brown's birth on July 25, 1978, was irrefutable proof that in vitro fertilization could produce a healthy baby. Her entry into the world by Cesarean section, filmed by a professional television crew, was cushioned by the financial deal that Steptoe arranged for the Browns: exclusive rights to their story for a British tabloid, an arrangement that made the Browns at least a half a million pounds wealthier. The day after the birth, a beaming Steptoe and Edwards held a news conference. The baby seemed absolutely normal, they noted, and by having the birth filmed and the absence of Lesley Brown's fallopian tubes clearly shown, they had documented their claim of having brought about the first successful in vitro fertilization. A few years earlier, another physician had announced that he had done so, but his assertion was never verified. In 1974 Douglas Bevis, a gynecologist and researcher at the University of Leeds, England, reported to the press that he had used in vitro fertilization successfully in three pregnancies that resulted in full-term births. But Bevis later refused to discuss the fertilizations further, and never published details of his research.[54]

In an ironic aside to the swirl of publicity that greeted the birth of Louise Brown, the lawsuit that the Del Zios had filed in 1974 against Columbia–Presbyterian Hospital and Raymond Van de Wiele for the destruction of the beaker holding what the Del Zios hoped would be *their* test-tube baby, came to trial at that very moment. As Mrs. Del Zio later remarked, the lawyers for Columbia–Presbyterian attempted to portray Landrum Shettles, who had a distinguished if controversial career, "as a quack." Since the recent birth of Louise Brown made it impossible for the hospital to argue that in vitro fertilization could not possibly work, they chose to contend that Shettles used "Model T" procedures that resulted in a "bloody gook" that "would have been almost a guarantee of peritonitis and a danger of death." Perhaps. More likely was the explanation Shettles gave Mrs. Del Zio: that Van de Wiele said he destroyed the material because "in vitro fertilization was against the policy of the National Institutes of Health." The jury found for the Del Zios, awarding them $50,000.[55]

Louise Brown's evident good health knocked out one prop of the opposition to test-tube fertilization, that it was likely any resulting baby would not be normal. "One fear," as *Newsweek* reported, "was that the fetus might have been damaged, or even altered genetically, by the dramatic procedures attending its creation." The news magazine quoted infertility expert Luigi Mastroianni, a former protégé of John Rock, who expressed concern about how the mother might react to a child conceived in such a manner. Even after the birth, some researchers complained that without an immediate report to the scientific community, how could they know it wasn't a hoax? Others, now that it had been done, called it a mere mechanical thing, and not of particular scientific importance.[56]

No doubt there were Americans who felt resentful that the success had not been theirs, and others who believed that the English researchers had been too reckless in trying the procedure on women before it had been perfected in animals. But as this book has shown, throughout the history of infertility research and treatment, clinicians have rarely waited for the verdict of the laboratory before offering possible solutions to their patients. From the intrauterine artificial insemination attempts of J. Marion Sims in the 1850s, through the testosterone pellets implanted in oligospermic men in the 1950s, infertility specialists were often "empirics" in the nineteenth-century sense, looking for anything that worked, even if the bench scientists had not conclusively proved its worth or determined its safety. Steptoe and Edwards were part of a long, if not necessarily hallowed, tradition.

As Robert Edwards said after the birth of Louise Brown, "We're at the end of the beginning—not the beginning of the end." One IVF birth had occurred, and one other pregnancy was proceeding smoothly, but neither these researchers nor others could predict a consistent success rate. For the technique to be useful, it had to be replicable. Researchers and clinicians all over the United States were eager to join their colleagues working on this subject in other countries. Also eager for their success were the estimated five hundred thousand or so infertile women with blocked fallopian tubes. Their numbers were increasing as a result of the disastrous experience of women who had used the Dalkon Shield, a flawed intrauterine contraceptive device that caused pelvic inflammatory disease and subsequent tubal blockage in hundreds of thousands of its users. For such women, IVF, however slim its chances of succeeding, offered their only hope of bearing children.[57]

Perhaps the most well-prepared researchers in the United States worked at Vanderbilt University in Nashville. Pierre Soupart, an accomplished researcher in the field of human fertilization, and his practitioner collaborator James Daniell hoped to serve as midwives to the first American baby conceived through IVF. Soupart's research had until the mid-1970s always received funding from the federal government. After the funding moratorium was promulgated, his was the first application to be received. When *People* magazine discovered him in the aftermath of the birth of Louise Brown, in August of 1978, he expressed hope that the promised advisory board on the funding of IVF research would quickly convene and approve his application. Although this particular project did not directly involve reimplantation, most American universities were reluctant to endanger their federal funding for other projects by allowing any IVF research until the advisory board convened and ruled.[58]

Given the birth of a healthy baby, which alleviated a number of concerns, Soupart and Daniell proceeded with their search for suitable couples for whom to replicate the success of Steptoe and Edwards. Unlike the working-class Browns, those seeking IVF in the United States appeared to be from the middle class. Daniell's patients included the wives of military officers and professionals. They were also racially diverse. Medical technician Mary Patton, married to a Nashville police sergeant, had acquired her adhesions after surgery for an ovarian cyst. The Pattons were African American, as were "a good percentage," according to Dr. Daniell, of the thirty or so Nashville couples who were under consideration for the procedure. In general, African Americans tended to hold conservative views on reproductive technology, principally on religious grounds, but Mary Patton did not consider that IVF violated her religious beliefs. Although she opposed abortion she asserted, "I don't believe an egg is a human being. . . . If I get pregnant I'll have a baby to worry about, and that's more important."[59]

Because Daniell expected the Pattons to be among the first to be brought into the proposed IVF program, the first American IVF birth could have been to an African American couple. But the Pattons, as well as Soupart and Daniell, were destined for disappointment. The advisory board equivocated, and the new National Commission for the Study of Ethical Problems in Medicine and Biomedical and Behavioral Research, set up in 1980, refused to become involved. As biologist Clifford Grobstein noted, "the Commission recognized a hot potato when it saw one."[60]

While established medical centers prepared to submit to a new bureaucratic process, one small, new, virtually unknown medical school in Norfolk, Virginia, simply plunged in. The Eastern Virginia Medical School owed its very existence to the political savvy of Mason Andrews, a local obstetrician/gynecologist with a long family history in the city and considerable public influence. Whether with astuteness or simple good luck, Andrews managed to lure the celebrated fertility experts Georgeanna Jones and her husband, Howard Jones, to the fledgling institution. Howard Jones was sixty-seven; Georgeanna Jones, sixty-five. They had spent a long and successful career at the Johns Hopkins School of Medicine, from which they were about to retire. Georgeanna Jones and her husband had worked together for most of their careers. A reproductive endocrinologist, she was a past president of the American Fertility Society.

Andrews attracted the Joneses by promising them facilities to pursue whatever research interests they chose. Arriving in Norfolk just after the announcement of the birth of Louise Brown, they decided to concentrate on in vitro fertilization. Steptoe and Edwards served as advisers, and private gifts supplied the funds. In early 1980, in spite of furious opposition from antiabortion activists, the state allowed the new clinic to open. The furor would perhaps astonish the men and women of the mid-1990s who have come to see in vitro fertilization as a regular option for treating infertility, but across the political spectrum doubts arose. *Washington Post* columnist Richard Cohen asked, "why, in a world full of unwanted babies," we want to make "new ones in a laboratory." Syndicated columnist Ellen Goodman, although confessing to "qualms," counseled a wait-and-see attitude. "Fertilization and transplant," she said, seemed to her "no more dehumanizing than artificial insemination. . . . I think we should neither fund such a clinic . . . nor prohibit it. We should, rather, monitor it, debate it, control it. We have put researchers on notice that we no longer accept every breakthrough and every advance as an unqualified good." While abortion foes declaimed over the embryos that would be lost in the transfer process, and Cohen, who noted that he was the father of a child born the "natural" way, wondered why the infertile could not just adopt, Goodman and others were more worried about

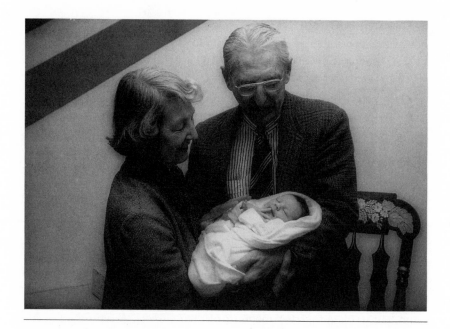

Drs. Georgeanna Jones and Howard Jones with Elizabeth Jordan Carr, the first baby born in the United States using the technique of in vitro fertilization. The Joneses, after a long and distinguished career at the Johns Hopkins School of Medicine, "retired" to the Eastern Virginia Medical School, where they founded this country's first in vitro fertilization center. Courtesy of Georgeanna Jones, M.D., and Howard Jones, M.D.

where the new technology was leading. As a *Washington Post* editorial noted, "Somewhere between 300,000 and 600,000 American women are infertile because of blocked fallopian tubes, and for many of them the inability to bear children is a constant personal tragedy. For these people the procedure would be a godsend. The problem with the clinic has nothing to do with them. Rather, the risks concern the road down which this procedure and the knowledge associated with it are taking society."[61]

In spite of the fury of some, the doubts of others, and start-up funds of only $5,000, donated by a former patient of Georgeanna Jones, the clinic began enrolling patients in March 1980. The patients paid up to $4,000 to be experimental subjects, and the Joneses donated their time for the first year, which did not produce any pregnancies. By the second year, they had made changes in their technique, including superovulation, meticulous monitoring of the patient's hormone levels, and delaying fertilization for some six to eight hours after removing the ova. Three days after Christmas, in 1981, Elizabeth Jordan Carr, the daughter of a teacher and an engineer, became the first American baby born as a result of in vitro fertilization, bringing the worldwide total up to 15.[62]

The Joneses found themselves, as a headline in the *Washington Post* exclaimed, at the "Forefront of [the] Test-tube Baby Boom" by 1982. Other medical centers, unwilling to let clinical opportunities pass them by, now opened in vitro fertilization centers. The federal government remained unwilling to fund research; indeed, a government embryologist was forbidden to speak at an IVF conference in 1982 on the grounds that it might violate the federal funding ban. However, some medical schools and, increasingly, private practices now decided to bypass the government. By the fall of 1982 the University of Pennsylvania, Yale, two branches of the University of Texas, the University of Southern California, and Vanderbilt (although too late for Pierre Soupart, who died of cancer in the early 1980s) opened IVF centers. All but the Texas universities were private institutions. And within years, health plans in a number of states began to fund, in whole or in part, IVF treatment. Without ever confronting as a society those "down the road" implications about which Ellen Goodman and others wrote, by the middle of the 1980s IVF became an accepted, if controversial, infertility treatment.[63]

In vitro fertilization was perhaps the most "invasive" of all procedures to date that physicians had invented to make the barren fertile; it was surely the most controversial. Over the next decade, opposition to it and to related reproductive technologies would come from feminists as well as social conservatives. In hindsight, it seems easy to argue that as a polity Americans should have attempted to consider the implications of reproductive technology before it became so widespread. But in fact, although research into human in vitro fertilization was a much more privatized endeavor than, for example, the development of fertility drugs, since both federal government and foundation support was lacking, it nevertheless bore important similarities to the way in which most infertility research and treatment had evolved.

Infertile women, and less often infertile men, have for more than a century served as research subjects and patients, very often paying for the opportunity to undergo experimental treatments that often did not help them and may have left them worse off than before they initiated treatment. Women, and sometimes couples, made decisions, occasionally based on full information, more often on a hope that this time something would work, to submit to surgery or take drugs because they wanted to bear children.

It was not the willingness of women to undergo experimental treatments for infertility, or their doctors to provide them, that differentiated this period from the postwar baby boom. Rather, it was the change in social attitudes toward the infertile and the treatment of their condition. In the early 1950s, when few actual technological breakthroughs took place, except in diagnosis, public attitudes toward both the infertile and those who treated the condition were almost uniformly positive. During the late 1960s and 1970s, when significant new discoveries such as fertility drugs became available and dramatic strides toward overcoming the condition of blocked fallopian tubes were taken, the American media instead focused their attention on birth control and overpopulation. Although infertile couples continued to seek solutions to their problem, they did so in a fundamentally different cultural climate, one which, at least in the view of some of them, was less sympathetic to their anguish and their desires.

In retrospect, the pervasive sense in the 1970s that a significant proportion of an entire generation might forgo parenthood entirely proved to have been exaggerated. Nevertheless, conflicts would continue within the society over the extent to which the quest for parenthood should take precedence over concerns about the ethics of new reproductive technologies. The concluding section of *The Empty Cradle* assesses these new technologies and the controversy over them in the context of a long history of seeking solutions for infertility.

The Past in
the Present

*Putting Reproductive
Technology in Perspective*

On Christmas Day, 1993, a fifty-nine-year-old Englishwoman gave birth
to twins. She was not a contemporary Sarah, becoming fruitful through
the will of the Lord, but a beneficiary of modern-day technology. Sperm
obtained from her forty-five-year-old husband were used to fertilize the
ova of a young Italian woman; the resultant embryos were then placed
into her uterus. This woman's decision notwithstanding, infertility experts
are not likely to see a rush of women in their late fifties and older seeking
pregnancies. "Realistically," as one writer puts it, "not many sixty-year-
old women crave new motherhood." But neither are such women complete anomalies. In California, for example, one fertility clinic has been
employing egg donation to impregnate postmenopausal women up to the
age of fifty-five since the early 1990s. More commonly, however, recipients of such technology are younger, either women in their forties whose
ova are no longer capable of fertilization or even younger women suffering from premature ovarian failure. Throughout the United States, it is no
surprise to obstetricians to find themselves caring for pregnant women
who are gestating children from other women's ova.[1]

Achieving pregnancy after menopause and breaking the genetic tie between mother and child through the use of donor eggs are among those practices that have made contemporary reproductive medicine controversial. Advocates of the new reproductive technologies argue that without such techniques, many couples desiring children will simply be unable to have them. In vitro fertilization, for example, provides the only means for a woman with irreversibly blocked (or absent) fallopian tubes to conceive. For a woman whose own ovaries fail to produce fertilizable ova, a donor egg is the only way in which she could experience pregnancy. Critics from a variety of political viewpoints, however, counter that such technology—as well as the use of surrogate and "gestational" mothers—is a perversion of human reproduction.[2] With the exception of the issue of surrogacy, on every side the technology itself has become the focus of the debate. If this study of the history of infertility offers any insight into this contemporary debate, however, it is that the use of these technologies, like those employed in the past to assist infertile couples to conceive, is socially and culturally conditioned.

"Assisted reproduction," as the use of the new technology has come to be called, has become an issue at a time when American culture is deeply divided over questions of reproduction, sexuality, and the meaning of family life. Indeed, the very term *family* has become hotly contested, with conservatives urging Americans to re-create what they view as the traditional family form of two parents with their own children, and liberals countering that at best such a goal is unrealistic. The dramatic transformation of women's roles over the past quarter of a century has contributed to the controversy. Although even many conservative politicians have come to recognize that most families need two earners to achieve or to hold a place in the middle classes, since the 1980s there has been an antifeminist backlash (among some women as well as men) that has attempted to encourage high-achieving women to abandon the "fast track" for the "mommy track." It would be possible, of course, to interpret all treatments for infertility, including some of the new reproductive technologies, as strengthening the family, since they promote childbearing. But because they challenge so provocatively conventional notions of family formation, they have become one of the lightning rods for the controversy over the meaning of family and the changing roles of women.

Our focus in this Epilogue on the new reproductive technologies should not be seen as a suggestion that such methods have subsumed all medical therapies for infertility. In fact, the majority of couples who seek medical advice pursue more conventional treatments such as medication for ovulatory disorders, conservative surgery, and artificial insemination. Assisted reproduction, however, is more than simply a way for the infertile to expand their options for attempting to achieve a pregnancy. It represents a particular way of conceptualizing reproductive choice, both for those seeking pregnancy and for society as a whole. A historical perspective contributes to an understanding and evaluation of the assumptions about the role of reproductive technology that underlie the controversy over its use.

A number of separate but related issues contribute to this controversy. In the first place, considerable concern has arisen over what is widely perceived as a rising infertility rate, which, depending on one's point of view, requires either the use of ever more advanced technological solutions or policies aimed at prevention. Observers disagree on exactly how great an increase has occurred. Just the same, the belief prevails that infertility is a more serious problem now than in the past. One author of a recent study argues that since the late 1960s, infertility has risen by 25 percent, while a guide for social workers on the subject of infertility and adoption claims that the rate of increase has been more than 100 percent.[3]

These perceptions do not reflect reality. Historically, precise infertility statistics are difficult to come by, but whether one takes a long or a short view, the nation is not experiencing anything like an "epidemic" of infertility. No reliable estimates of the incidence of infertility existed before the second half of the nineteenth century. Beginning in the 1870s and 1880s, American physicians accepted the figures of Scottish physician J. Matthews Duncan, who had conducted the most extensive analysis of what was then called sterility. Summarizing the results of a number of studies of various small populations, Duncan discovered that estimates ranged from about 8 to 14 per cent. He concluded, based on these researches plus his own data, that rates of involuntary childlessness probably stood at about 10 percent. Readers will recall that although alarmists throughout the first two-thirds of the twentieth century contended that primary infertility afflicted as many as 17 per cent of American couples, more sober analysts generally set the figure at between 10 and 13 percent.[4]

Data from 1965 to the present conform to these earlier estimates. In our introduction, we noted that 11.2 percent of married women in the 1960s declared that they had experienced an infertility problem; in the 1980s, that figure had dropped to about 8.5 percent. It is true, however, that primary infertility has increased over this period, while secondary infertility has declined.[5]

In spite of the attempts of demographers in the early 1990s to put to rest the idea that infertility was on the increase, the idea remains firmly entrenched, as does its corollary, that it is a particularly middle-class problem. And despite the publication of contemporary demographic studies that show poor and working-class women enduring higher rates of infertility than their highly educated counterparts, the belief that middle-class women are the principal victims of infertility remains potent, with as little validity as it had in the past.[6]

Public opinion also holds women responsible for bringing infertility upon themselves by delaying childbearing in order to pursue careers. Even one writer highly sympathetic to the plight of infertile women nevertheless states flatly, "Infertility was the unexpected fallout of the women's revolution."[7] The issue of age came to the forefront in the early 1980s. Until then, conventional medical wisdom held that although women's fertility was highest at the age of twenty-five, until the age of thirty-five very little decline occurred.

One of the few studies that attempted systematically to assess the relationship between age and fecundity had shown only that women over thirty-five seeking a first pregnancy had a median conception time of approximately four months, which was two months greater than women under twenty-five. But in 1982 the *New England Journal of Medicine* published the results of a French study based on approximately two thousand women who underwent artificial insemination, which showed a decline in fecundability for women over the age of thirty rather than thirty-five. The authors called the decline "slight but significant after 30 years of age," and "marked" after thirty-five.[8]

Although the French study dealt with artificial insemination (which has a longer mean conception time than natural fertilization), and although it found only a slight decline in fertility after the age of thirty, an editorial in the *Journal* suggested that the results called for women to reevaluate any decision to postpone childbearing to satisfy their professional ambitions. The authors of the editorial specifically denied that they were suggesting that women eschew careers altogether. Rather, they suggested, women ought to consider having their children in their twenties and begin to build their professional lives in their thirties, an equally unrealistic idea for large numbers of women.[9]

Such recommendations give no hint of the fact that the only age group for which infertility has actually risen since 1965 is young women between the ages of 20 and 24, who have seen their rates of infertility jump from 4 to 11 percent. Researchers attribute much of that increase to the "tripled gonorrhea rate of this age group between 1960 and 1977." But the idea of women forgoing the opportunity to be mothers because they have put their career interests first has gained considerably more public attention. The 1980s were not the first time, readers will recall, that women were told that seeking worldly success could result in infertility. One scholar, in fact, has argued that the medical profession has a long history of viewing infertility as in some way "volitional." However, the idea of volition in illness is fairly widespread in the late twentieth century; whether the disease is AIDS or heart disease or cancers of various kinds, often the first question asked is what behavior of the afflicted individual might have brought on the condition. The fact that medical authorities today would cite behavior such as delaying the decision to marry or bear children as major factors in infertility should come as no surprise in such a context.[10] The evidence in this book, however, suggests that to make the argument that infertile women have always been blamed for their predicament oversimplifies the views of infertility practitioners in the past.

It is true that during the late nineteenth century, women were castigated for educating themselves into sterility. And in the post–World War II era, some psychoanalytically inclined "experts" suggested that a woman's rejection of her appropriate feminine role could make her infertile. Indeed, this idea was prevalent enough to form a new rationale for the idea that adopting a child often enabled a woman to conceive. However, among gynecological infertility specialists, as we suggest, the psychoanalytic model was ridiculed at least as often as it was embraced. Even some of those who believed in psychological causes of infertility did not necessarily assume that abandoning a career was the answer.[11]

With the exception of these two earlier periods and the present, explanations for the etiology of infertility have not highlighted female behavior. In the mid–nineteenth century, J. Marion Sims and the surgeons of the Woman's Hospital attributed most sterility to a mechanical failure of the cervix; men came in for their share of the blame in the 1910s and 1920s; and the most advanced practitioners of the 1930s considered that blockages of the fallopian tubes as well as various endocrinological disorders were the principal causes of female infertility.

Sexually transmitted diseases have been considered important causes of infertility in contemporary America as well as in the first three decades of the century. When early-twentieth-century physicians insisted that gonorrhea was perhaps the major cause of infertility in the United States, however, they saw men as the culprits and their wives and fiancées as the victims. Only recently—as a result of the sexual revolution of the 1960s and 1970s—have women been perceived as responsible for their own infertility as a result of their sexual behavior. The notion of male responsibility has receded into the background.[12] In short, the idea that women bring infertility upon themselves has not been a constant refrain of the medical profession or the society over time.

One could accept the idea that certain life choices—for example, the decision to postpone childbearing until one's thirties in favor of a career—may reduce one's chance of a prompt pregancy without coming to the conclusion that women are somehow "at fault" for waiting. An argument could be made—although it is not one we would make—that one solution to the problem of infertility in the contemporary world is to embrace technology more fully. Conversely, one might argue, as did two Harvard Medical School students in response to the aforementioned editorial in the *New England Journal of Medicine* that encouraged women to postpone their careers in favor of early motherhood, that a proposal "for universal day care and equal parenting by father and mother" was at least as appropriate a social policy suggestion as the one the editorial made. "Scientific facts," these students concluded, "in themselves do not lead to social conclusions."[13]

This society has clearly not taken this route, but in many ways it has chosen to embrace technology. Dramatic innovations in assisted reproduction have taken place since the 1980s. Conventional in vitro fertilization—in which the wife provides the ova and her husband the sperm—has come to seem almost routine. In 1987, the use of donor ova became an available option in the United States. And although the most sensational news stories have involved women in their fifties and sixties, more commonly women in their forties whose ovaries are not producing fertilizable ova and younger women suffering from premature ovarian failure are the principal consumers of such services. Most of the recipients have been trying unsuccessfully to conceive with their own eggs, sometimes for years.[14]

Egg donation and its counterpart, embryo donation (for the couple in which both partners have an infertility problem), have been joined by new in vitro fertilization techniques that attempt to overcome sperm inadequacies. One new procedure, called intracytoplasmic sperm injection, or ICSI, devised by Andrew Van Steirteghem of the Free University in Brussels, involves the injection of a single sperm into an egg. All of these high-technology procedures are not only expensive but for the woman they require a major investment of time as well as the endurance of invasive procedures preceded by hormonal injections, usually Pergonal or some preparation that combines a number of ovulation-inducing drugs.[15]

Couples embark on infertility treatment with high hopes. But although success rates overall—measured by the birth of a baby—range at around 50 percent, it is more conventional therapies such as hormonal treatment for ovulatory dysfunction and artificial insemination (with either husbands' or donor sperm) that form the basis for these statistics.[16] The new reproductive technologies have so far disappointed most of those who have tried them. If one measures the success of conventional IVF treatments in terms of how many couples who initiate treatment actually have a child, the overall figure is somewhere between 10 and 15 percent, although in some centers the figures are considerably higher. Success rates are greater when donor eggs are used, ranging at between 25 and 30 percent.[17] It is clear that more infertile couples can be assisted to conceive today than in the past. But since most of the success comes from hormonal therapies, conservative surgery, and refinements in techniques of artificial insemination rather than new technologies of assisted conception, the principal effect of the publicity over the most advanced reproductive technologies has been not so much to report reality as to create a perception of progress. Such a perception has always been one of the key forces in encouraging the infertile to seek treatment.

Since the middle of the nineteenth century, scientific and technological advances both in the understanding of the human reproductive system and in therapies for infertility have been important in the long run to increasing the success of treatment. However, such advances have never in themselves fueled surges in demand for such treatment. J. Marion Sims's therapies for infertility, considered bold strides in his day, were more significant for giving women the feeling that their infertility could be cured than in actually enabling them to become pregnant. In the twentieth century, the most important genuine advances in understanding the male and female reproductive cycles took place in the 1920s and 1930s, during which time a number of new diagnostic and therapeutic procedures were developed. Physician interest in infertility increased, and practitioners encouraged the infertile to seek treatment.

To some extent, clinicians' urgings were successful, but the enormous expansion in treatment demand occurred in the 1950s. By then, although progress in the ability to diagnose the causes of infertility was unquestionable, in terms of methods of treatment practitioners could do little more than they had been able to do two decades earlier. What had changed, however, was the public belief that dramatic advances had taken place and were still continuing, combined with an intensely pronatalist culture. In contemporary America, the increase in demand for treatment stems from a similar belief that new scientific discoveries are clinically efficacious, combined with a return to pronatalist values, albeit not so intensely as in the 1950s.[18]

This use of the term *pronatalism* should not be taken to mean that only during these eras have Americans valued having children. Reproduction, to belabor the obvious, is the bedrock of human existence. Without denying the coercive aspects of what psychologists have called the "motherhood mandate," we should recognize that for most Americans, becoming a parent is viewed as a normal rite of passage from youth to full adulthood. In fact, such values were not openly questioned by a significant proportion of this society until the 1970s. To describe the 1950s as intensely pronatalist and the 1980s and 1990s as relatively so ought to be viewed in the context of a society in which marriage and parenthood have always been valued. For women, this has been particularly true, because until very recently in our history motherhood was viewed as a goal for most women, although not all achieved it, and as the primary vocation for those who married. As stifling as such attitudes could be for those who did not wish to conform, they also posed problems for those who wanted to conform and could not.

In the 1980s and 1990s, infertile couples have been the focus of considerable media and scholarly attention. Most studies agree that the experience of infertility affects women more deeply than it does men.[19] The "motherhood mandate" remains a strong force in many women's lives. As Margarete Sandelowski has argued, women perceive their infertility "as a social impediment preventing them from gaining admission into . . . 'the special club of motherhood.' Although women now have greater opportunities than ever before to pursue life goals other than motherhood, . . . biological maternity remains a critical factor in a woman's sense of herself as a normal woman." As a result, for many women, in the words of sociologist Arthur Griel, "infertility present[s] itself as intolerable, identity threatening." His study of infertile couples demonstrated that, in contrast to their wives, "the majority of husbands viewed the experience [of infertility] as disappointing but not devastating." As one husband said, "My personal infertility has . . . never eaten away at me."[20]

Psychotherapist Aline Zolbrod also found that "women [infertility] patients are obsessed to an extraordinary extent with getting pregnant . . . , much more than are their partners." Even when the husband rather than the wife is afflicted with the medical condition causing the couple's inability to conceive, the wife apparently takes responsibility for the problem. Among Griel's couples, wives took the lead in seeking treatment and making decisions about what therapies to accept. In another study, a husband diagnosed as the sole cause for a couple's infertility said that he had "not felt the involved party."[21]

Until the 1980s, most of the condemnation of in vitro fertilization and the technologies that emerged out of it came principally from the Catholic Church, which opposed any method of conception that did not result from the sexual act, and from antiabortion forces, who disapproved of a technique that involved the destruction of at least some of the embryos created. In an even more sensational way than had artificial insemination, these new techniques subverted the link between sex and reproduction and challenged traditional verities.

Such criticism has not abated, but to it has been added the voices of a number of feminists, in particular a group united internationally as FINRRAGE (Feminist International Network of Resistance to Reproductive and Genetic Engineering). These feminists have formulated a position—vastly different from that of the religious conservatives—which nevertheless adamantly opposes the use of the new reproductive technologies. From Renate D. Klein's pithy denunciation, "Reproductive Technology Fails Women: It's a Con," to medical ethicist Janice Raymond's extended argument that the new reproductive technologies "violate the integrity of a woman's body in ways that are dangerous, destructive, debilitating, and demeaning, [and] are a form of medical violence against women," members of FINRRAGE have articulated a powerful critique of what in much of American society has become a set of increasingly acceptable measures to achieve pregnancy.[22]

The members of FINRRAGE and like-minded critics of the new reproductive technologies make six interrelated arguments: First, that such technologies, requiring the use of powerful drugs and invasive procedures, are inherently harmful to women; second, that many women who undergo these procedures do so not because they are infertile themselves but in order to enhance the procreative power of their male partners' inadequate sperm; third, that the success rates of these techniques, given the risks, are very low; fourth, that they uphold a patriarchal system under which a woman's only value rests on her ability to raise children; fifth, that their use is controlled by a male medical establishment and enforced upon women; and finally, that they perpetuate a class-based hegemony, with less advantaged women serving as the egg donors and gestational mothers for more advantaged women.[23]

One can agree with some of these points—especially that a relatively small proportion of infertile women conceive through these methods, and that many women who are fertile themselves undergo high-technology procedures in order to enhance the capabilities of a partner's weakly motile sperm—without accepting the view that the technologies are inherently antagonistic to women. As this book has documented, at least since the 1850s infertile women have served as both patients and experimental subjects. When feminist opponents of reproductive technology argue that "women are submitting to pressure to have children at any cost because their lives are devalued without children," however, they oversimplify the desire to bear and rear children and devalue women's capacity to choose a reproductive strategy for themselves.[24]

Women in infertile relationships are not merely passive victims of a medical establishment that preys on their desire for a child but are active agents in seeking out medical solutions. Griel describes women who insisted, in spite of their gynecologists' unwillingness, on undergoing diagnostic procedures. Zolbrod characterizes women infertility patients as "obsessed." Writer Anne Taylor Fleming recalled her own inability to give up after treatments repeatedly failed. Such active participation in the "medicalization" of infertility on the part of women is evident throughout this book. By seeking treatment, women made an active choice to confront their childlessness. By challenging their doctors and making decisions about what treatments they would and would not accept, they demonstrated the limits of their willingness to put their fate in another's hands.[25]

To argue that women actively participate in therapy does not suggest, however, that there is no pressure to seek it. As this book illustrates historically and as a number of contemporary studies have documented, the pressure comes less from some "medical establishment" than from the cultural expectation that most women will be mothers and women's own internalization of that belief. In this sense, the desire for a child is "socially produced," but only in the sense, as one scholar notes, that "all needs and desires are socially produced." One should not construe a woman's persistent seeking of medical treatment as a sign that she is unable to make rational and informed choices about that treatment.[26]

These arguments, from feminists and conservatives alike, do in fact add a new dimension to the discussion of infertility and its treatment, one for which no true historical parallel exists. In the middle of the nineteenth century, the health reform movement, particularly hydropathy, opposed all invasive therapies for women's reproductive disorders. In the 1870s and 1880s, the criticism by women physicians and women's rights advocates of the views held by a male medical profession of the relationship between women's biology and behavior targeted a particular medical orientation, but it did not openly challenge the importance of motherhood to the lives of most women. And for most of the history of reproductive technology, from Robert Morris's "ovarian transplantations" to John Rock's attempts at in vitro fertilization, approbation rather than condemnation was the most common societal reaction to such developments.

Some observers are less concerned with the ethics of the new technologies per se than with the increasingly class-stratified nature of infertility treatment. Previous generations of infertile couples who were poor—as long as they lived in or near a large city where teaching hospitals were located—could often receive the most advanced treatments, at little or no cost, at gynecological clinics or infertility centers located at teaching hospitals.[27] The high-technology treatment of the late twentieth century, in contrast, is largely privatized and generally not covered by medical insurance. For the first time since infertility treatment became available at the Woman's Hospital and others like it in the nineteenth century, those without substantial financial resources are excluded from advanced therapies. Undergoing one attempt at in vitro fertilization costs between about $6,000 and $10,000. Medical insurance usually covers little to none of the cost. By the early 1990s, in an attempt to make infertility treatment more accessible, at least to those who are insured, ten states mandated insurance coverage for infertility treatments. In most cases, however, the limits of coverage fall short of the costs, and the laws do not cover treatments considered experimental, which means that a couple would be covered for one or two cycles of a routine IVF. Under these laws, insurers are not required to cover additional cycles of IVF or the utilization of more experimental procedures. Assisted reproduction, therefore, is restricted to the lucky few with outstanding medical coverage or to those who can afford the high price, which can range to $70,000 and beyond.[28]

Inequities prevail in the new high-technology medicine. Since the 1970s, when the federal government determined that its agencies would observe a "moratorium" on human embryo research, it has been left up to individual researchers and practitioners to decide what techniques are acceptable and appropriate, to set their own standards for determining success, and to charge whatever fees they either believe fair or think the traffic will bear. A significant number of centers for reproductive medicine are profit-making enterprises which are free to choose or not to follow the guidelines set down by the American Society for Reproductive Medicine. One consequence of the federal government's refusal to fund clinical research on reproductive technologies is that only affluent patients have access to the technology.

The World Health Organization, among others, has been critical of the "profit-driven proliferation" of reproductive technology around the world. More clinical trials, it insists, are necessary. Maria Bustillo, in 1994 president of the Society for Assisted Reproductive Technology and a reproductive endocrinologist in New York, however, declared that it is wishful thinking to expect underwriting for clinical trials in this current era of government parsimony in granting funds for scientific research. "We can't even get money for doing basic research on endometriosis. Where would we get the dollars to do this?"[29] The privatization of reproductive technology has had significant consequences.

Inequities in the availability of these new technologies arise, at least in part, from the way in which this culture defines the problem of infertility today. We began this Epilogue with a discussion of the ways in which the media, the public, and even many members of the medical profession misconceive or ignore the demographic analyses of the extent and causes of infertility in favor of an explanation that unduly emphasizes women of the upper middle classes who have postponed childbearing until their thirties. This gap between the demographic realities of infertility and the way it is defined culturally enables Americans simultaneously to castigate women for careerism and to provide those who are well insured or well-to-do an ever-expanding array of technological resources with which to combat the condition.

Focusing on infertility among the educated also permits the society to ignore the public health dimensions of the problem. Given the outcry over attempts to use the media to educate Americans about precautions against AIDS, it is hard to imagine a massive public health campaign that would explain how to avoid sexually transmitted diseases (unless it called for abstinence). And given the current trends in national government to reduce subsidies for health care, any major new initiative aimed at prompt treatment of such diseases seems equally improbable.

As much as infertility may be defined as a medical condition, we have argued in this book, it can never be isolated from its cultural context. And part of that context is a historical one. Because contemporary analysts have lacked a historical perspective in dealing with the complex questions and controversies surrounding reproductive medicine today, it seems clear, Americans have come to see these issues as having sprung fully formed from the technologies themselves. It is important to recognize, however, that both the determination of the infertile to find solutions to their problems and the desire of physicians to seek technological means of alleviating infertility are not recent inventions. The medicalization of infertility began nearly two centuries ago, not in the 1970s. Furthermore, as early as the late nineteenth century, at least some practitioners and their patients, for example, believed that the biological tie between parents and children was less important than making it possible for a woman to bear a child. History, of course, cannot resolve current dilemmas, but it can, and should, provide a frame of reference within which they can be understood.

appendix   # How Reproduction
             Occurs

This Appendix is offered as a simple explanation of the process of reproduction as physicians currently explain it to their patients. From "How Reproduction Occurs," in H. C. Visscher, M.D., and R. D. Rinehart, eds., *The ACOG Guide to Planning for Pregnancy, Birth, and Beyond* (1990), published by the American College of Obstetrics and Gynecology, 409 12th Street, S.W., Washington, DC 20024-2118. Used with permission.

The Menstrual Cycle

A woman's fertility revolves around her menstrual cycle. Each month her ovaries produce an egg. The uterus is prepared for pregnancy by development of a thick lining in which the egg will grow if it is fertilized. If the egg is not fertilized, the lining is shed during the menstrual period and the cycle begins again. The changes that take place in the menstrual cycle are caused by hormones, substances normally produced by the body to control certain functions.

Days 1–5 of the menstrual cycle are called menstruation, during which

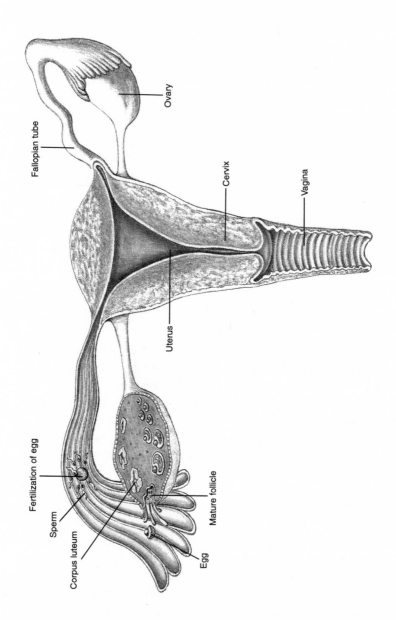

The female reproductive system
Illustration by Robert Colleluori

the endometrium (lining of the uterus) breaks down and is shed through the vagina. This shedding is triggered by a drop in the levels of the hormones estrogen and progesterone, which occurs when an egg is not fertilized.

The drop in estrogen and progesterone signals the pituitary to send a surge of the hormone FSH (follicle stimulating hormone) to the ovaries. During days 1–13 of the menstrual cycle FSH stimulates follicles in the ovaries to produce estrogen. The follicles are structures that produce the egg inside the ovary. Each month one dominant follicle is the source of the egg for that cycle. The estrogen produced by the follicle causes the endometrium to begin to thicken and develop. At this time cervical mucous becomes thinner and clearer.

Ovulation is the release of an egg from one of the ovaries. This generally occurs on day 14 in the average 28 day cycle. The increased amount of estrogen produced by the follicles in addition to stimulating the endometrium also causes an increase in LH (luteinizing hormone) from the pituitary, which in turn triggers the follicle to release the egg. After ovulation the follicle is changed into the corpus luteum. During the second half of the cycle the corpus luteum produces progesterone which causes further thickening of the lining of the uterus. When fertilization does not occur, estrogen and progesterone production drop sharply. This drop triggers the endometrium to shed, marking the beginning of another menstrual cycle.

Fertilization

About every 28 days an egg is released from one of the ovaries into the nearby fallopian tube. Once the egg is in the tube it moves slowly towards the uterus. If a man's sperm does not fertilize the egg while it is in the tube, the egg continues down the tube to the uterus and is absorbed by the body.

Sperm cells are made in a man's testes. When the sperm cells mature they leave the testes through the vas deferens. The vas deferens carry the sperm from the testes to the penile urethra. As sperm travel from the testes they mix with fluid from the seminal vesicles and prostate gland (which produces most of the fluid for ejaculation). The mixture of sperm and fluid is the semen. When the man ejaculates during intercourse semen travels through the urethra in the penis into the vagina.

Pregnancy can occur during sexual intercourse on or near the time of ovulation. At the time of ejaculation the sperm are released into the vagina. They then travel up through the cervix into the uterus and out into the fallopian tubes. If live sperm meet a ripe egg in one of the fallopian tubes, fertilization can occur. The ripe egg can survive only about 12–24 hours but sperm normally can live 2–3 days or longer. The fertilized egg then moves through the tube into the uterus and becomes attached there to grow and develop.

Note on Sources

To our knowledge, *The Empty Cradle* is the first book-length history of infertility to appear in the United States. Other works with a historical perspective include the thoughtful essay by Margarete Sandelowski, "Failures of Volition: Female Agency and Infertility in Historical Perspective," *Signs* 15 (spring 1990): 475–99. She covers the same ground in her book, *With Child in Mind: Studies of the Personal Encounter with Infertility* (Philadelphia: University of Pennsylvania Press, 1993). Naomi Pfeffer's book, *The Stork and the Syringe: A Political History of Reproductive Medicine* (Cambridge, England: Polity Press, 1993), contains some information about the history of reproductive medicine in the United States but is mostly about England. Elaine Tyler May's book on the history of childlessness, *Barren in the Promised Land: Childless Americans and the Pursuit of Happiness* (New York: Basic Books, 1995), appeared after this book went to press. We have relied on a number of secondary works on the history of childbirth, demographic history, and the history of medicine, as well, all of which appear in the endnotes, but a few should be mentioned here. Judith Walzer Leavitt's compelling history of childbirth, *Brought to Bed: Childbearing in America, 1750–1950* (New York: Oxford University Press, 1986), influenced the way in which we approached the relationship between physicians and patients. Susan Householder Van Horn, *Women, Work, and Fertility* (New York: New York University Press, 1988), and Claudia Goldin, *Understanding the Gender Gap* (New York: Oxford University Press, 1990), were important sources for understanding demographic data. Works which we drew upon in our interpretations of nineteenth-century medicine in general and gynecology in particular included Regina Morantz-Sanchez, *Sympathy and Science: Women Physicians in American Medicine* (New York: Oxford University Press, 1985); Paul Starr, *The Social Transformation of American Medicine* (New York: Basic Books, 1982); John Harley Warner, *The Therapeutic Perspective: Medical Practice, Knowledge, and Identity in America* (Cambridge: Harvard University Press, 1986); Charles Rosenberg, *The Care of Strangers: The Rise of America's Hospital System* (New York: Basic Books, 1987); and Deborah Kuhn McGregor, *Sexual Surgery and the Origins of Gynecology: J. Marion Sims, His Hospital, and His Patients* (New York: Garland, 1989).

Most of our research relied on primary sources. The extant Casebooks of the Woman's Hospital, located in the Bolling Medical Library, St. Lukes–Roosevelt Hospital Center in New York City, contain patient records, both inpatient and outpatient, for the first fifteen years of the hospital's existence. In keeping with common practice, we have not used the real names of the patients whose stories we tell. For understanding the early-twentieth-century development of endocrinology, particularly in terms of how it was conducted and funded, the records of the Committee for Research in Problems of Sex, located in the Bureau of Social Hygiene Archive at the Rockefeller Archive Center, Tarrytown, New York, are essential. The Papers of John Rock, located in the Countway Medical Library, Harvard University Medical School, are in pretty much the same state that they were when Richard Wolfe persuaded Rock to give them to the library. Although they are in no particular order, they contain a wealth of material, not only about Rock's own career, but also about the development of twentieth century reproductive medicine. Other manuscript collections that we used less extensively appear in the endnotes, as do the numerous medical journals, memoirs, and popular periodicals from which we constructed our interpretation.

In order to understand more clearly the nature of the experience of infertility from the mid- to late twentieth century, in addition to relying on the numerous contemporary sociological studies and popular accounts, we also conducted our own small survey. We asked Lucia Herndon, the family life columnist for the *Philadelphia Inquirer,* if she would ask readers of her column who had experienced infertility from the 1940s through the 1970s to contact us. In the end, twenty-three women, whose years of infertility ranged from the 1940s to the 1980s, filled out questionnaires and discussed their feelings. In recounting their stories, we have changed their names and other identifying information to protect their privacy.

Notes

Introduction

1. William D. Mosher and William F. Pratt, "Fertility and Infertility in the United States," *Advance Data* (December 4, 1990): 3–5; Ellen Hopkins, "Tales from the Baby Factory," *New York Times Magazine* (March 15, 1992): 78. For a somewhat different interpretation of the same data, with a higher figure of two million for infertility visits, see John A. Robertson, *Children of Choice: Freedom and the New Reproductive Technologies* (Princeton: Princeton University Press, 1994), 97–99. Margarete Sandalowski, *With Child in Mind: Studies of the Personal Encounter with Infertility* (Philadelphia: University of Pennsylvania Press, 1993), 8–9, has noted as well the historical consistency of infertility estimates and suggests that the "rediscovery of infertility," as she calls it, in the 1980s resulted principally from the development of assisted reproduction.

2. Readers may be surprised at such an inexact figure; but there are many variables that affect the outcome of infertility treatment, ranging from the nature of the diagnoses to the length of time conception has been attempted. For further explanation, see Daniel R. Mishell Jr. and Val Davajan, eds., *Infertility, Contraception, and Reproductive Endocrinology,* 2d ed. (Boston: Blackwell Scientific Publications, 1991), 559–62, 566–69.

1. Denied "a Blessing of the Lord"

1. Martin Duberman, "Male Impotence in Colonial Pennsylvania," *Signs* 4 (winter 1978): 399, 401 (transcription of entire trial); Merrill D. Smith, *Breaking the Bonds: Marital Discord in Pennsylvania, 1730–1830* (New York: New York University Press, 1991), 80–82.

2. There is a voluminous literature that traces this shift. Recent works that have influenced our interpretation include, for the colonial period, Helena M. Wall, *Fierce Communion: Family and Community in Early America* (Cambridge: Harvard University Press, 1990); for the late eighteenth century, Gordon S. Wood, *The Radicalism of the American Revolution* (New York: Knopf, 1992), 145–50; for changes in family life in the nineteenth century, Anne C. Rose, *Victorian Americans and the Civil War* (New York: Cambridge University Press, 1992), pp. 145–83. Margaret Marsh deals extensively with changes in middle-class family life from the mid–nineteenth to the mid–twentieth century in *Suburban Lives* (New Brunswick: Rutgers University Press, 1990).

3. Mary Vial Holyoke's diary is available in printed form, along with diaries of other Holyoke family members, in George Francis Dow, ed., *The Holyoke Diaries* (Salem, Mass.: Essex Institute, 1911). Only three of her children lived into adulthood, all daughters. They died at the ages of 62, 67, and 81, respectively. Mary Vial Holyoke Diary, entries for May 14 through May 23, 1770; April 13, 1763; February 12, 1765; March 4, 1765; September 14, 1766; April 28, 1782.

4. Judith Walzer Leavitt, *Brought to Bed: Childbearing in America, 1750–1950* (New York: Oxford University Press, 1986), 14.

5. Laurel Thatcher Ulrich, *A Midwife's Tale: The Life of Martha Ballard, Based on Her Diary, 1785–1812* (New York, Vintage Books, 1991.)

6. Ever since the early twentieth century, writers have been citing as fact that colonial Americans had a childless marriage rate of only 2 percent. This percentage, as far as we can figure out, seems to have been derived from one very flawed study: Frederick S. Crum, "The Decadence of the Native American Stock," *American Statistical Association Journal* 14 (1916–17): 215–22. The 2 percent figure seems to have taken on a life of its own, although at least one physician did his best to debunk it. Samuel Meaker, a noted infertility specialist of the 1930s, recognized the flaw of using genealogical studies to track infertility: "It is obvious that those who were sterile in the eighteenth century are the very ones most unlikely to come to the notice of the genealogists." Samuel Meaker, *Human Sterility: Causation, Diagnosis, and Treatment* (Baltimore: Williams and Wilkins, 1934), 9. Still, as late as the 1980s Crum was still being cited as *the* authority on colonial childlessness. See, for example, the study by Robert Wells, *Revolutions in Americans' Lives: A Demographic Perspective on the History of Americans, Their Families, and Their Society* (Westport, Conn.: Greenwood Press, 1982). The source for the 8 percent figure is Steven Mintz and Susan Kellogg, *Domestic Revolutions: A Social History of American Family Life* (New York: Free Press, 1988),

12; for the 23 percent figure, Joyce Goodfriend, *Before the Melting Pot: Society and Culture in Colonial New York City, 1664–1730* (Princeton: Princeton University Press, 1991), 30.

7. Benjamin Wadsworth, *The Well-Ordered Family; or, Relative Duties* (1712; reprinted in *The Colonial Family: Collected Essays,* New York: Arno Press, 1972), 25–26.

8. Michael Etmuller, *Etmullerus Abridg'd: A Compleat System of the Theory and Practice of Physic* (London: E. Harris, 1699); François Mauriceau, *The Diseases of Women with Child, and in Child-Bed,* 3d ed., trans. Hugh Chamberlen the Elder (London: Andrew Bell, 1697).

9. Nicholas Culpeper, *A Directory for Midwives: or, A Guide for Women, in Their Conception, Bearing, and Suckling Their Children* (London: John Streater, 1671).

10. *Aristotle's Master Piece* and the *Masterpiece Compleated* are available in numerous editions, and, until 1766, when the first American printing occurred, colonists used imported English editions. We looked at a number of them; citations indicate the edition and year from which any quotes were taken. For a study of the influence of the *Master Piece* in America, see Otho J. Beall Jr., "*Aristotle's Master Piece* in America: A Landmark in the Folklore of Medicine," *William and Mary Quarterly* 20 (1963): 207–22. See also Angus McLaren, *Reproductive Rituals: The Perception of Fertility in England from the Sixteenth Century to the Nineteenth Century* (London: Methuen, 1984), 19; and Steven Nissenbaum, *Sex, Diet, and Debility in Jacksonian America: Sylvester Graham and Health Reform* (Westport, Conn.: Greenwood Press, 1980), 27–28.

11. McLaren, *Reproductive Rituals,* 17–18; Mauriceau, *Diseases of Women* (in the 1697 English translation, above), 8–9. See also the English edition of Jakob Rueff, *The Expert Midwife* (London: E. G. for S. B., 1637), 10; and Peter Chamberlen, *Dr. Chamberlain's [sic] Midwifes Practice* (London: Thomas Rooks, 1665), 65–66.

12. F. J. Cole, *Early Theories of Sexual Generation* (Oxford: Oxford University Press, 1930), 10, 43.

13. McLaren, *Reproductive Rituals,* 22–23; Cole, *Early Theories,* 54, 163–66.

14. McLaren, *Reproductive Rituals,* 26.

15. Etmuller, *Etmullerus Abridg'd,* 595; Mauriceau, *Diseases of Women,* 7; John Marten, *A Treatise of All the Degrees and Symptoms of the Venereal Disease in Both Sexes* (London: S. Crouch, 1708); *Aristotle's Master Piece Compleated* (London, 1731), 22. (The 1720 edition evaded the question of two seeds, but the 1731 edition explicitly stated that women had no seed.) Female sexual pleasure, however, was still considered essential to conception. Indeed, this not only was the dominant medical and popular opinion, but it was embodied in the law. (A woman who became pregnant after claiming to have been raped, for example, could be branded a false accuser.) Further, there was religious as well as medical support for the importance of women's sexual pleasure. Seventeenth- and

early-eighteenth-century ministers reminded their hearers that husbands and wives had the duty of giving "due benevolence" to one another. Wives, therefore, had as much right to demand conjugal rights as did husbands. Wadsworth, *Well-Ordered Family*, 24.

16. *Aristotle's Master Piece Compleated*, 1731 edition. Readers should take careful note of the "Grass seldom grows" quote: This idea was used by numerous medical authorities all the way up to the twentieth century as evidence that having sex too often was a cause of infertility.

17. Ulrich, *Midwife's Tale*, 55–56.

18. See Charles Rosenberg, "The Therapeutic Revolution," in Morris Vogel and Charles Rosenberg, eds., *The Therapeutic Revolution: Essays in the Social History of Medicine* (Philadelphia: University of Pennsylvania Press, 1979), 3–25. The term *injection* as used in the eighteenth century refers to the introduction of a liquid into the vagina (or, more rarely, into the uterus) with a syringe.

19. McLaren, *Reproductive Rituals*, 14. McLaren says that in using artificial insemination, Hunter was the first to separate pleasure from reproduction, but that may be only partially accurate. As late as the early twentieth century, husbands were in fact encouraged either to have intercourse, then aspirate the semen for insemination, or to otherwise stimulate their partner in order to improve the chances for artificial insemination to work.

20. *Elizabeth Marvin's Recipe Book* (handwritten, c. 1770s, College of Physicians, Philadelphia); Marilyn Thornton Williams, *Washing "the Great Unwashed": Public Baths in Urban America, 1840–1920* (Columbus: Ohio State University Press), 11; Nicholas Culpeper, *A Directory for Midwives* (London: George Sawbridge, 1681), 78–80. The evidence is very murky about the issue of whether childless women were more likely to be accused of witchcraft themselves. One cannot tell, for example, whether those accused witches who did not have children were actually infertile, or bereaved mothers. John Winthrop, *Winthrop's Journal*, vol. 1, ed. James Kendell Hosmer (New York: Scribner, 1908).

21. James Graham, *A Lecture on Love: or, Private Advice to Married Ladies and Gentlemen* (London: privately printed, c. 1784), 70–71; *Aristotle's Master Piece Compleated* (London, 1720), 13.

22. Wood, *Radicalism*, 46; for one example, see William M. Fowler Jr., *The Baron of Beacon Hill: A Biography of John Hancock* (Boston: Houghton Mifflin, 1980), 10–11. A good summary of the changes in adoption practice from a legal perspective remains Helen L. Witmer et al., *Independent Adoptions* (New York: Russell Sage Foundation, 1963). The first chapter, written by a legal expert, details changes in adoption practice and law from the colonial period through the mid-twentieth century. See esp. 19–30.

23. Wood, *Radicalism*, 47; Wall, *Fierce Communion*, 86–87, 90–91, 204n1.

24. Goodfriend, *Melting Pot*, 38, 44.

25. Wall, *Fierce Communion*, 99 (the name was variously spelled as Lathrop

and Lothrop); Goodfriend, *Melting Pot,* 44; Wood, *Radicalism,* 47; Fowler, *Baron of Beacon Hill,* 10–11, 18.

26. Ulrich, *Midwife's Tale,* passim; also, Wall, *Fierce Communion,* 8, 86. Mintz and Kellogg seem to go further and suggest that the family/household was self-sufficient, indeed almost to say that the family *was* the community. *Domestic Revolutions,* 44.

27. Wall, *Fierce Communion,* 8, 86.

28. Wood, *Radicalism,* 146–49; Mary Ryan, *Cradle of the Middle Class* (New York: Cambridge University Press, 1981); see also Edward Shorter, *The Making of the Modern Family* (New York: Basic Books, 1975); and Randolph Trumbach, *The Rise of the Egalitarian Family* (New York: Academic Press, 1976).

29. In colonial America, most "adoptions" were of relatives' children, as this chapter makes clear, and in some cases one parent was alive and a part of the child's life. The definition of a family, and the line separating it from the community, would increasingly harden over the course of the nineteenth century, although this would be a slow, uneven, and incomplete process.

30. Harvey Graham [pseud. of Harvey Flack, M.D.], *The Eternal Eve* (Garden City, N.Y.: Doubleday, 1951), 370–71.

31. James Graham, *Lecture on Love,* 68.

32. Ibid., 71.

33. Harvey Graham, *Eternal Eve,* 371–74.

34. As late as 1989, infertility experts encouraged practitioners to recommend such dietary changes as elimination of caffeine to women seeking pregnancy. Course notes from "Managing the Infertile Couple," 1989, in authors' possession.

35. James Walker, *An Inquiry into the Causes of Sterility in Both Sexes; with Its Method of Cure* (Philadelphia: E. Oswald, 1797). The title is misleading. As far as Walker was concerned, impotence or deformity caused male sterility; a man who could complete the act of intercourse was, in his view, a fertile man. See Leavitt, *Brought to Bed,* 40–41, for a discussion of physicians attending at childbirth during this period.

36. Walker, *Inquiry,* 7–8.

37. Ibid., 13. It was the nineteenth-century popular physician and lecturer Frederick Hollick who, although not truly an animalculist, declared that in the individual sperm one could see the beginnings of the spinal column and the brainstem. Hollick, *The Origin of Life* (New York, 1845), 59.

38. Walker, *Inquiry,* 13.

39. Ibid., 19–20; Alexander Hamilton, *A Treatise on the Management of Female Complaints,* 4th ed. (Edinburgh: Peter Hill, 1797), 108. American physicians knew about Hamilton; an earlier edition of this work was published in New York by Samuel Campbell in 1795.

40. Walker, *Inquiry,* 21; see also Hamilton, *Treatise,* 98–104.

41. Walker, *Inquiry,* 21.

42. William Buchan, *Domestic Medicine* (New York: Richard Scott, 1812). According to Paul Starr, *The Social Transformation of American Medicine* (New York: Basic Books, 1982), 32–33, this work, which first appeared in the colonies in the eighteenth century, went through at least thirty editions. In the early nineteenth century, it had a number of American "adaptors" and successors. See John B. Blake, "From Buchan to Fishbein: the Literature of Domestic Medicine," in Guenter Risse et al., eds., *Medicine without Doctors: Home Health Care in American History* (New York: Science History Publications, 1977), 15–17.

43. Buchan, *Domestic Medicine*, 319.

44. Joseph Brevitt, *Female Medical Repository and Treatise on the Primary Diseases of Infants* (Baltimore: Hunter and Robinson, 1810), 72–75; Horatio Gates Jameson, *American Domestic Medicine* (Baltimore: author, 1818). See also *American Lady's Medical Pocketbook and Nursery Advisor* (Pittsburgh: James Kawson and Bro., 1833).

45. Joseph Ralph, *Domestic Guide to Medicine* (New York: author, 1835), 126–27.

46. James Hamilton, *Outlines of Midwifery for the Use of Students* (London: Bell and Bradfute, 1826), 162.

47. James C. Mohr, *Doctors and the Law: Medical Jurisprudence in Nineteenth-Century America* (New York: Oxford University Press, 1993), 40, 20; John W. Francis, "Facts and Inferences, chiefly relating to Medical Jurisprudence," *New York Medical and Physical Journal* 2 (January–March 1823): 9–30.

48. A. C. Freeman, ed., *The American Decisions* (San Francisco: Bancroft and Whitney, 1910), 14: 563–68; 28: 447–51, quotation on 447.

49. Ibid., 28: 448–49.

50. Ibid., 449–50; Michael Ryan, *Lectures on Population, Marriage, and Divorce: Comprising an Account of the Causes and Treatment of Impotence and Sterility*, 1st American ed. (Baltimore: Lucas and Wright, 1835), 6, 62–63.

51. Catharine Beecher, *Letters to the People on Health and Happiness.* (New York: Harper and Bros., 1855), 121–33, 1*–16*.

52. Susan Cayleff, *Wash and Be Healed: The Water Cure Movement and Women's Health* (Philadelphia: Temple University Press, 1987); quotation from James H. Cassedy, *Medicine and American Growth, 1800–1860* (Madison: University of Wisconsin Press, 1986), 175.

53. Cassedy, *Medicine and American Growth*, 173, 175.

54. See ibid., 174–75; James C. Mohr, *Abortion in America: The Origins and Evolution of National Policy* (Oxford: Oxford University Press, 1978); and William A. Alcott, *The Physiology of Marriage* (New York: Selden, Lamport, and Blakeman, 1856), 121. William Alcott took an M.D. degree, but for the most part concentrated on health reform, not on practicing medicine. Some of these ideas may have prefigured the "race suicide" theory that we will tackle later, but mid-century writers were more benign in their attitudes toward immigrants, perhaps because most newcomers in this era were from northern and western Europe.

Catharine Beecher, for example, said that "the mingling of the races is the surest mode of achieving the highest physical development of the human family. The superiority of the Anglo-Saxon race is always traced to the happy combination of the British, Celtic, Saxon, and Norman races. In America a new development is to be made, by the union of almost every civilized race, and the eventual result must be the highest type of human physical development, so far as any single cause shall have its influence." Beecher, *Letters,* 164.

55. Leavitt, *Brought to Bed,* 3: Sylvia Hoffert, *Private Matters: American Attitudes toward Childbearing and Infant Nurture in the Urban North, 1800–1860* (Urbana: University of Illinois Press, 1989), 2.

56. Ulrich, *Midwife's Tale,* 30–33; on the meaning of republican motherhood, see Linda Kerber, *Women of the Republic: Intellect and Ideology in Revolutionary America* (Chapel Hill: University of North Carolina Press, 1980); on the differences between republican motherhood and the ideology of domesticity, see Marsh, *Suburban Lives,* esp. 8–11.

57. Nancy Cott, *The Bonds of Womanhood* (New Haven: Yale University Press, 1977), 200; Kathryn Kish Sklar, *Catharine Beecher: A Study in Domesticity* (New Haven: Yale University Press), 1973.

58. (Mrs.) L. H. G. Abell, *Woman in Her Various Relations* (New York, 1851), 209. For a fuller discussion of this issue, see Marsh, *Suburban Lives,* 22–25; and Hoffert, *Private Matters,* 2.

59. Catharine Beecher and Harriet Beecher Stowe, *The American Woman's Home* (New York: J. B. Ford, 1869), 216; Ryan, *Cradle of the Middle Class,* 230–42, quotation on 232.

60. There are several biographies of Lydia Maria Child, including Milton Meltzer, *Tongue of Flame: The Life of Lydia Maria Child* (New York: Crowell, 1965); Bernice Grieves Lamberton, "A Biography of Lydia Maria Child," (master's thesis, University of Maryland, 1952); Helene Gilbert Baer, *The Heart Is Like Heaven* (Philadelphia: University of Pennsylvania Press, 1964); and Deborah Clifford, *Crusader for Freedom: A Life of Lydia Maria Child* (Boston: Beacon Press, 1992).

61. Marsh, *Suburban Lives,* 33–35; Baer, *The Heart Is Like Heaven,* 59; Meltzer, *Tongue of Flame,* 76; Clifford, *Crusader for Freedom.* Clifford suggests (84) that David and Maria may have had sexual difficulties, but he neither elaborates nor gives a citation, and while we found evidence of great tension in the relationship, we could not pinpoint any specific sexual dysfunction. They may have wanted to adopt. One Christmas, she and David took in a homeless boy and spent the holiday with him. She intimates, but never exactly says, that they considered adopting him, except that he really wanted to have brothers and sisters, and she and David could not provide that.

62. Lydia Maria Child to Lydia (Bigelow) Child, June 23, 1831, p. 2, letter 48, Microfilm Collection, Library of Congress.

63. Lydia Maria Child to Louisa (Gilman) Loring and Ellis Gray Loring, April

30, 1839, p. 2, letter 179, Microfilm Collection, Library of Congress. She expressed her disappointment yet again to the Lorings in a later letter: Lydia Maria Child to Ellis Gray Loring and Louisa (Gilman) Loring, May 14, 1849, letter 751, Microfilm Collection, Library of Congress. Letter to Mrs. H. B. Shaw in Lydia Maria (Francis) Child, *Letters of Lydia Maria Child* (1883; reprint, New York: Arno Press, 1969), 140.

64. After Amelia Bloomer died, her husband, Dexter Bloomer, published a memorial to her, which included a biography and a selection of her writings and letters. Dexter Bloomer, *Life and Writings of Amelia Bloomer* (1895; reprint, New York: Schocken Books, 1975).

65. Williams, *Washing "the Great Unwashed,"* 11; Bloomer, *Life and Writings,* 17–18, 128–29.

66. Bloomer, *Life and Writings,* 299–300.

67. Ibid., 189, 241–42.

68. The Mary Chesnut diaries that were published posthumously as *A Diary from Dixie* were heavily revised and edited. Although Chesnut seems to have had literary ambitions, she did not publish during her lifetime. Mary Boykin Chesnut, *A Diary from Dixie* (Boston: Houghton Mifflin, 1949), all quotations from this edition. In 1984, C. Vann Woodward and Elisabeth Muhlenfeld, Chesnut's biographer, edited and published the original diaries as *The Private Mary Chesnut: The Unpublished Civil War Diaries* (Oxford University Press, 1984).

69. Elisabeth Muhlenfeld, *Mary Boykin Chesnut: A Biography* (Baton Rouge: Louisiana State University Press, 1981), 62–63, 235n.34; Chesnut, *Diary from Dixie,* xvii.

70. Chesnut, *Diary from Dixie,* 22; Muhlenfeld, 64, 127.

71. Chesnut, *The Private Mary Chesnut,* xx.

72. Vincent Marie Mondat, *On Sterility in the Male and Female: Its Causes and Treatment,* trans. from 5th French ed. (New York: J. S. Redfield, 1844).

73. Ibid., 41.

74. Ibid., 147, 180, 198.

75. Ibid., 160–80, 93. Mondat held to the pervasive view that men were never sterile unless they were impotent.

76. James Whitehead, *On the Causes and Treatment of Abortion and Sterility* (Philadelphia: Lea and Blanchard, 1848).

77. We discuss this movement more thoroughly in Chapter 2. Fueled by distrust of the heroic medicine practiced by the medical establishment in the 1830s and 1840s, the new democratic medicine had itself become an established phenomenon by the 1850s. With the universal repeal of medical licensure laws, almost anyone could call himself or herself a physician. Thomsonianism and hydropathy were two of the most popular systems that competed with regular medicine for patient loyalty and fees. See Starr, *Social Transformation of American Medicine,* 52–57; and Regina Markell Morantz-Sanchez, *Sympathy and Sci-*

ence: Women Physicians in American Medicine (New York: Oxford University Press, 1985), 31, 60–70.

2. "Purely Surgical"?

1. Thomas Addis Emmet, *Reminiscences of the Founders of the Woman's Hospital Association* (New York: American Gynecological Association, 1899), 2; reprinted, with additional information, from the *American Gynecological and Obstetrical Journal* (April 1899). On male sterility, see James Whitehead, *On the Causes and Treatment of Abortion and Sterility* (Philadelphia: Lea and Blanchard, 1848), 346, who said, "The non-existence of the procreative power in the [male] sex [is], in reality, extremely rare." J. Marion Sims was one of the few who was convinced that some men were indeed sterile and that some cases of male sterility were curable. J. Marion Sims, *Clinical Notes on Uterine Surgery, with Special Reference to the Management of the Sterile Condition* (New York: William Wood, 1866), 355–57.

2. John Harley Warner, "Medical Sectarianism, Therapeutic Conflict, and the Shaping of Orthodox Professional Identity in Antebellum American Medicine," in W. F. Bynum and Roy Porter, eds., *Medical Fringe and Medical Orthodoxy: 1750–1850* (London: Croom Helm, 1987), 236.

3. Amelia Bloomer, for example, who was childless and who ultimately adopted two children, was a regular visitor at hydropathic spas, which may have been related to her childlessness. See Dexter Bloomer, *Life and Writings of Amelia Bloomer* (1895; reprint, New York: Schocken Books, 1975), 17–19. On the Thomsonians, see Paul Starr, *The Social Transformation of American Medicine* (New York: Basic Books, 1982), 52–57; on sectarian medicine and women, see Regina Markell Morantz-Sanchez, *Sympathy and Science: Women Physicians in American Medicine* (New York: Oxford University Press, 1985), 31, 60–70.

4. Starr, *Social Transformation of American Medicine,* 54–58, 96–97; Morantz-Sanchez, *Sympathy and Science,* 32–46. The homeopaths, who constituted the largest group of sectarians at midcentury (Starr, 96), would end up differing hardly at all from the regulars on the issue of sterility by the 1880s.

5. Starr, *Social Transformation of American Medicine,* 54–55. Our overall views on this issue have been largely shaped by the arguments of John Harley Warner, *The Therapeutic Perspective: Medical Practice, Knowledge, and Identity in America, 1820–1885* (Cambridge: Harvard University Press, 1986), who reminds us (186–91) that Americans adopted French scientific methods but used them in a context of American therapeutics. The French, American doctors claimed, cared more about understanding than treating disease. Augustus Gardner left a memoir of his student days in Paris, *Old Wine in New Bottles; or, Spare Hours of a Student in Paris* (New York: Francis Publishing, 1848).

6. Warner, *Therapeutic Perspective,* 191–96.

7. See Ann Dally, *Women under the Knife: A History of Surgery* (New York: Routledge, 1991), 48–51; for the new French infertility therapeutics, see Vincent Mondat, *On Sterility in the Male and Female, Its Causes and Treatment*, trans. from 5th French ed. (New York: J. S. Redfield, 1844). James V. Ricci surveyed the nineteenth-century medical literature in *One Hundred Years of Gynecology, 1800–1900* (Philadelphia: Blackston, 1945).

8. Augustus K. Gardner, *On the Causes and Curative Treatment of Sterility, with a Preliminary Statement of the Physiology of Generation* (New York: DeWitt and Davenport, 1856).

9. Ibid., 127, 137, 144–53, 158.

10. Augustus K. Gardner, *Conjugal Sins against the Laws of Life and Health* (New York: G. J. Moulton, 1870); a second edition appeared under the same title in 1874. See also Gardner, *Sterility*, 123–25. The best work on abortion in the nineteenth century remains James C. Mohr, *Abortion in America: The Origins and Evolution of National Policy* (New York: Oxford University Press, 1978).

11. Gardner, *Sterility*, 52.

12. Jacob A. Rose, *Family Medical Advisor* (Philadelphia: author, c. 1854), 4, 21. Charles Lohman wrote under the pseudonym of A. M. Mauriceau (see Mohr, *Abortion in America*, 62–63). His *Married Woman's Private Medical Companion* (New York: author, 1850) promoted his proprietary medicines for fertility as well as purported abortifacients.

13. J. H. Robinson, *Brief Review of the Two Systems of Medicine* (Bangor, Maine, 1844); Simon M. Landes, *Improved Family Physician* (Lancaster, Pa.: Independent Whig Printer, 1853); Orson Fowler, *Creative and Sexual Science* (n.p., n.d. [1850s]).

14. Joel Shew, *Midwifery and Diseases of Women* (New York: Fowler and Wells, 1856), 226–27.

15. See Warner, *Therapeutic Perspective*, esp. 20–21, 50–55.

16. The new treatment of women's diseases would be surgical in nature, but it was surgery of a different sort than that commonly performed. Although the practice of surgery did not suffer from the controversy that medicine faced in the middle of the nineteenth century, surgery was understood to be a procedure of last resort, and only in extreme circumstances would a surgeon consider invading the bodily cavities. William G. Rothstein, *American Physicians in the Nineteenth Century: From Sects to Science* (Baltimore: Johns Hopkins University Press, 1972; reprint, 1992), 250–51. Gynecological surgery was different in two respects: First, it was invasive in a way that amputations and surgery for facial deformities, for example, were not. And second, it involved women's sexual organs, which brought it into the whole realm of controversy over women's health. The hydropathists and Thomsonians, who encouraged women to take charge of their own health and who dismissed the efficacy of any invasive treatments for the sexual organs, did not consider what the "women's surgeons" were advocating to be legitimate treatments for reproductive disorders.

17. The best recent work on the Woman's Hospital is Deborah Kuhn Mc-Gregor's *Sexual Surgery and the Origins of Gynecology: J. Marion Sims, His Hospital, and His Patients* (New York: Garland, 1989); see esp. 29.

18. Seale Harris, *Woman's Surgeon: The Life Story of J. Marion Sims* (New York: Macmillan, 1950); McGregor, *Sexual Surgery*. In characterizing Sims as we do in this chapter, we have drawn on these biographies, as well as Sims's and Emmet's memoirs, to create our own portrait.

19. According to McGregor, *Sexual Surgery*, 14, Philadelphia had been a mecca for southern medical students since the 1760s, when the medical college at the University of Pennsylvania was founded.

20. J. Marion Sims, *The Story of My Life* (New York: Appleton, 1884), 231.

21. Emmet, *Reminiscences of the Founders*, 17. McGregor argues, in *Sexual Surgery*, 176–77, that rickets probably caused deformed pelvises in many women, which could have resulted in prolonged labors and subsequent fistulas; Dally, *Women under the Knife*, 22, agrees with McGregor. Fistulas remain a common complication of childbirth in some areas of the world today, and hospitals continue to be devoted to their cure.

22. Harris, *Woman's Surgeon*, 99.

23. Martin S. Pernick, *A Calculus of Suffering: Pain, Professionalism, and Anesthesia in Nineteenth-Century America* (Ithaca: Cornell University Press, 1985), esp. 151–53, but discussions about the medical risks of anesthesia and its moral and ethical implications appear throughout the work. In the specific case of Sims, McGregor, *Sexual Surgery*, 47–48, both quotes from Sims's "Silver Sutures" speech and gives an additional explanation for the lack of anesthesia in the early years. As performed in the early years, the surgery required the active cooperation of the patient, who had to hold herself in position for the surgery. That this was not an insuperable obstacle to anesthesia, however, is underlined by the fact that they did anesthetize the patients by the late 1860s, and nevertheless with a nurse's help managed to keep them in the proper position.

24. McGregor, *Sexual Surgery*, 82–83; Sims, *Story of My Life*, 269, 295.

25. Emmet, *Reminiscences of the Founders*, 6; Mary S. Benson, "Sara Platt Doremus," in Edward T. James, ed., *Notable American Women* (Cambridge: Harvard University Press, 1971), 1:500–501.

26. Emmet, *Reminiscences of the Founders*, 14.

27. Sims, *Story of My Life*, 299–300; McGregor, *Sexual Surgery*, 90–93.

28. See McGregor, *Sexual Surgery*, 207–12; and Woman's Hospital Casebooks. In keeping with common practice, we have changed the names of the patients. The casebooks are in the collection of the Bolling Medical Library at St. Luke's–Roosevelt Hospital Center in New York. There are three surviving manuscript casebooks from the Woman's Hospital, which cover the period 1855–70. Some patients appear in more than one casebook for the same dates and same surgery, so it is difficult to figure out the method that was used in taking case histories. A number of casebooks were lost; it is unclear how many. However, the inpatient

and outpatient population of the hospital in these years numbered in the thousands, and these cases only in the hundreds. Clitoridectomy in no. 2, case 226.

29. According to Emmet, the Woman's Hospital in its early years refused to take women whose conditions were considered incurable. Emmet, *Reminiscences of the Founders*, 4–5, tells Mary Smith's story. Sims never mentioned her eventual fate, or even the number of her operations, in his autobiography.

30. Sims, *Story of My Life*, 338; Woman's Hospital Casebooks. Sims, *Clinical Notes*, 323, noted that "the hospital [is] the legitimate field for experimental observations," a phrasing that, taken alone, would suggest that all his experiments were done on hospital patients. We are not so sure, for in the paragraphs immediately following, he discussed his experimental treatment of a private patient. When her mother objected, he told the mother that if his treatment failed to work, a divorce was probable, and therefore experimenting was justified. The mother disagreed, prevailing upon the daughter to stop treatments. See *Clinical Notes*, 323–24.

31. Peter Knights, *Yankee Destinies: The Lives of Ordinary Nineteenth-Century Bostonians* (Chapel Hill: University of North Carolina Press, 1991), 57.

32. *Lancet* 1 (1849): 529, cited in Ricci, *One Hundred Years of Gynecology*, 379.

33. James V. Ricci, *The Development of Gynecological Surgery and Instruments* (Philadelphia: Blackston, 1949), 442; Sims, *Clinical Notes*, 142.

34. Emmet, *Reminiscences of the Founders*, 15.

35. Sims, *Clinical Notes*, 140–41.

36. Gardner, *Sterility*, 144–53; McGregor, *Sexual Surgery*, 218, for Gardner's change of heart, and 228–33 for an excellent discussion of medical opposition to cervical surgery; Hugh Hodge, *On Diseases Peculiar to Women, Including Displacements of the Uterus* (Philadelphia: Blanchard and Lea, 1860), 207–9.

37. Sims, *Clinical Notes*, 140–46.

38. Woman's Hospital Casebooks, passim. It was not until the 1870s that any physician believed that gonorrhea was a serious disease. In 1872, Emil Noeggerath began to note the connection between what we now call pelvic inflammatory disease in women and the fact that their husbands had been "cured" of gonorrhea. See *Transactions of the American Gynecological Society* 1 (1876): 268–300. He was not taken seriously at first. Chapter 3 discusses this issue in full.

39. See, for example, Woman's Hospital Casebook, no. 1, pp. 380, 386.

40. Sims, *Clinical Notes*, 209.

41. Quantitative conclusions are impossible, given what a small portion of cases we have. Inpatients numbered between 100 and 150 per year in the 1860s, but the outpatient population soared by 1863 to over 600 annually. *Constitution and Ninth Annual Report of the Woman's Hospital Association* (New York: Baker and Godwin, 1864), 14–15; Woman's Hospital Casebooks, nos. 1 and 2, 1855–70.

42. Woman's Hospital Casebook, no. 1, p. 60.

43. Ibid.

44. Ibid.

45. We now refer to this technique, still widely used, as a D&C. Woman's Hospital Casebook, no. 2, case 148.

46. Woman's Hospital Casebook, no. 1, p. 76.

47. Woman's Hospital Casebook, no. 1, p. 380; see also p. 425 for a similar case.

48. Up until about 1868, it appears, mostly women with definable physical symptoms—generally dysmenorrhea—seemed to be candidates for surgery. Even in the one clitoridectomy we found, the indication for the surgery was "dysmenorrhea." Clitoridectomy, when done in this era, was usually performed to "cure" masturbation, but such a diagnosis did not appear here. Woman's Hospital Casebook, no. 2, case 226.

49. For example Sims, *Clinical Notes,* 46.

50. Harris, *Woman's Surgeon,* 247, has a good discussion of the negative reaction to Sims.

51. We discuss ovariotomy in Chapter 3; on Thomas, see McGregor, *Sexual Surgery,* 229.

52. Sims, *Story of My Life,* 300. The best work on the nineteenth-century hospital is Charles Rosenberg, *The Care of Strangers: The Rise of America's Hospital System* (New York: Basic Books, 1987).

53. Emmet did not need to give these women a title simply to clarify their marital status, which was discussed in the case notes. Woman's Hospital Casebooks, passim. Emmet discussed his attitude toward his private patients in his memoirs, *Incidents of My Life* (New York: Putnam, 1911), 210.

54. Emmet, *Reminiscences of the Founders,* 14; Emmet, *Incidents of My Life,* 205–6.

55. It is not clear why Sims, in particular, would place his private patients in the Woman's Hospital, unless it was because his private "hospital" was full, but occasionally he did. See Woman's Hospital Casebook, no. 1, p. 76.

56. Sims, *Clinical Notes,* 143–44.

57. Ibid., 360, 365–71. John Hunter was the first to perform a recorded successful artificial insemination in 1776; however, that insemination was vaginal, not uterine.

58. Sims, *Clinical Notes,* 369–70.

59. We cannot tell from any of the evidence whether the artificial insemination cases involved private or hospital patients. McGregor, *Sexual Surgery,* 273, believes that they were hospital patients, but we think she inferred this from Sims's statement, cited in n. 21, above, that the hospital was the place to experiment. But he himself violated that rule. Because artificial insemination required the doctor to be on hand when intercourse occurred, and because Sims appears to us to have been mostly at the homes of his private patients, we think it equally likely that his artificial insemination patients came from his private practice. We have no idea

where the secondary sources who refer to Sims as having had a baby born through artificial insemination got their information. In the *Clinical Notes,* 368–70, Sims says definitively that the closest he got was a miscarriage at four months.

60. This patient tried other remedies from 1860 to 1862, when she agreed to surgery. Woman's Hospital Casebook, no. 2, case 174.

61. Leavitt, *Brought to Bed,* chap. 4; James White quoted in McGregor, *Sexual Surgery,* 234.

62. Frederick Hollick, *The Origin of Life* (New York, 1845), 207; James Reed, *From Private Vice to Public Virtue: The Birth Control Movement and American Society since 1830* (New York: Basic Books, 1978), 11–13.

63. Edward Bliss Foote, *Plain Home Talk about the Human System* (New York: Murray Hill, 1870); Reed, *Private Vice,* 15–16.

64. "Temperamental Inadaptation" was said to occur when men and women with incompatible physical characteristics married. Foote, *Plain Home Talk,* 495, 502, 512, 515–17.

65. Sims, *Story of My Life,* 330.

66. Sims, *Clinical Notes,* 141–42.

67. McGregor, *Sexual Surgery,* 258–62; Buck cited and quoted in Reed, *Private Vice,* 17; Ricci, *One Hundred Years of Gynecology.* Sims's penchant for taking what his peers considered undue credit for some of his innovations may have caused more of the hostility to him than did his operations themselves. Even when he acknowledged that he had adapted a therapeutic technique pioneered by others—after all, James Y. Simpson had invented the operation of cervical incision, although he had not used it for infertility per se—Sims always declared that his own technique was better, that he had invented a superior instrument, or that his patients had many fewer complications. And when compelled to admit that one or another of his experiments failed to work, as in the case of his trial of artificial insemination, he predicted (correctly, in that instance) the circumstances under which such an experiment would work. Sims, *Clinical Notes,* 370.

68. Sims did not apologize for his frankness but came close to doing so when he discussed women and orgasm. Debunking what he said remained a rampant error among the public, shared as well by many practitioners, that for pregnancy to occur the woman, as well as the man, required "exhaustive satisfaction," Sims explained that nothing could be further from the truth. All that was necessary was "that semen with the proper fructifying principle be placed in the vagina at the right moment." Then, sensing that he might have offended, he said that if he had he was sorry, but "I justify myself by the fact, that a false philosophy has gained almost universal credence," and it was his duty to overthrow it. Sims, *Clinical Notes,* 359.

69. Take, for example, his discussion of vaginismus, which is the medical term for an involuntary contraction of the vaginal muscles, which absolutely prevents intercourse. Although many of Sims's colleagues believed that vaginismus resulted from a "hysterical" fear of intercourse, Sims believed it was purely a physiologi-

cal disorder. Since the contraction relaxed when a woman was under anesthesia, some French physicians repeatedly etherized women in order for their husbands to have intercourse with them. Sims demurred. He dealt with vaginismus by surgical removal of the hymen and gradual enlargement of the vagina by means of dilators. Still, if a woman refused surgery, or if the operation failed, he did occasionally himself resort to anesthesia if his patient expressed a strong desire to become pregnant. Sims, *Clinical Notes,* 330–36, 354–55, 362. The editor of the *Medical Times* is quoted in Harris, *Woman's Surgeon,* 247.

70. McGregor, *Sexual Surgery,* 265; Sims, *Story of My Life,* 330. There was also disagreement over Sims's interest in the new operation of "normal ovariotomy," or Battey's operation, which is discussed in detail in the next chapter. See Lawrence Longo, "The Rise and Fall of Battey's Operation: A Fashion in Surgery," in Judith Walzer Leavitt, ed., *Women and Health in America* (Madison: University of Wisconsin Press, 1984), 273–77. Both Thomas Addis Emmet and T. Gaillard Thomas stayed on at the Woman's Hospital after Sims left, and the hospital continued to play an important role in the emergent specialty of gynecology.

71. Sims, *Story of My Life,* 330; also McGregor, *Sexual Surgery,* 265.

72. Beyond this circle of elite practitioners as well, affecting the practice of medicine in general, the tide was just beginning to turn, and it was turning in favor of regular medicine and its claim to expertise. The process would take some thirty or forty years to complete, but licensure laws resurfaced in the 1870s, and the term *medical specialty* began to be used to denote a legitimate field of expertise rather than serving as a euphemism for charlatanism. Beginning in the 1870s and 1880s as well, the adoption of the germ theory of disease, and the development first of antiseptic and later of aseptic techniques, would make surgery safer. Then, too, as more and more regularly trained practitioners began to write for popular as well as medical audiences, both their cultural and their medical influence grew. Medical expertise, not self-help, was the wave of the future for treating reproductive problems.

3. The "Degeneracy of American Womanhood"

1. Regina Markell Morantz-Sanchez provides the most balanced summary of the cultural role of physicians in late-nineteenth-century America in *Sympathy and Science: Women Physicians in American Medicine* (New York: Oxford University Press, 1985), 203–8, quotation on 207.

2. This subject has a voluminous literature, of which the following are illustrative: Sheila Rothman, *Woman's Proper Place: A History of Changing Ideals and Practices, 1870 to the Present* (New York: Basic Books, 1978); Ruth Bordin, *Woman and Temperance: The Quest for Power and Liberty* (Philadelphia: Temple University Press, 1981); Nancy Cott, *The Grounding of Modern Feminism* (New Haven: Yale University Press, 1987); Karen Blair, *The Clubwoman as Fem-*

inist: True Womanhood Redefined, 1868–1914 (New York: Holmes and Meier, 1980).

3. Radicals did challenge the family, and often with vehemence, but they were a minority. See Margaret S. Marsh, *Anarchist Women, 1870–1920* (Philadelphia: Temple University Press, 1981); Judith Walzer Leavitt, *Brought to Bed: Childbearing in America, 1750–1950* (New York: Oxford University Press, 1986), 19; Susan Householder Van Horn, *Women, Work, and Fertility* (New York: New York University Press, 1988), 17–18; Margaret Marsh, *Suburban Lives* (New Brunswick: Rutgers University Press, 1990), 51; and Peter Filene, *Him/Her/Self: Sex Roles in Modern America*, 2d ed. (Baltimore: Johns Hopkins University Press, 1986), 41.

4. Martin Pernick, *A Calculus of Suffering: Pain, Professionalism, and Anesthesia in Nineteenth-Century America* (New York: Columbia University Press, 1985), 238–39; Charles Rosenberg, *The Care of Strangers: The Rise of America's Hospital System* (New York: Basic Books, 1987), 145–49; William G. Rothstein, *American Physicians in the Nineteenth Century* (Baltimore: Johns Hopkins University Press, 1972; reprint, 1992), 250–58, 261–67.

5. See Paul Starr, *The Social Transformation of American Medicine* (New York: Basic Books, 1982), chap. 3.

6. This is not to suggest that gynecologists were the only ones to accept this view, but their adoption and promotion of it had important implications for the development of the specialty. Primary sources cited as applicable below. For overviews, see Morantz-Sanchez, *Sympathy and Science*, 204–8; and Cynthia Eagle Russett, *Sexual Science: The Victorian Construction of Womanhood* (Cambridge: Harvard University Press, 1989), chap. 4, quotation on 10. For somewhat more pointed interpretations, see John S. Haller and Robin M. Haller, *The Physician and Sexuality in Victorian America* (New York: Norton, 1974), chap. 2; and Carroll Smith-Rosenberg, "From Puberty to Menopause: The Cycle of Femininity in Nineteenth-Century America," in *Disorderly Conduct: Visions of Gender in Victorian America* (New York: Knopf, 1985), 182–96.

7. Edward H. Clarke, *Sex in Education; or, a Fair Chance for the Girls* (Boston: James R. Osgood, 1873).

8. Ibid., quotation on 139; Edward H. Clarke, *The Building of a Brain* (Boston: James R. Osgood, 1874). For reviews, see "Clarke's Sex in Education," *Nation* 17 (November 13, 1873): 324–25; "Dr. Clarke's 'Sex in Education' " *North American Review* 118 (January 1874): 140–41; "Sex in Education," *Religious Magazine and Monthly Review* 50 (December 1873): 552–59; and "Sex in Education," *Old and New* 9 (March 1874): 379–83.

9. M. Carey Thomas, "Present Tendencies in Women's College and University Education," *Educational Review* 25 (1908): 58, quoted in Morantz-Sanchez, *Sympathy and Science*, 55; Filene, *Him/Her/Self*, 28.

10. Horace Bigelow, "The Moral Significance of Sterility," *Obstetric Gazette of Cincinnati* (January 1883): 9, 13.

11. Rickie Solinger, *The Abortionist: A Woman against the Law* (New York: Free Press, 1994), 6–7; Leavitt, *Brought to Bed,* 19; James C. Mohr, *Abortion in America: The Making of National Policy* (New York: Oxford University Press, 1978), esp. 226, 230. After 1880, most women having abortions appear to have been young and single, according to Mohr; when married women had abortions in this era, they tended to be among the poor and immigrant populations (241). When Clelia Mosher began to survey married women about their sexual habits in 1892, she found that most of her respondents had attempted to limit births. Nearly all, for example, had practiced periodic abstinence. A few relied on condoms, one careful respondent listing their price by the dozen; others preferred douches. "Hygiene and Physiology of Women: Notes on the Physiology of Marriage with Some Consideration of Its Relation to the Birth Rate," vol. 10, "Marriage," Manuscript Case Records, Mosher Collection, Clelia Mosher Papers, Stanford University Library.

12. Edward Stewart Taylor, *History of the American Gynecological Society, 1876–1981, and American Association of Obstetricians and Gynecologists, 1888–1981* (St. Louis: Mosby, 1985), 9–11, 79–80; circulation figures from *American Medical Advertisers* (Philadelphia: Hummel and Parmele, 1892), 78–92.

13. "Review of Literature Pertaining to Diseases of Women," *American Journal of Obstetrics* (hereafter *Am. J. Obstet.*) 2 (1870): 549 (condensation of Joseph Kammerer, "Pathological Conditions Causing Sterility in the Female); see, e.g., for discussion of treating malpositions with "adjusters," Alexander J. C. Skene, *Treatise on the Diseases of Women* (New York: Appleton, 1890), 311.

14. Russett, *Sexual Science,* 5; John P. Reynolds, "Presidential Address," *Transactions of the American Gynecological Society* (hereafter *Transactions*) 15 (1890): 19; see also Theophilis Parvin, "Presidential Address," *Transactions* 18 (1894): 15.

15. Margarete Sandelowski, "Failures of Volition: Female Agency and Infertility in Historical Perspective," *Signs* 13 (spring 1990): 475–99.

16. Bigelow, "Moral Significance of Sterility," 8; Joseph Kammerer, "On the Treatment of Uterine Catarrh," *Am. J. Obstet.* 2 (August 1869): 191; Clarke, *Sex in Education,* 139; George J. Engelmann, "The Increasing Sterility of American Women," *Journal of the American Medical Association* 37 (October 5 and December 7, 1901), esp. 895.

17. J. Marion Sims apparently named the operation. See Lawrence D. Longo, "The Rise and Fall of Battey's Operation: A Fashion in Surgery," in Judith Walzer Leavitt, ed., *Women and Health in America* (Madison: University of Wisconsin Press, 1984), 269–84, esp. 273; Lillian Towslee, "From 1771 to 1898," *Women's Medical Journal* 7 (1898): 340.

18. Paul Mundé, "Report on the Progress of Gynecology," *Am. J. Obstet.* 4 (1876): 140–41.

19. Thomas quoted in ibid.; Mary Dixon-Jones, "Oophorectomy in Diseases of the Nervous System," *Women's Medical Journal* 4 (1895): 1–8.

20. Longo, "Rise and Fall," 277; Mundé, "Report," 141. Disagreements over performing this procedure, notes Longo, were a factor in the resignation of J. Marion Sims from the Woman's Hospital.

21. Longo claims that many of the patients were middle or upper class. While that may have been true of Battey's patients themselves, in reviewing the literature it seems to us that few middle- and upper-class wives underwent the procedure. We have seen instances of poor women undergoing it, however. As late as the 1890s, just as many leading gynecologists were repudiating the so-called normal ovariotomy, practitioners nevertheless continued to insist that in cases of actual ovarian disease it was acceptable to resort to ovariotomy on "the working class of women" at a much earlier stage of treatment than among women "in the better class of society." Anna Fullerton, "Gonorrhea of the Uterus and Its Appendages —a Surgical Survey," *Women's Medical Journal* 7 (1898): 176; see also "Discussion" following Thomas Ashby, "Laparotomy for Intra-Pelvic Pain," *Transactions* 15 (1890): 332.

22. See Longo, "Rise and Fall," 280. For an example of the new views on surgery, see W. M. Polk, "Operations upon the Uterine Appendages with a View to Preserving the Functions of Ovulation and Menstruation," *Transactions* 18 (1894): 175–99.

23. See Mundé, "Report," 127–39; A. Reeves Jackson, "The Ovulation Theory of Menstruation: Will It Stand?" *Am. J. Obstet.* 9 (October 1876): 529–60; and "Quarterly Report," *Am. J. Obstet.* 8 (1875): 724–26.

24. Mundé, "Report," 127–39.

25. Ibid., 127–28.

26. Thomas Laqueur, *Making Sex: Body and Gender from the Greeks to Freud* (Cambridge: Harvard University Press, 1990), 107.

27. George Engelmann, "The American Girl of Today [Presidential Address]," *Transactions* 25 (1900): 4–21.

28. A few examples from an extensive literature include Horace Bigelow, "An Aggravated Instance of Masturbation in the Female," *Am. J. Obstet.* 15 (1882): 436–41; Charles Fayette Taylor, "Effect on Women of Imperfect Hygiene of the Sexual Function," *Am. J. Obstet.* 15 (1882): 161–77; and Thomas More Madden, "Observation on Certain Cerebro-Nervous Disorders Peculiar to Women," *Am. J. Obstet.* 16 (1883): 1150–59.

29. Joseph H. Beck, "How Do the Spermatozoa Enter the Uterus?" *Am. J. Obstet.* 3 (November 1874): 353–91. See also Ely Van de Warker, "Impotency in Women," *Am. J. Obstet.* 11 (January 1878): 36–47; and Bigelow, "Masturbation in the Female."

30. Parvin, "Presidential Address," 15. It may be true, as William G. Rothstein has argued, that specialization in the late nineteenth century required "medically valid knowledge," but in the case of gynecology, "medically valid" knowledge, at least until the 1890s, seemed overshadowed by social explanations (*American Physicians*, 208).

31. See Morantz-Sanchez, *Sympathy and Science*, 55, for a discussion of Jacobi's 1876 prize. Clelia Mosher, "The Hygiene and Physiology of Women: Experimental Studies," box 2, folder 1, Mosher Papers, contains some of Mosher's published work on the subject, including "Normal Menstruation and Some of the Factors Modifying It," *Johns Hopkins Hospital Bulletin* (1901); "Functional Periodicity of Women and Some of the Modifying Factors," *California State Journal of Medicine* (1911): 2–9; and *Health and the Woman Movement* (New York: Young Women's Christian Association, 1916). Although historians have paid the most attention to her sex survey, Mosher's papers, housed at the Stanford University Library, devote much greater attention to her studies of menstruation. See also "Clelia Duel Mosher: The Questioner," typescript, 1902 and later, Mosher Papers.

32. Alumni Association of the Woman's Medical College of Pennsylvania, *Report of Proceedings, 11th Annual Meeting* (Philadelphia: Jas. B. Rogers, 1886), 16–18.

33. Taylor, *History of the American Gynecological Society,* 28.

34. Allan Brandt, *No Magic Bullet* (New York: Oxford University Press, 1985), 11–12; Sarah Stage, *Female Complaints: Lydia Pinkham and the Business of Women's Medicine* (New York: Norton, 1979), 82; Augustus K. Gardner, *Gonorrhea: A Non-Specific Disease* (New York: Written for and Reprinted from "The Medical Independent," 1864), esp. 6.

35. Emil Noeggerath, "Latent Gonorrhea, Especially with Regard to Its Influence on Fertility in Women," *Transactions* 1 (1876): 268–300.

36. Ibid., 287–89.

37. Ibid., 270, 285–86.

38. Ibid., 300; John D'Emilio and Estelle B. Freedman, *Intimate Matters: A History of Sexuality in America* (New York: Harper and Row, 1988), 148; William Goodell, "A Case of Sterility," *Am. J. Obstet.* 10 (1877): 122.

39. "Abstract of [J. Matthews] Duncan's Lectures on Sterility," *Am. J. Obstet.* 16 (1883): 980–81.

40. Thomas Ashby, "The Influence of Minor Forms of Ovarian and Tubal Disease in the Causation of Sterility," *Transactions* 19 (1894): 260–71.

41. Claudia Goldin, *Understanding the Gender Gap* (New York: Oxford University Press, 1990), 140–41; Engelmann, "Increasing Sterility," 891. Although we argue in this book as a whole that infertility rates *since* approximately the last third of the nineteenth century appear to have been consistent, there are simply no good data for the first half of the century. It seems plausible that gonorrhea was on the rise and was the cause of more infertility, but it cannot be proved.

42. Goodell, "Case of Sterility," 121–22.

43. A. D. Hard, "Artificial Impregnation," *Medical World* (April 1909): 163–64. For related stories, see N. J. Hamilton, "Artificial Impregnation," *Medical World* (June 1909): 253; Ernest Barton, "Impregnation and Religion," *Medical World* (July 1909): 305; and response by A. D. Hard and editorial comment,

Medical World (July 1909): 306. See E. B. Foote, *Plain Home Talk,* rev. ed. (New York: Murray Hill, 1899), 514–15; and Frederick Hollick, *The Male Generative Organs in Health and Disease* (New York: American News, 1877), 48.

44. Samuel W. Gross, *A Practical Treatise on Impotence, Sterility, and Allied Disorders of the Male Sexual Organs,* 4th ed. (Philadelphia: Lea Brothers, 1890), 108; R. W. Taylor, *A Practical Treatise on Sexual Disorders of Male and Female* (New York: Lea, 1897), 141; Edward Martin, *Impotence and Sexual Weakness* (Detroit: George Davis, 1893), 12. See also the posthumously published George Beard, *Sexual Neurasthenia* (New York: E. B. Treat, 1891).

45. Martin, *Impotence and Sexual Weakness,* 28–29.

46. Gross, *Treatise on Impotence,* 108.

47. Although it seems reasonable to believe that advances in pathology assisted in the demise of Battey's operation, it is also not rare to find physicians continuing to defend ideas that no longer seem scientifically valid. Embarrassment over the excesses of some practitioners was perhaps the most important factor. See Longo, "Rise and Fall," 277; and Alexander J. C. Skene, "The Status of Gynecology in 1876 and 1900," *Transactions* 25 (1900): 425–38. Battey's operation was also omitted from Howard Kelly's highly regarded *Operative Gynecology,* 2 vols. (New York: Appleton, 1898).

48. The *Transactions of the American Gynecological Society* for the years 1890 through the turn of the century covered these issues intensively. For a defense of radical surgery, see in particular S. C. Gordon, "Conservative Gynecology," *Transactions* 24 (1899): 402–16. For the other, and increasingly dominant, point of view, see Thomas Ashby, "Laparotomy for Intra-Pelvic Pain," *Transactions* 15 (1890): 323–42; and A. Reeves Jackson, "Presidential Address," *Transactions* 16 (1891): 3–19. See also Alexander J. C. Skene, *Medical Gynecology* (New York: Appleton, 1895).

49. See W. M. Polk, "Operations," 175–99.

50. Arthur W. Johnstone, "Internal Secretion of the Ovary," *Transactions* 25 (1900): 269. There were some exceptions: Robert Morris, whom we discuss in Chapter 5, which deals with the development of endocrinology, was one.

51. Jackson, "Presidential Address," 9. The new ideas can even be traced in the career of a single practitioner, the distinguished Alexander J. C. Skene. In his *Treatise on the Diseases of Women,* he still believed "that the ovaries give to woman all her characteristics of body and mind" (448), and he chastised colleagues such as William Goodell for suggesting that "the psychological influence of the ovaries upon women has been greatly overstated." Skene also was still defending Battey's operation. By 1895, while he still believed strongly in differences in mind based on gender, as did nearly all his colleagues, he had reversed his earlier stand against women in the professions, instead suggesting that they should be able to do whatever they liked in terms of work (*Medical Gynecology,* 89). By 1900, to judge from his retrospective on the field of gynecology, "The Status of Gynecology," a reader would think he had never even heard of Battey's operation.

See also Walter B. Chase, "Remarks on Primitive Amenorrhea: With Report of Case and Presentation of Pathological Specimen," *Transactions of the American Association of Obstetricians and Gynecologists* 11 (1898): 155–63. For discussion of the surgical suspension of the uterus, see C. C. Frederick, "Which Is the Preferable Operative Method of Holding the Uterus in Position?" *Transactions of the American Association of Obstetricians and Gynecologists* 10 (1897): 326–21; and Herman E. Hayd, "Sterility Depending upon Retrodisplaced Uteri, and Their Relief by the Alexander Operation, with Report of Twelve Subsequent Pregnancies," *Transactions of the American Association of Obstetricians and Gynecologists* 17 (1904): 183–97.

52. Filene, *Him/Her/Self,* 26. For an especially lucid exploration of the conflicts over the question of marriage felt by accomplished women of the late nineteenth and early twentieth centuries, see Joyce Antler, *Lucy Sprague Mitchell: The Making of a Modern Woman* (New Haven: Yale University Press, 1986), especially the introduction and 163. Nancy Cott, *Grounding of Modern Feminism,* quotation on 180. Cott argues convincingly that even as late as the 1920s, the idea of women combining home and family was viewed as "extraordinarily iconoclastic" (179). See also Julia Ward Howe, "The Joys of Motherhood," *Delineator* 71 (May 1908): 806, 879. Charlotte Perkins Gilman's views are represented in *The Home: Its Work and Influence* (New York, 1903). See also Dolores Hayden, *The Grand Domestic Revolution* (Cambridge: MIT Press, 1981), 188–92.

53. Mary Ryan, *Cradle of the Middle Class* (New York: Cambridge University Press, 1981), 232.

54. Harriet Beecher Stowe, *My Wife and I* (New York: J. B. Ford, 1871), 478. One of us has explored the domestic role of men extensively, and we refer readers to the following works: Margaret Marsh, "Suburban Men and Masculine Domesticity, 1870–1915," *American Quarterly* (summer 1988): 165–86; "From Separation to Togetherness: The Social Construction of Domestic Space in American Suburbs, 1840–1915," *Journal of American History* (September 1989): 506–27; and *Suburban Lives,* esp. 35–40, 74–83.

55. Jennie June [Jane Cunningham Croly] considered herself a suffragist and reformer, but her attitudes about voluntarily childless women reflected the dominant view of the culture. *Jenny Juneiana* (Boston: Lee and Shepard, 1869), 63.

56. For what remains one of the best summaries of views of motherhood in the late nineteenth century, see Rothman, *Woman's Proper Place,* 97–134. On sterility among the poor, and quotation, see "Report from the Woman's Hospital," *Transactions of the Alumni Association of the Woman's Medical College of Pennsylvania,* 16th Annual Report, May 7 and 8, 1891, 92–93. See also case records for the "Hospital and Dispensary of the Alumnae of the Woman's Medical College of Pennsylvania," bk. 1, Dr. Griscom, 1895–96, esp. pp. 5, 21, 73, 146, Archives of the Medical College of Pennsylvania.

57. The literature on the changing dimensions of the family is voluminous and often contradictory, but the disagreements are more often over the timing and

cause of the transformation than over the changes themselves. Scholars tend to agree that the transformation began among upper- and middle-class Europeans and Americans in the eighteenth and nineteenth centuries, and that it was in place by the second half of the nineteenth century. They also agree that the shift toward closer and more loving familial relationships is in some way connected to the declining birthrate. But whether the smaller families were the cause or the result of new attitudes remains a matter of controversy. See Edward Shorter, *The Making of the Modern Family* (New York: Basic Books, 1975); Laurence Stone, *The Family, Sex, and Marriage in England, 1500–1800* (London: Weidenfeld and Nicolson, 1977); Randolph Trumbach, *The Rise of the Egalitarian Family* (New York: Academic Press, 1976); J. A. Banks, *Victorian Values* (London: Routledge and Kegan Paul, 1981); Anne C. Rose, *Victorian Americans and the Civil War* (New York: Cambridge University Press, 1992), chap. 4; and Marsh, *Suburban Lives*, 39–40.

58. We say this with some confidence because we made an intensive search among the memoirs and papers of dozens of nineteenth-century women whom we speculated were infertile. We located them using various biographical guides. Although we did not come up entirely empty, we came up nearly so. See Otto Friedrich, *Clover* (New York: Simon and Schuster, 1979), 215; Leavitt, *Brought to Bed,* chap. 2; and Diana Reep, *Margaret Deland* (Boston: Twayne, 1985), preface.

59. Kate Douglas Wiggin, *My Garden of Memory* (Boston: Houghton Mifflin, 1923); Nora Archibald Smith, *Kate Douglas Wiggin as Her Sister Knew Her* (Boston: Houghton Mifflin, 1925), 313–14.

60. Reep, *Deland,* 3; Ella Wheeler Wilcox, *The Worlds and I* (New York: Doran, 1918), 69, 118–24, 134–35.

61. Friedrich, *Clover,* 214.

62. Patricia O'Toole, *The Five of Hearts: An Intimate Portrait of Henry Adams and His Friends* (New York: Clarkson Potter, 1990), 83–84.

63. Ibid., 84.

64. "From the Transactions of the Philadelphia Obstetrical Society: A Case of Sterility," *Am. J. Obstet.* 10 (1877): 121; A. W. Edis, *Sterility in Women, Including Its Causation and Treatment* (London: H. K. Lewis, 1895), 95.

65. H. Marion Sims, "Sterility, and the Value of the Microscope in Its Diagnosis and Treatment," *Transactions* 13 (1888): 291–300; see also Max Huhner, *Sterility in the Male and Female* (New York: Rebman, 1913), 60. J. Marion Sims, his son H. Marion, and Max Huhner have given the name to the postcoital test to determine whether sperm survive in the cervical mucous (the Sims-Huhner test), which physicians today use as a part of their routine diagnostic workup in infertility cases.

66. See Starr, *Social Transformation of American Medicine,* 136–37; and John B. Blake, "From Buchan to Fishbein: The Literature of Domestic Medicine," in

Guenter B. Risse et al., eds., *Medicine without Doctors* (New York: Science History Publications, 1977), 11–30.

67. Mundé, "Report," 159.

68. Woman's Hospital Casebook, no. 1, p. 380; Goodell, "Case of Sterility," 121. Thomas Ashby, in a revealing comment on the doctor-patient relationship, was referring to all surgery and not simply infertility treatment when he argued that physicians should "abide by the wishes of the patient" insofar as doing so was compatible with good medical practice. "With a woman [surgery] becomes a question of debt and credit, and she should be assisted in making the account balance by judicious medical advice." Ashby, "Laparotomy for Intra-Pelvic Pain," 325.

69. Harriet Jones, "The Treatment of Stenosis of the Uterine Canal," *Women's Medical Journal* 4 (1895): 225.

70. Goodell, "Case of Sterility," 121–22; Gustavus M. Bleck, *The Practitioners' Guide to the Diagnosis and Treatment of Diseases of Women* (Chicago: M. Robertson, 1903); Huhner, *Sterility in the Male and Female,* 116; Noeggerath, "Latent Gonorrhea," 300; D'Emilio and Friedman, *Intimate Matters,* 148. See also A. W. Edis, *Sterility in Women,* 95.

71. Edis, *Sterility in Women,* 95.

72. Huhner, *Sterility in the Male and Female,* 60.

73. It is also possible, although evidence is lacking that would allow us to say definitively, that not all of the indigent patients treated for sterility were actually interested in pregnancy. Joseph Kammerer, for example, defined as "sterile" all his married patients who had not borne children after four years of marriage, but apparently some of his sterile clinic patients presented themselves not for "relief of the sterile condition" but for freedom from pain. Kammerer, "Pathological Conditions," 549.

74. Ashby, "Ovarian and Tubal Disease."

75. See Goodell, "Case of Sterility," 121–22; and Noeggerath, "Latent Gonorrhea," 300.

76. Kammerer, "Pathological Conditions," 546–49. Huhner, *Sterility in the Male and Female,* 56, notes that a few practitioners did try to ascertain their success rates in the late nineteenth and early twentieth centuries, but that it was almost impossible for a reader to judge these studies, in part because there were no agreed-upon definitions for many of the conditions alleged to cause infertility, and also because it was rarely clear that the treatment was the reason for the subsequent pregnancy. T. Gaillard Thomas quoted in William B. Atkinson, *The Therapeutics of Gynecology and Obstetrics* (Philadelphia: D. G. Brinton, 1881), 213.

77. On Lydia Pinkham, see Stage, *Female Complaints;* and James Harvey Young, "Patent Medicines and the Self-Help Syndrome," in Risse et al., *Medicine without Doctors,* esp. 102–3.

78. Julie Berebitsky, " 'To Raise as Your Own': The Growth of Legal Adoption in Washington," *Washington History* 6 (spring/summer 1994): 4–27.

79. See Helen L. Witmer et al., *Independent Adoptions* (New York: Russell Sage Foundation, 1963), 30.

80. Jamil Zainaldin and Peter Tyor, "Asylum and Society: An Approach to Institutional Change," *Journal of Social History* 13 (fall 1979): 27–29.

81. Ibid., 31.

82. Berebitsky, "To Raise as Your Own," 5–19.

83. Correspondence 1905–6, box 680, Papers of the Breckinridge Family, Library of Congress. Madeline Breckinridge left no clue in these papers to the reason for her childlessness. Although she suffered from tuberculosis, it seemed not to inhibit her tireless reform activity. She might, of course, have been voluntarily childless. However, it seems telling that in her sister-in-law Sophonisba Breckinridge's detailed and laudatory biographical tribute to Madeline's reform career, which was ruthlessly pruned of almost all personal information, there is not a word about the Kentucky Children's Home Society. Sophonisba Preston Breckinridge, *Madeline McDowell Breckinridge: A Leader in the New South* (Chicago: University of Chicago Press, 1921). See 23–24 for very veiled hints of a medical reason for her childlessness.

84. Margaret Deland, *Golden Yesterdays* (New York: Harper and Bros., 1941), 138; Reep, *Deland*, 6–7.

Entr'Acte: 4. Framing Infertility

1. Viviana Zelizer, *Pricing the Priceless Child: The Changing Social Value of Children* (New York: Basic Books, 1985).

2. The term *framing disease* is from Charles E. Rosenberg, "Framing Disease: Illness, Society, and History," in Charles E. Rosenberg and Janet Golden, eds., *Framing Disease: Studies in Cultural History* (New Brunswick: Rutgers University Press, 1992), xii–xxvi.

3. By making such a generalization, we contend that *normative* values were undergoing a change. We recognize that there are always deviations from the norm, but those who refuse to conform know that they are going against the grain. Even during their heyday, Victorian values did not embrace everyone in the society, but those who rebelled knew perfectly well that they had set themselves in opposition to a dominant culture. By the same token, Americans in the twentieth century who held fast to an older set of values fully realized that they faced a struggle against what in their view was an ever-rising tide of permissiveness.

4. Margaret Marsh, among others, has studied this phenomenon: see *Suburban Lives* (New Brunswick: Rutgers University Press, 1990), esp. chaps. 5, 6. See also Robert L. Griswold, *Fatherhood in America: A History* (New York: Basic Books, 1993), chap. 5; and Zelizer, *Pricing the Priceless Child,* esp. 188–94.

5. Zelizer, *Pricing the Priceless Child,* 188–94.

6. Works that contain excellent overviews of this change and its challenge include Griswold, *Fatherhood in America;* and John D'Emilio and Estelle B. Freed-

man, *Intimate Matters: A History of Sexuality in America* (New York: Harper and Row, 1988).

7. Speech reprinted in Charles Morris, *The Marvelous Career of Theodore Roosevelt* (n.p.: W. E. Scull, 1910), 364.

8. Ethel Wadsworth Cartland, "Childless Americans," *Outlook* 105 (November 15, 1913): 587; see also Holt A. Milton [pseud.], "Race Suicide," *Independent* 56 (March 4, 1904): 661–65.

9. Cartland, "Childless Americans," 587; Susan Householder Van Horn, *Women, Work, and Fertility* (New York: New York University Press, 1988), 15; E. A. Ross, "Slow Suicide," *Century Magazine* 107 (February 1924): 509. By the mid-1920s the "race suicide" hysteria had dissipated somewhat, but not because the United States had turned back the nativist and ethnocentric tide. Instead, it had succumbed to it. After 1924, immigrants from Asia and southern and eastern Europe were welcome only in very small numbers, if at all.

10. George Engelmann, "The Increasing Sterility of American Women," *Journal of the American Medical Association* 27 (October 5, 1901): 893.

11. Ibid., 895.

12. Ibid.

13. Laura Richards, "The Postponement of Motherhood," *Good Housekeeping* 54 (January 1912): 84–85; Letters to the Editor, *Good Housekeeping* 53 (October 1911): 460–61, and 54 (January 1912): 88–89. Only one writer, physician John Getz, signed a name.

14. As readers will recall from Chapter 3, gonorrhea causes sterility in one of two ways: an infected man can become azoospermic, or an infected woman can develop a pelvic inflammation occluding the fallopian tubes and spreading to the ovaries.

15. Prince Albert Morrow, *The Social Diseases and Marriage* (New York: Lea, 1904), 25.

16. See, e.g., Gustavus M. Bleck, *The Practitioners' Guide to the Diagnosis and Treatment of the Diseases of Women* (Chicago: M. Robertson, 1903); and Mark Thomas Connelly, "Prostitution, Venereal Disease, and American Medicine," in Judith Walzer Leavitt, ed., *Women and Health in America* (Madison: University of Wisconsin Press, 1984), 197–99.

17. Allan M. Brandt, *No Magic Bullet: A Social History of Venereal Disease in the United States since 1880* (New York: Oxford University Press, 1985), 24, claimed that the *Ladies Home Journal's* discussion of venereal disease also brought about the cancellation of seventy-five thousand subscriptions. Abraham L. Wolbarst, "The Tragedy of the Marriage Altar," *Ladies Home Journal* 25 (October 1908): 26. Magazines discussed in Linda W. Rosenzweig, *The Anchor of My Life: Middle-Class American Mothers and Daughters* (New York: New York University Press, 1993), 30–31.

18. William A. McKeever, "Instructing Adolescents in Regard to Sex," *Good Housekeeping* 53 (November 1911): 602.

19. Morrow, *Social Diseases and Marriage;* Engelmann, "Increasing Sterility," 891; McKeever, "Instructing Adolescents," 602; Claudia Goldin, *Understanding the Gender Gap* (New York: Oxford University Press, 1990), 141; Connelly, "Prostitution," 201–2. Some physicians continued to discuss gonorrhea and sterility in public forums into the 1920s. For one example, see Gulielma F. Alsop, "Social Hygiene—A Public Problem," *Woman Citizen* 9 (November 29, 1924): 25.

20. Allan M. Brandt, *No Magic Bullet,* 11; on 49–50, Brandt suggests that anxieties over sexuality caused an overreaction to the dangers of venereal disease. See also Connelly, "Prostitution," 197–200. The proportion of women who actually do develop pelvic disease following gonorrheal infection is unknown. In addition, because physicians in this period *believed* that gonorrhea caused most pelvic infections, they tended to underplay the other possible causes.

21. Brandt, *No Magic Bullet,* chaps. 2, 3, esp. pp. 85–91, 149.

22. Most of Clelia Mosher's research volumes in the Stanford University Library are devoted to studies of menstruation. In England, the principal of Newnham College, Cambridge (a woman's college) conducted a statistical analysis of women college graduates and their sisters, demonstrating, as Daniel Kevles has remarked, that such women "were just as healthy, just as likely to be married, and just as fertile as their less educated female relatives; the degree of spinsterhood and childlessness was a mark of their social class, not their higher learning." In the United States, the definitive study appeared in 1900. Among other findings, it demonstrated that controlling for years married, college women bore more children than noncollege women. Daniel Kevles, *In the Name of Eugenics: Genetics and the Uses of Human Heredity* (New York: Knopf, 1985), 89; Margaret M. Caffrey, *Ruth Benedict: Stranger in This Land* (Austin: University of Texas Press, 1989), p. 44.

23. Sheila Rothman, *Woman's Proper Place: A History of Changing Ideals and Practices, 1870 to the Present* (New York: Basic Books, 1978); John Modell, *Into One's Own: From Youth to Adulthood in the United States* (Berkeley: University of California Press, 1989), 114.

24. D'Emilio and Freedman, *Intimate Matters,* 223.

25. Carl M. Degler, "What Ought to Be and What Was: Women's Sexuality in the Nineteenth Century," *American Historical Review* 79 (1974): 1479–90. That Victorians were more sexual than they seemed is demonstrated in the Mosher study. See also D'Emilio and Freedman, *Intimate Matters,* esp. chap. 10; and Peter Gay, *The Education of the Senses* (New York: Oxford University Press, 1984), 71–95.

26. See Nancy Cott, *The Grounding of Modern Feminism* (New Haven: Yale University Press, 1987), 156–59; and D'Emilio and Freedman, *Intimate Matters,* 288.

27. Letters, *Good Housekeeping* 54 (January 1912): 88.

28. Ernest Groves quoted and discussed in Griswold, *Fatherhood in America,* 92; Walter Lippmann, *A Preface to Morals* (New York: Macmillan, 1929), 308.

29. Those who sought to combine a demanding career with marriage and a family invariably found their advancement stalled or blocked entirely. Women scientists, academics, and physicians almost inevitably found that if they married, their careers suffered irretrievable losses. For women professionals, see Penina Glazer and Miriam Slater, *Unequal Colleagues: The Entrance of Women into the Professions* (New Brunswick: Rutgers University Press, 1987).

30. Marsh, *Suburban Lives*, 136–37; Mary Roberts Coolidge, typewritten biographical notes re: Mosher, p. 18, Clelia Mosher Papers, Mosher Collection, Stanford University Library; Cott, *Grounding of Modern Feminism*, 174.

31. Goldin, *Understanding the Gender Gap*, 204–5; see also Van Horn, *Women, Work, and Fertility*, 33–35.

32. Katharine Bement Davis, *Factors in the Sex Life of Twenty-two Hundred Women* (1928; reprint, New York: Arno Press, 1972), 15, 44.

33. Ibid., 14–22.

34. Cott, *Grounding of Modern Feminism*, 158–62; see also Allen F. Davis, *American Heroine: The Life and Legend of Jane Addams* (New York: Oxford University Press, 1975).

35. Griswold, *Fatherhood in America*, 90–91, 93.

36. Letters, *Good Housekeeping* 52 (April 1911): 532.

37. Letters, *Good Housekeeping* 52 (July 1911): 21–22, 132; Letter, *Good Housekeeping* 52 (October 1911): 460–61; Richards, "Postponement of Motherhood," 84–85; Julia Ward Howe, "The Joys of Motherhood," *Delineator* 71 (May 1908): 806.

38. Candace Falk, *Love, Anarchy, and Emma Goldman* (New York: Holt, Rinehart and Winston, 1984), 30. On Ellen Key, see Cott, *Grounding of Modern Feminism*, 46–49.

39. Grace Ellery Channing, "The Children of the Barren," *Harper's Monthly Magazine* 114 (March 1907): 511–19.

40. Anna Hamlin Wikel, "The Childless Kindergartner," *Education* 22 (April 1902): 481.

41. Julie Berebitsky, " 'To Raise as Your Own': The Growth of Legal Adoption in Washington," *Washington History* 6 (spring/summer 1994): 4–26; Zelizer, *Pricing the Priceless Child*, 185–95.

42. Letters, container 3, files 255 and 263, Hillcrest Children's Center Papers, Library of Congress. Both letters were written to the Washington City Orphan Asylum, the first dated January 31, 1913, and the second undated but in file dated 1906–13. In order to protect confidentiality, we do not list the writers here.

43. Berebitsky, "To Raise as Your Own," 16–17. The *Delineator* campaign ran from 1907 through 1911. Numerous articles appeared: a few examples are Lydia Kingsmill Commander, "The Home without a Child," 70 (November 1907): 720–23ff.; "The Delineator Child-Rescue Campaign—For the Child That Needs a Home and the Home That Needs a Child," 71 (February 1908): 249–53; "Child Rescue," 71 (April 1908): 607–8; "What the Children Think of the Child-Rescue

Campaign," 72 (September 1908): 407–8ff.; and "The Gift of Life," 72 (August 1908): 262–63.

44. Letter to Washington City Orphan Asylum, container 3, file 255, Hillcrest Children's Center Papers.

45. Julie Berebitsky, "True Families: Adoption and the Children's Aid Society of Philadelphia, 1882–1900," paper, Temple University, 5 (used with permission).

46. See the *Delineator* articles in n. 43, above ("The Homeless Child and the Childless Home," *Charities and the Commons* [February 22, 1908]: 1612, is critical of the *Delineator*'s campaign); and Zelizer, *Pricing the Priceless Child*, 189–95.

47. See Judith Walzer Leavitt, *Brought to Bed: Childbearing in America, 1750–1950* (New York: Oxford University Press, 1986), 3, on the importance of childbearing. But culturally, childrearing was equally significant.

5. Degrees of Infertility

1. Robert T. Morris, *Lectures on Appendicitis and Notes on Other Subjects,* 3d ed. (New York: Putnam, 1899).

2. Ibid., 176; Robert Tuttle Morris, *Fifty Years a Surgeon* (New York: Dutton, 1935).

3. Victor Medvei, *A History of Endocrinology* (Boston: MTP Press, 1982), 296; Morris, *Lectures,* 176.

4. Morris, *Lectures,* 177–79; Robert T. Morris, "Case of Heteroplastic Ovarian Grafting, Followed by Pregnancy and the Delivery of a Living Child," *Medical Record* 69 (May 5, 1906): 697–98; Morris, *Fifty Years a Surgeon,* 218. Medvei, *History of Endocrinology,* 371, notes that whether the patient who gave birth conceived "because of the ovarian graft or whether some ovarian tissue had been left . . . is very difficult to prove."

5. Morris, "Case of Ovarian Grafting," 697; Morris, *Lectures,* 180.

6. Morris, *Lectures,* 180; Morris, "Case of Ovarian Grafting," 698.

7. Jean D. Wilson and Daniel W. Foster, eds., *Williams Textbook on Endocrinology* (Philadelphia: Saunders, 1992), 489; Thomas Addison, *On the Constitutional and Local Effects of Disease of the Supra-Renal Capsules* (London: Highly Publishers, 1855).

8. The English were skeptical about the efficacy of testicular extracts. See Merriley Borell, "Organotherapy, British Physiology, and the Internal Secretions," *Journal of the History of Biology* 9 (fall 1976): 235–68, at 238; and Medvei, *History of Endocrinology,* 189.

9. Medvei, *History of Endocrinology,* 336–37; John G. Gruhn and Ralph R. Kazor, *Hormonal Regulation of the Menstrual Cycle* (New York: Plenum Medical, 1989), 37.

10. Gruhn and Kazor, *Menstrual Cycle,* 43; Medvei, *History of Endocrinology,* 500–501; Merriley Borell, "Organotherapy and the Emergence of Repro-

ductive Endocrinology," *Journal of the History of Biology* 18 (spring 1985): 1–30, esp. 2.

11. Harold B. Shaw, *Organotherapy* (London, 1905), 2, 200–203, 205; Aleksandr V. Poehl, *Rational Organotherapy* (London: Churchill, 1906), 60–61, 150–68.

12. Samuel M. McCann, ed., *Endocrinology: People and Ideas* (Bethesda, Md.: American Physiological Society, 1988), 11.

13. Morris, *Lectures,* 176; Morris, *Fifty Years a Surgeon,* 217–19.

14. Henry R. Harrower, *The Internal Secretions in Practical Medicine* (Chicago: Chicago Medical Book, 1917), 115; Henry R. Harrower, *Practical Hormone Therapy* (New York: Paul Hoeber, 1914), 466.

15. Follicle-stimulating hormone is abbreviated FSH; luteinizing hormone is LH.

16. We have conflated this process into one paragraph so that the nonmedical reader will be able to follow the discussion.

17. There are a number of fascinating works detailing the scientific discoveries as they were in progress. Among the best are William P. Graves, *Female Sex Hormonology: A Review* (Philadelphia: Saunders, 1931); and George W. Corner, *The Hormones in Human Reproduction* (Princeton: Princeton University Press, 1942). Albert Q. Maisel, *The Hormone Quest* (New York: Random House, 1965), and Loretta McLaughlin, *The Pill, John Rock, and the Church* (Boston: Little, Brown, 1982), are more recent popular accounts.

18. First Annual Report of Committee for Research on Sex Problems, March 1, 1923, typescript, series 3, box 8, folder 189, p. 1, Bureau of Social Hygiene Archives (hereafter BSH), Rockefeller Archive Center.

19. Ibid.

20. Ibid.

21. Sophie Aberle and George Corner, *Twenty-five Years of Sex Research: A History of the National Research Council Committee for Research in Problems of Sex, 1922–1947* (Philadelphia: Saunders, 1953), 16–18, 32, 104. Lillie also was generously funded by the committee, receiving the second highest total amount of money for the entire twenty-five-year period covered by this history.

22. Ibid., 82–93.

23. James Reed, *From Private Vice to Public Virtue: A History of Birth Control in America* (New York: Basic Books, 1978), 313.

24. Aberle and Corner, *Twenty-five Years,* 90.

25. The involvement of pharmaceutical houses in research in reproductive endocrinology was an international phenomenon. See Nelly Oudshoorn, "Endocrinologists and the Conceptualization of Sex, 1920–1940," *Journal of the History of Biology* 23 (summer 1990): 163–86, at 166–68.

26. Gruhn and Kazor, *Menstrual Cycle,* 63–64; Corner, *Hormones in Human Reproduction,* 87.

27. Maisel, *Hormone Quest,* 34; Gruhn and Kazor, *Menstrual Cycle,* 77.

28. George Papanicolau developed the vaginal smear test. Maisel, *Hormone Quest,* 46–47; Reed, *Private Vice,* 314.

29. Frank Lillie, Report of Progress, 1929–30, series 3, box 8, folder 188, p. 1, BSH; Medvei, *History of Endocrinology,* 403.

30. Charles Gardner Child, *Sterility and Conception* (New York: Appleton, 1922), 21. See also Lewis Berman, *The Glands Regulating Personality* (New York: Macmillan, 1928); Thomas Scott, *Endocrine Therapeutics* (London: H. K. Lewis, 1922); and Theodore van de Velde, *Fertility and Sterility in Marriage* (New York: Random House, 1931), esp. 200–201.

31. Nancy Cott, *The Grounding of Modern Feminism* (New Haven: Yale University Press, 1987), 165–66; Claudia Goldin, *Understanding the Gender Gap* (New York: Oxford University Press, 1990), 140–42.

32. Susan Householder Van Horn, *Women, Work, and Fertility* (New York: New York University Press, 1988), 70.

33. Ibid., 77.

34. Samuel Meaker, *Human Sterility: Causation, Diagnosis, and Treatment: A Practical Manual of Clinical Procedure* (Baltimore: Williams and Wilkins, 1934), 244–45.

35. Gladys Denny Shultz, "Maybe You Can Have a Baby," *Better Homes and Gardens* 18 (August 1940): 46.

36. Meaker, *Human Sterility,* 253–56; Samuel Lewis Siegler, *Fertility in Women: Causes, Diagnosis, and Treatment of Impaired Fertility* (Philadelphia: Lippincott, 1944), 25.

37. For discussion of the Rubin test, see the comments following N. Sproat Heaney, "A Simple Method of Testing the Patency of the Fallopian Tubes," *Gynecological Transactions* 48 (1923): 218.

38. Child, *Sterility and Conception,* 75–79; Edward Reynolds and Donald Macomber, *Fertility and Sterility in Human Marriage* (Philadelphia: Saunders, 1924), 84–86; Robert A. Gibbons, *Sterility in Woman* (London: Churchill, 1923), 27, 97.

39. The English, by contrast, retained a stronger faith, although no higher a success rate, in the possibility of pregnancy after surgery. Meaker, *Human Sterility,* 227.

40. Van de Velde, *Fertility and Sterility in Marriage,* 35; Gibbons, 138.

41. Van de Velde, *Fertility and Sterility in Marriage,* 201.

42. Reed, *Private Vice,* 181–93. See Linda Gordon, *Woman's Body, Woman's Right* (New York: Viking, 1976), 262, for discussion of Dickinson's relationship with Margaret Sanger.

43. Reed discusses Dickinson and the Committee on Maternal Health (ibid., 168–91, quoted material from 184–85). According to files in the Rockefeller Archive Center, during the period 1929 to 1932, the Bureau of Social Hygiene contributed $46,900 to the committee. Individual donations at the nadir of the depression included $1,000 from Gertrude Minturn Pinchot; other women gave amounts ranging from $250 to $2,000. These contributions were less than usual,

the memo went on to say, because the depression had cut into the benefactors' incomes. Memo from Ruth Topping to Lawrence Dunham, January 17, 1933, and File Memorandum RT, June 29, 1932, both in series 3, box 7, folder 174, BSH.

44. See Louise Bryant, "Appeal to the Bureau of Social Hygiene from the Committee on Maternal Health," December 8, 1928, series 3, box 7, folder 173, BSH.

45. This memo describes the nature of the committee's interest in researching infertility problems. Some of the staff members at the Bureau of Social Hygiene did not share Dickinson's enthusiasm for linking birth control and research on infertility. See, for example, memo from Lawrence Dunham to Raymond Fosdick, December 14, 1927, and Fosdick's December 22 reply, series 3, box 7, folder 173; also letter from R. L. Dickinson to K. B. Davis, January 14, 1925, folder 172; and a memo that says only "Topping" in upper right, n.d., folder 175, all in BSH. The Committee for Maternal Health funded Moench's research. See File Memorandum RT, November 28, 1932, folder 174, BSH.

46. Robert L. Dickinson, "Investigation of Human Sterility: Memorandum of Project to Be Undertaken by the Committee on Maternal Health," December 5, 1927, series 3, box 7, folder 173, BSH; Meaker, *Human Sterility*, 8–10.

47. Meaker, *Human Sterility*, 8–10; Samuel R. Meaker, "Two Million American Homes Childless," *Hygieia* 5 (November 1927): 346–48.

48. Meaker, *Human Sterility*, 19, 36, 43–44.

49. Ibid., vii, 9. Meaker's reasoned argument cut no ice with some of his colleagues. Sam Gordon Berkow, writing for a general audience in *Childless: A Study of Sterility, Its Causes, and Treatment* (New York: Lee Furman, 1937), used those very genealogical studies to say (28–29) that sterility had increased 600–fold since the late eighteenth century.

50. Meaker, *Human Sterility*, 9.

51. Ibid., 46, 227, 245, 18–25.

52. Ibid., 76.

53. Molly Ladd-Taylor, *Raising a Baby the Government Way: Mothers' Letters to the Children's Bureau, 1915–1932* (New Brunswick: Rutgers University Press, 1986), 66.

54. Ibid., 64–68.

55. Ibid., 67–68.

56. See, e.g., *Hygieia* 5 (February 1927): 100–101; Meaker, "Two Million Homes Childless," 346–48; Helen Huntington Smith, "Making It Possible to Have a Baby," *Parents* 9 (November 1934): 18–19ff.; James A. Tobey, "The Control of Human Sterility," *Scribner's Magazine* 89 (April 1931): 421–24; *Reader's Digest*, "Test-Tube Babies" (February 1937): 18–20; and Maxine Davis, "Why Don't We Have a Baby?" *Pictorial Review* 40 (January 1939): 12–13ff. Quotations from Smith, 19, and Davis, 13. We mean, in this instance, childlessness among married couples, not the total number of women, married or single, who never bore children.

57. Comment by Asta Wittner following Sophia Kleegman, "Recent Advances

in the Diagnosis and Treatment of Sterility," *Medical Women's Journal* 46 (January 1939): 10; Davis, "Why Don't We Have a Baby?" 12.

58. Meaker, *Human Sterility,* 74–76, 79; Cedric Lane-Roberts et al., *Sterility and Impaired Fertility* (New York: Hoeber, 1939), 17.

59. Deborah Dwork, "Sophia Josephine Kleegman," in Barbara Sicherman and Carol Hurd Green, eds., *Notable American Women: The Modern Period* (Cambridge: Harvard University Press, 1980), 399–400; Kleegman, "Recent Advances," 1–10; and see Margaret C. Sturgis, "Fertility," *Transactions of the 52nd Annual Meeting of the Alumnae Association of the Woman's Medical College of Pennsylvania* (1927): 63, for a similar view.

60. Wittner, commenting on Kleegman, "Recent Advances," 10.

61. Davis, "Why Don't We Have a Baby?" 12–13; Meaker, *Human Sterility,* 83–86.

62. Smith, "Making It Possible," 67–68; Berkow, *Childless,* 248–49; Samuel L. Siegler, *Fertility in Women* (Philadelphia: Lippincott, 1944), 200.

63. Meaker, *Human Sterility,* 11, 79.

64. See, e.g., Kleegman, "Recent Advances," pp. 1–10. The next chapter provides an extensive discussion of the clinic at the Free Hospital in the post–World War II era.

65. We discuss Rock extensively in the next chapter. See John Rock, "Harvard 50th Report," November 5, 1964, typescript, pp. 1–3, John Rock Papers, Rare Books and Manuscripts Division, Countway Library of Medicine, Harvard University; Patient Records, handwritten, 1932–35; "Report on Sterility Cases," n.d., but internal evidence suggests the early 1950s and the cases are from the 1940s, typescript, n.p., Rock Papers. The Rock Papers are as yet uncatalogued.

66. Meaker, *Human Sterility,* 14, 237–41.

67. Lane-Roberts et al., *Sterility and Impaired Fertility,* 122. British physicians sometimes did surgical grafts of pituitary tissue to increase sperm count, but Americans do not seem to have taken up the practice to any great extent.

68. Siegler, *Fertility in Women,* 238, 262, discusses the successes of Rubin and others.

69. Frances Seymour, "A Simple Method of Tubal Insufflation for Treatment of Sterility," *Medical Woman's Journal* (May 1938): 120–22; Siegler, *Fertility in Women,* 238, 262, emphasis in original.

70. Kleegman, "Recent Advances," 5; Meaker, *Human Sterility,* 74–76; Case Records of Laparotomies, 1933, Rock Papers.

71. Kleegman, "Recent Advances," 5; Meaker, *Human Sterility,* 74–76.

72. Edgar Allen et al., *Sex and the Internal Secretions* (Baltimore: Williams and Wilkins, 1932), 1292.

73. Davis, "Why Don't We Have a Baby?" 12, 13ff.

74. "Ghost Fathers," *Newsweek* (May 12, 1934): 16; *New York Times,* May 1, 1934, 25.

75. See, e.g., Herman Rohleder, *Test Tube Babies: A History of the Artificial Impregnation of Human Beings* (New York: Panurge Press, 1934), 26, 40, 169.

76. Berkow, *Childless,* 251–52; van de Velde, *Fertility and Sterility in Marriage,* 164; Rohleder, *Test Tube Babies,* 159; Edward Fyfe Griffith, *The Childless Family: Its Cause and Cure* (London: Kegan Paul, 1939, 123.

77. John Harvey Caldwell, "Babies by Scientific Selection," *Scientific American* 150 (March 1934): 124–25.

78. *National Cyclopaedia of American Biography,* vol. C (New York: James T. White, 1930), s.v. "Holmes, John Haynes"; "Ghost Fathers," 16; Allen et al., *Sex and the Internal Secretions,* 1292.

79. Kleegman, "Recent Advances," 10; Anne Lockhart Needham, "Artificial Insemination and the Emergence of Medical Authority in Twentieth-Century America" (bachelor's thesis, Harvard University, 1988), 64–65, 84–85.

80. Quotation from Joseph Francis Fletcher, *Morals and Medicine* (Princeton: Princeton University Press, 1954), 103–4; Frances Seymour and Alfred Koerner, "Artificial Insemination: Present Status in the United States as Shown by a Recent Survey," *Journal of the American Medical Association* 116 (June 21, 1941): 2747–49; Clair E. Folsome, "The Status of Artificial Insemination," *American Journal of Obstetrics and Gynecology* 45 (June 1943): 915–27; Needham, "Artificial Insemination," 83.

81. "Test-Tube Babies: A Medico-Legal Discussion," *Scientific American* 156 (January 1937): 40–41ff.; Needham, "Artificial Insemination," 91–98.

82. Needham, "Artificial Insemination," 85–87.

83. J. D. Ratcliff, "Clinics for the Childless," *Hygieia* 19 (October 1941): 854.

84. *Newsweek* (September 13, 1943): 87–88; Marie Beynon Ray, "Fathers Anonymous: Artificial Insemination," *Woman's Home Companion* 72 (January 1945): 20.

85. *Newsweek* (September 13, 1943); "Test-Tube Babies" (*Scientific American*); Albert Horlings, "Can They Have Children?" *Harper's Magazine* 184 (January 1942): 184.

86. "Gracie's Own Story, as Told to Jane Kessner Morris," *Woman's Home Companion* (March 1953), 40ff., does not mention that her children were adopted; George Burns, *Gracie: A Love Story* (New York: Putnam, 1988), 120–23.

87. Paula F. Pfeffer, "Homeless Children, Childless Homes," *Chicago History* (spring 1987): 50–62; George Walsh, *Gentleman Jimmy Walker* (New York: Praeger, 1974), 336–339.

88. *New York Times,* March 20, 1936, 25; *New York Times,* March 24, 1936, 25; *New York Times,* March 29, sec. 2, p. 1; Benson Jaffee and David Fanshel, *How They Fared in Adoption: A Follow-up Study* (New York: Columbia University Press, 1970), esp. 62–64. See also Tobey, "Control of Human Sterility," 422; Shultz, "Maybe You Can," 59; Griffith, *Childless Family,* 12; *Hygieia* article cited

in Ratcliff, "Clinics for the Childless," 854; and McLaughlin, *John Rock,* 49. John Rock conducted the studies debunking the relationship between adoption and fertility, which are discussed in the next chapter.

89. Jaffee and Fanshel, *How They Fared,* 62–64.

90. Ibid., 49–52; "Adoptions in Pennsylvania," Public Charities Association of Pennsylvania, Philadelphia, 1939, typescript, p. 9, Library of Congress.

91. Rickie Solinger, *The Abortionist: A Woman against the Law* (New York: Free Press, 1994), 44; Pfeffer, "Homeless Children," 63.

92. Quoted in Viviana Zelizer, *Pricing the Priceless Child: The Changing Social Value of Children* (New York: Basic Books, 1985), 192.

93. Case Records of Laparotomies, 1933, Rock Papers.

6. "Such Great Strides"

Epigraph from Grace Naismith, "Helping the Childless," *Today's Health* 32 (February 1954): 21.

1. John Rock and Miriam F. Menkin, "In Vitro Fertilization and Cleavage of Human Ovarian Eggs," *Science* 100 (August 4, 1944): 105–7. The full report was published later, as Miriam F. Menkin and John Rock, "In Vitro Fertilization and Cleavage of Human Ovarian Eggs," *American Journal of Obstetrics and Gynecology* 55 (March 1948): 440–51. Letter to Miriam Menkin from P. D., August 4, 1944; letter to John Rock from Carl Hartman, June 8, 1954, both in John Rock Papers, Rare Books and Manuscripts Division, Countway Library of Medicine, Harvard University; Sam Gordon Berkow, "After Office Hours: A Visit with Dr. John Rock," *Obstetrics and Gynecology* 15 (May 1960): 665–72, at 668.

2. Miriam Menkin, "Notes for Lecture, American Association of Anatomists," 1948, typescript, p. 3, Rock Papers.

3. Berkow, "After Office Hours"; John Rock, "Harvard 50th Report," November 5, 1964, typescript, Rock Papers. Loretta McLaughlin, *The Pill, John Rock, and the Church* (Boston: Little, Brown, 1982), is the only book-length biography of Rock, although James Reed, *Birth Control in America: From Private Vice to Public Virtue* (New York: Basic Books, 1978), also has some biographical information.

4. McLaughlin, *John Rock,* 68–71. We have reviewed some forty boxes of Rock's papers, which he does not appear to have censored (or organized), and which remain pretty much in the state they arrived in at the Countway Library. The cumulative impact of these papers was to convince us that Rock deserved the affection that both his patients and his staff bestowed on him.

5. John Rock, "The Problem of Sterility," *New England Journal of Medicine* (hereafter *NEJM*) 199 (July 12, 1928): 79–85; "Incomplete Survey of Sterility Patients Made by Dr. Fleck in 1939," 1939, handwritten, Rock Papers. By the end of the 1930s, Rock had become skeptical of the animal gonadotropins currently available, although when new ones were developed, he seemed always to give

them a try. Henry W. Erving, Christine Sears, and John Rock, "Clinical Experience with Equine Gonadotropic Hormone," draft of paper, typescript [1939]; Stephen Fleck, "Human Fertility . . . in the Light of Public Health," 1939, typescript, pp. 45–54, both in Rock Papers.

6. Fleck, "Human Fertility," 47.

7. William L. Estes, "A Method of Implanting Ovarian Tissue in Order to Maintain Ovarian Function," *Pennsylvania Medical Journal* (May 1910): 610–13; William L. Estes Jr., "Further Results with Ovarian Implantation," *Journal of the American Medical Association* 83 (August 30, 1924): 674–77. Hans Simmer, "After Office Hours: Robert Tuttle Morris: Pioneer in Ovarian Transplants," *Obstetrics and Gynecology* 35 (February 1970): 324, mentions the Estes operation and notes that "ovarian autotransplants did enable women to become pregnant, [but] the success rate was . . . 6% or less." He does not mention the source of his figure; it may have been the 4 out of 95 cited by Estes Jr.

8. Some biographical information on Menkin is in McLaughlin, *John Rock,* 70–78; quotation from Miriam Menkin, "Lecture Prepared for Delivery at Cold Spring Harbor," July 26, 1949, typescript, Rock Papers.

9. The following story was pieced together from these sources: "Plans for Ova Research," November 9, 1940, typescript; "Human Ova," January 22, 1942, typescript; "Figures on Number of Patients Studied," March 24, 1948, typescript; Menkin, "Cold Spring Harbor," all in Rock Papers.

10. They obtained a total of 800 ova from 245 patients, but most of them for one reason or another were not deemed suitable for fertilization. The 138 came from 47 women. Rock Papers.

11. Menkin, "Cold Spring Harbor," 14.

12. Ibid.

13. Ibid., last page.

14. See clipping, newspaper unknown but probably Boston, August 4, 1945, Rock Papers; letters cited below.

15. Mrs. G. P. H. to Miriam Menkin, November 23, 1944; Mrs. P. C. H. to Miriam Menkin, November 21, 1944; Mrs. H. M. D. to "Dear Sirs," August 17, 1944, all in Rock Papers.

16. John Rock to Mrs. P. C. H., November 30, 1944; John Rock to Mrs. T. R. N., October 16, 1944; John Rock to Mrs. H. M. D., August 31, 1944, all in Rock Papers.

17. Mrs. J. R. to John Rock, n.d.; John Rock to Mrs. J. R., March 19, 1945; John Rock to Mrs. L. C., April 28, 1945, all in Rock Papers.

18. J. D. Ratcliff, "Babies by Proxy," *Look* (January 31, 1950): 44.

19. Mrs. E. M. to John Rock, January 1950; Mrs. B. S. to John Rock, March 19, 1950, both in Rock Papers.

20. Mrs. L. W. to John Rock, October 11, 1950; John Rock to Mrs. L. W., October 16, 1950, both in Rock Papers.

21. Typewritten abstract of findings of "A. Westman, *Acta. Obst. et Gynec.*

Scandinav. 30: 186–202, reported in *Yr. Bk. Obstet. and Gyn.*, 1951, 313–14"; notes probably taken by Menkin, and part of a series of abstracts on surgical treatment of sterility, especially tuboplasty, 1951, both in Rock Papers.

22. Mrs. R. T. to John Rock, July 13, 1951, August 6, 1951; Rock's replies, July 23, 1951, August 9, 1951, all in Rock Papers.

23. See clipping dated August 4, 1944, Boston newspaper, unidentified further, Rock Papers, for Rock's hope that IVF would prove a practical way around blocked fallopian tubes.

24. McLaughlin, *John Rock*, 87, states that opposition from the Catholic Church to this and Rock's embryo study with C. Hertig, for which he and Hertig won an award from the American Gynecological Society in 1949, was what caused them to stop. However, neither any information in the Rock Papers nor the director's reports in the Free Hospital's annual reports supports that idea. Perhaps McLaughlin, or perhaps Rock himself, whom she interviewed toward the end of his life, conflated the later intense opposition to such research with this earlier period. Landrum Shettles is discussed in more detail in Chapter 6.

25. Paul Starr, *The Social Transformation of American Medicine* (New York: Basic Books, 1982), 352–53.

26. Albert Q. Maisel, "Beware the Fertility Racketeers," *Park East* (April 1952): 17–20, quotation on 17; Albert Q. Maisel, "The Truth about Sterility," *Parents* 28 (January 1953): 44ff.

27. Maisel, "Truth about Sterility," 44; Isabella Taves, "New Advance in Female Fertility," *Look* 28 (May 19, 1964): 93; Fred A. Simmons, "Medical Progress in Human Infertility," *NEJM* 255 (December 13, 1956): 1145.

28. Simmons, "Medical Progress," 1191; letters to John Rock, 1945–1960, Rock Papers. Rock either sent his correspondents the name of a specialist or, if he knew no one in their area, asked Planned Parenthood to provide a referral.

29. See McLaughlin, *John Rock*, 41. Rock's reports in the annual reports of the Free Hospital, available for most of the 1940s through his retirement in 1955, provide details of each year's funding. Rock Papers.

30. Beginning in the 1950s, the Rock Papers are full of notes to, from, and about all the students, fellows, and practitioners who worked or observed at Rock's clinic. See, for example, Anthony Cominos to John Rock, July 18, 1957; John Rock to Anthony Cominos, October 29, 1957; "the Mastroianni Family" to John Rock, May 4, 1957; Celso-Ramon Garcia to Luigi Mastroianni, June 25, 1958; John Rock from Angeliki Tsacona, September 30, 1965; and John Rock to Angeliki Tsacona, December 11, 1965.

31. Fibroids can cause infertility if their location in the uterus obstructs the opening into the fallopian tubes. Janet Schwartz's story was obtained through the Marsh/Ronner Infertility Survey.

32. Susan Householder Van Horn, *Women, Work, and Fertility* (New York: New York University Press, 1988), 92; National Center for Health Statistics, *Vital Statistics of the United States, 1989*, vol. 1, *Natality*, DHHS Pub. no. (PHS)

93-1100 (Washington, D.C.: U.S. Government Printing Office, 1993), 1–2, 33–37, 47–48.

33. Margaret Marsh, *Suburban Lives* (New Brunswick: Rutgers University Press, 1990), 184–85; Elaine Tyler May, *Homeward Bound* (New York: Basic Books, 1988), 160; Robert Griswold, *Fatherhood in America: A History* (New York: Basic Books, 1993), 188–89.

34. May, *Homeward Bound*, 139; Van Horn, *Women, Work, and Fertility*, 95–96; *Vital Statistics*, 35, 37.

35. P. Cutright and E. Shorter, "The Effects of Health on the Completed Fertility of Non-white and White U.S. Women Born from 1867 to 1935," *Journal of Social History* 13 (winter 1979): 201; Van Horn, *Women, Work, and Fertility*, 151.

36. Judy Seabaugh, "Please Stop Telling Me That I Have to Have a Baby," *Redbook* 121 (May 1963): 6; Marsh/Ronner Infertility Survey.

37. See *Vital Statistics*, 34. Fred Simmons, in "Medical Progress," 1140, put the infertility rate at about 15 percent, but popular articles sometimes put it as high as 17 percent. See, for example, Lawrence Galton, "What Every Husband Should Know about Sterility," *Better Homes and Gardens* 28 (October 1949): 42; Clarissa Lorenz, "Hope for the Childless," *Today's Health* 29 (October 1951): 20; Maisel, "Truth about Sterility," 71; I. C. Rubin, as told to Margaret Albrecht, "Childlessness and What Can Be Done about It," *Parents* 32 (March 1957): 46.

38. Galton, "What Every Husband Should Know," 42; Maisel, "Truth about Sterility," 44; Joseph Wassersug, "More Help for the Childless," *Hygieia* 25 (November 1947): 835; Maxine Davis, "Infertility," *Good Housekeeping* 137 (August 1953): 154. Edward Tyler was somewhat more cautious, saying in 1957 that cure rates were at about one-third but were continuing to rise. Edward Tyler as told to Roland Berg, "Childless Couples Can Have Babies," *Look* 21 (September 17, 1957): 41–42ff.

39. "Desire Was My Downfall," *Tan Confessions* 1 (March 1951): 21–22ff.; Julian Lewis, "Babies for Childless Couples," *Tan Confessions* 1 (October 1951): 48–49ff.; "We Had to Have a Baby," *Tan Confessions* 2:3 (January 1952): 22–23ff. This magazine was published by an African American–controlled corporation and was designed to appeal principally to women. *Childless* advertisement in *Ebony* 3 (July 1948): 46; see "How to Plan a Family," *Ebony* 3 (July 1948): 13–17; David Toth, letter to the editor regarding the infertility services of Planned Parenthood in Delaware, *Ebony* 4 (November 1948).

40. As readers will recall from the last chapter, some practitioners claimed a 33 percent pregnancy rate in the 1930s as well. But in the immediate postwar era, 25 percent seemed to be the common estimate. Dorothy Schotton, "The Management of Pregnancy in the Previously Infertile Woman," *Proceedings of the Society for the Study of Sterility* 6 (1954): 1; S. Bender, "End Results in Treatment of Primary Sterility," *Fertility and Sterility* (hereafter *Fertil. Steril.*) 4:1 (1953): 42; Robert Wilson, "One Thousand Cases of Infertility: Clinical Review of a Five Year Series," *Fertil. Steril.* 4 (1953): 292–99; "Infertility Clinics Report 1-in-4 Success

Ratio," *Planned Parenthood News* (summer 1954): 2. Figures for the Rock Clinic in unidentified 1949 newspaper clipping, "Brookline Group Seeks Solution to Infertility," Rock Papers. The Brookline clinic still compared favorably with rates obtained by other hospital clinics. Rock's rate of pregnancy among private patients, due in part "to a closer watch of the patients and a higher degree of cooperation," was 25 percent (ibid.). In the 1950s the rate improved for a couple of years, to nearly 30 percent, but then it dropped to 21 percent. The drop after a two-year rise, Rock believed, occurred because he was seeing greater numbers of patients who came to him after being unsuccessfully treated elsewhere. *Free Hospital For Women,* Annual Report (Boston, 1953), 17, Rock Papers.

41. Patient statistics attached to letter from Frederick Hanson to John Rock, n.d., probably early 1950s. At the end of the decade, he was reporting about a one-third pregnancy rate in his new practice. Rock Papers.

42. Maisel, "Beware the Fertility Racketeers," 17–20.

43. *Free Hospital for Women,* Annual Reports, 1940 through 1956, Rock Papers.

44. Patient Records, 1950s, Rock Papers.

45. Stephen Fleck, "Incomplete Survey of Sterility Patients Made by Dr. Fleck in 1939," handwritten, 1939; *Free Hosital for Women,* Annual Report [1950]; Patient Records, 1950s, all in Rock Papers.

46. The information about low-income patients and Blue Cross is in a typescript draft of an article by Grace Naismith that appeared in *Today's Health* in 1953. The draft contains more detailed financial data than the published piece. Untitled draft, beginning, "She was a pretty . . . ," 1953, 14–15; Patient Billing Records sample, 1951, 1954–55, both in Rock Papers.

47. Clipping, n.d., Rock Papers.

48. *Seventieth Annual Report of the Free Hospital for Women* (Boston, 1945), 19; *Free Hospital for Women,* Annual Report (Boston, 1955), 16; *Free Hospital for Women,* Annual Report (Boston, 1956), 18, all in Rock Papers.

49. *Free Hospital for Women,* Annual Report (Boston, 1955), 18.

50. Simmons, "Medical Progress," 1140, 1145.

51. R. W. Noyes, A. T. Hertig, and J. Rock, "Dating the Endometrial Biopsy," *Fertil. Steril.* 1 (1950): 3–25. This important article eventually became the most cited of all articles from this journal. See Edward E. Wallach and Serena H. Chen, "Five Decades of Progress in Management of the Infertile Couple," *Fertil. Steril.* 62 (October 1994): 665–85; records of ovarian resections, Rock Papers. Fred Simmons discussed the current use of such treatments in "Medical Progress," 1190–91. A fellow Harvard faculty member who treated infertility at Massachusetts General Hospital, Simmons also argued that too many physicians misdiagnosed endometriosis and performed unnecessary surgery on young women. "I have seen young women deprived of their gonads," he noted, "by well meaning surgeons who did not recognize that this disease could be resected from the ovary, with functioning ovarian tissue left behind" (1191).

52. "Tuboplasty," typescript abstract of studies to 1951, 20 pp.; Simmons, "Medical Progress," 1142–43.

53. C. Mazur and S. L. Israel, considered eminent authorities, cautioned that only a woman with a bilateral, total occlusion, with the occlusion at the fimbriated extremity (the end at which the egg enters the tube) of at least one tube, in whom "all other . . . factors" that might cause infertility had been ruled out, should be considered a candidate for tubal surgery. At that, they argued, the couple should be willing to accept "a 5 per cent chance of pregnancy as a result of the operation." Others were a little less pessimistic, but still cautious. Simmons, "Medical Progress," 1142–43.

54. John Rock, "Surgery for Infertility," page proofs of an essay based on a paper read in Washington, D.C., in March 1956, p. 2, Rock Papers. A review of the articles that appeared in the first decade of the publication of *Fertil. Steril.* (1950–59), which was the U.S.'s most important infertility journal, demonstrates the surgical conservatism of the infertility elite.

55. John V. Kelly and John Rock, "Culdoscopy for Diagnosis in Infertility," *American Journal of Obstetrics and Gynecology* 72 (September 1956): 523–27; John Rock, "Surgery for Infertility," p. 7, Rock Papers; John Rock et al., "Polyethylene in Tuboplasty," *Obstetrics and Gynecology* 3 (January 1954): 21–29.

56. Casebook Records, 1950s, Rock Papers; Simmons, "Medical Progress," 1143.

57. For example, Clarissa Lorenz, "Hope for the Childless," *Today's Health* 29 (October 1951): 21; I. C. Rubin, "Childlessness and What Can Be Done about It," *Parents* 22 (December 1947): 70; and W. S. Kroger, "Evaluation of Personality Factors in the Treatment of Infertility," *Fertil. Steril.* 3 (1952): 548.

58. Earle M. Marsh and Albert M. Vollmer, "Possible Psychogenic Aspects of Infertility," *Fertil. Steril.* 2:1 (1951): 75–76.

59. Simmons, "Medical Progress," 1141, 1188.

60. John Rock, "Diagnosis and Treatment of Infertility," lecture, postgraduate course in infertility, 1956, typescript, pp. 9–10, Rock Papers. Earlier, on the basis of thirty-two cases, he had indeed reported very good results with antibiotic therapy. Herbert Horne Jr. and John Rock, "Oral Terramycin Therapy of Chronic Endocervicitis in Infertile Women," *Fertil. Steril.* 3:4 (1952): 321–27.

61. Rock, "Diagnosis and Treatment of Infertility," 1956, 12. These compounds were, of course, the prototypes of the famous birth control pill.

62. Lawrence Galton, "What Every Husband Should Know about Sterility," *Better Homes and Gardens* 28 (October 1949): 42ff.

63. Genevieve Parkhurst, *American Mercury* 64 (June 1947): 713; Galton, "Every Husband," 42.

64. Bruce Bliven Jr., "Fertility Miracle for Childless Couples," *Woman's Home Companion* (June 1953): 92.

65. Fred A. Simmons, "The Treatment of Male Sterility," *Fertil. Steril.* 1 (1950): 193–98.

66. Simmons, "Male Sterility," 193; Abner I. Weisman, "End Results of the Treatment of Male Infertility," *Fertil. Steril.* 1 (1950): 216–22. See also the issue of vol. 2, no. 2, of this journal, which is devoted entirely to male infertility. Its major thrust is the frustration of researchers and clinicians over the intractability of the problem.

67. Simmons, "Male Sterility," 193.

68. See Edward Henderson, "Testosterone and Testicular Function," 1956[?], typescript, p. 5; "Rebound from Azoospermia Tied to Pregnancy Increase," *New York Herald Tribune* clipping marked "filed 1/28/58," both in Rock Papers. See also Simmons, "Medical Progress," 1145.

69. Rock, "Diagnosis and Treatment of Infertility," [1956], pp. 2, 6–7.

70. For artificial insemination in Rock's practice, see Ledger Books 2 (early 1950s), 7 (late 1950s), and 9 (1960s); Rock, "Diagnosis and Treatment of Infertility," [1956], p. 8, all in Rock Papers. The concentrate/cap technique was earlier advocated by James Whitelaw, "Use of the Cervical Cap to Increase Fertility in the Case of Oligospermia," *Fertil. Steril.* 1:1 (1950): 22–99. Last quote from an early draft of an article by Frederick Hanson and John Rock, "Artificial Insemination with Husband's Sperm," [1950], typescript, p. 1, Rock Papers.

71. Simmons, "Medical Progress," 1146.

72. See, e.g., ibid., 1146–47.

73. Sophia Kleegman, "Therapeutic Donor Insemination," *Fertil. Steril.* 5:1 (1954): 11–12.

74. Allan Morrison, "Test-tube Babies," *Ebony* 5 (July 1950): 65–69.

75. Milton Golin, "Paternity by Proxy," *Medico-Legal Digest* (May 1960): 17–20; Emily Patt, "A Pathfinder on Artificial Insemination," *Legal Reference Services Quarterly* 8:1/2 (1988): 131–32.

76. The following discussion of adoption is focused specifically on the connections between adoption and infertility. There is no attempt to consider any of the extensive literature on the institutional or legal history of adoption itself in the 1950s.

77. Helen L. Witmer et al., *Independent Adoptions* (New York: Russell Sage Foundation, 1963), 85, 96.

78. Quoted in Frederick H. Hanson and John Rock, "The Effect of Adoption on Fertility and Other Reproductive Functions," typescript [March 1949], p. 7, Rock Papers.

79. Hanson and Rock went on to note that surgical treatment of endometriosis was known to be followed by pregnancy "within a year or two" without adoption. Ibid., 3–4.

80. The Marsh/Ronner Infertility Survey was the result of a request we made to *Philadelphia Inquirer* family life columnist Lucia Herndon. We received twenty-three responses to our request for letters from women who had experienced difficulty conceiving. Twenty-one of them filled out questionnaires, which included

personal narratives of their experiences. This is one of those experiences. The name is a pseudonym.

81. Ibid. This name too is a pseudonym.

82. Ibid.

83. Hanson and Rock, "Effect of Adoption," 12. After their findings were published in the *American Journal of Obstetrics and Gynecology,* other studies, including one by Edward Tyler, confirmed their conclusions. John Rock et al., "Effect of Adoption on Infertility," page proofs of article for *Fertility and Sterility;* "Have Few Children Following Adoptions," *Science News Letter* 80 (July 8, 1961): 25.

84. The Grace Fuschetto story is in Alan Levy, "The Baby She'd Always Wanted," *Good Housekeeping* (February 1967): 48ff.

85. Ibid.

86. Taves, "New Advance," 93.

87. C. Lee Buxton et al., "The Effect of Human FSH and LH on the Anovulatory Ovary," typescript of paper presented at the annual meeting of the American Gynecological Society, May 13–15, 1963, p. 3, Rock Papers; see, e.g., John Rock, "Discussion of Paper by C. Lee Buxton," 1963, typescript, n.p. In his comments on this report, which was delivered to an audience of gynecologists, John Rock cautioned Buxton both not to be too quick to attribute ovulation to his therapy, since he got only two pregnancies and in his experience women often began to ovulate unexplainedly even after long anovulatory periods, and to be very careful about multiple births.

88. For accounts aimed at a general audience, see, e.g., Taves, "New Advance," 91–96; Alan Levy, "Now! Many Women Can Have the Babies They Want," *Good Housekeeping* 157 (October 1963): 79ff.; Levy, "Baby She'd Always Wanted," 48ff.; and "Fertility Drug Has Double Action," *Medical World News* (April 13, 1962): 87. Domini was not the only researcher to have this idea: see E. C. Jungck and W. E. Brown, "Human Pituitary Gonadotropin for Clinical Use: Preparation and Lack of Antihormone Formation," *Fertil. Steril.* 3 (1952): 224–29.

89. Aloys H. Naville et al., "Induction of Ovulation with Clomiphene Citrate," *Fertil. Steril.* 15:3 (1964): 290–309; Elliot Rivo and John Rock, "The Clinical Use of Clomiphene Citrate," *Pacific Medicine and Surgery* 73 (November–December 1965): 419.

90. We discuss both drugs more fully in Chapter 7.

7. "The End of the Beginning"?

1. Marsh/Ronner Infertility Survey.

2. Susan Householder Van Horn, *Women, Work, and Fertility* (New York: New York University Press, 1988), 151–54. These 63.5 million babies were born during the period 1946–60. During the previous fifteen years, only 41.5 million

babies were born in the United States. See Mary Beth Norton et al., *A People and a Nation*, 2d ed. (Boston: Houghton Mifflin, 1986), A-17; Stephanie Coontz, *The Way We Never Were: American Families and the Nostalgia Trap* (New York: Basic Books, 1992), 24; and Victor Fuchs, *How We Live: An Economic Perspective on Americans from Birth to Death* (Cambridge: Harvard University Press, 1983), 259. Note that the childlessness rate included all women, divorced, widowed, and single, as well as married. Women born in later years of the baby boom have not yet ended their childbearing years. Since the fertility statistics continued to show an increase in childbearing among women in their thirties as late as the early 1990s, we cannot give a figure for their overall childlessness, but it is estimated to be around 16–17 percent. See Amara Bachu, "Fertility of American Women," *Current Population Reports: Population Characteristics* (June 1992): xx–xxi.

3. Norton et al., *People and a Nation*, 882.

4. Fuchs, *How We Live*, 22. See also Claudia Goldin, *Understanding the Gender Gap: An Economic History of American Women* (New York: Oxford University Press, 1990), 140–41; Norton et al., *People and a Nation*, 976–77; and Van Horn, *Women, Work, and Fertility*, 157.

5. James Reed, *From Private Vice to Public Virtue* (New York: Basic Books, 1978), 369, 373.

6. Unsigned article in *Look* 34 (September 22, 1970): 17; see also "Make Love, Not Babies," *Newsweek* 75 (June 15, 1970): 111. A few "antichild" articles appeared in the 1960s, but in the 1970s they became pervasive and did not really moderate until the end of the decade. We surveyed popular magazines as well as social science–oriented publications such as the *Journal of Marriage and the Family*. See "Childless Bliss," *Newsweek* 84 (December 9, 1974): 87; Ann Landers, "If You Had It to Do Over Again—Would You Have Children?" *Good Housekeeping* 182 (June 1976): 100–101ff.; and Tilla Vahanian and Sally Wendkos Olds, "Will Your Children Break . . . or Make . . . Your Marriage?" *Parents* 49 (August 1974): 79. J. E. Veevers, who studied voluntary childlessness throughout the decade, argued in 1979 that such a state was stigmatized, although her data do not necessarily support that idea. See "Voluntary Childlessness: A Review of Issues and Evidence," *Marriage and Family Review* 2 (summer 1979), esp. 11–14.

7. "Make Love, Not Babies," 111.

8. For NON membership, see, e.g., Margaret Fisk, ed., *Encyclopedia of Associations*, 10th ed. (Detroit: Gale Research, 1976), 663; Nancy Yakes and Denise Akey, eds., *Encyclopedia of Associations*, 14th ed. (Detroit: Gale Research, 1980), 730; and Denise Akey, ed., *Encyclopedia of Associations*, 16th ed. (Detroit, Gale Research, 1981), 767. In 1976, NON had two thousand members and forty-five local chapters. In an apparent attempt to increase membership, it enlarged its staff from four to eight in 1979 and produced more publications. This having failed, it changed its name to the National Alliance for Optional Parenthood in 1980. By 1982, the staff had dropped to 6; by 1983, to 4. By 1984, the organization was defunct. For examples of coverage, see "Down with Kids," *Time* 100 (July 3,

1972): 35; "Kidding You Not," *Newsweek* 82 (November 5, 1973): 82; "Childless Bliss," 87; and "Those Missing Babies," *Time* 104 (September 1974): 54. The 1970s witnessed, as one scholar phrased it, a decline in "the taste for children." Susan Householder Van Horn, surveying such factors as the kinds of toys produced, the treatment of juvenile offenders in court, and the use of "contemptuous terminology such as 'rug rats' to describe young children," believes that in fact children did become "less valued" in the 1970s (*Women, Work, and Fertility,* 160). At the end of the 1970s, however, there appeared to be a shift. See, e.g., "Wondering If Children Are Necessary," *Time* 113 (March 5, 1979): 42–43.

9. During the 1970s, a large body of scholarship appeared on voluntary childlessness, since some sociologists seemed to believe, as did the popular press, that a major cultural shift was under way. In fact, as we suggest in the Epilogue, the 1970s were something of an antinatalist aberration. By the 1980s, very little scholarship was being done on the voluntarily childless, and once again the infertile became the focus of research. For two overviews of the scholarship on the involuntarily childless, see Veevers, "Voluntary Childlessness," 2–26; and Eleanor D. Macklin, "Nontraditional Family Forms: A Decade of Research," *Journal of Marriage and the Family* (November 1980): 905–21.

10. 1965 was the year of the first-ever national fertility study and hence the beginning of somewhat more accurate statistical analyses of infertility. These figures were extrapolated from the same kinds of polling techniques used for other kinds of surveys. Fertility surveys were repeated three times, in 1976, 1982, and 1988. Because sampling techniques differed and new categories, such as the surgically sterile, were added, the figures are not entirely comparable. For a summary of all the data, See William D. Mosher and William F. Pratt, "Fertility and Infertility in the United States," *Advance Data* 192 (December 4, 1990): 3–5.

11. Elizabeth Connell, M.D., "The Causes—and Cures—of Infertility," *Redbook* 139 (May 1972): 36, 39; Andrea Thompson, "Help for Couples Who Can't Conceive," *McCall's* 104 (August 1977): 72; Virginia Masters and William Johnson, "Advice for Women Who Want to Have a Baby," *Redbook* 144 (March 1975): 70; David Rorvik, "Hope and Help for the Infertile," *Good Housekeeping* 171 (October 1970): 79. Not until the end of the decade did this attitude shift once more.

12. The infertile themselves continued to seek answers. In 1970, after *Good Housekeeping*'s laudatory account of the work of the New York Fertility Research Foundation, in which the author asserted that within the last decade cure rates for infertility had increased by 50 percent, readers besieged the foundation's offices. In a follow-up article three years later, author Jean Libman Block said that "GH had hardly hit the newsstands when the switchboard at the foundation lit up and hundreds of letters poured in. 'The ladies were breaking down the doors—I never saw anything like it,' " said one foundation officer. Rorvik, "Hope and Help," 79; Jean Libman Block, "The Babies They'd Always Wanted," *Good Housekeeping* 177 (August 1973): 36; Susan T. Viguers, *With Child: One Couple's Journey to*

Their Adopted Children (New York: Harcourt Brace Jovanovich, 1986), 22–24, 42; Marsh/Ronner Infertility Survey. See also Barbara Eck Menning, *Infertility: A Guide for Childless Couples* (Englewood Cliffs, N.J.: Prentice-Hall, 1977). Menning is the founder of RESOLVE.

13. Viguers, *With Child*, 2.

14. Even when the husband had a low sperm count, the infertility was often still defined as "her" problem. And it was wives who continued to make the first attempts at medical treatment. One of our respondents, whose husband had an inadequate sperm count, made herself the expert on infertility in the family. Marsh/Ronner Infertility Survey; Robert L. Wolk and Arthur Henley, *The Right to Lie: A Psychological Guide to the Uses of Deceit in Everyday Life* (New York: Wyder, 1970), 172–73. The single article by an infertile man for this period is anonymous:it is untitled but begins, "More than a third . . ." *Good Housekeeping* 176 (January 1973): 73ff.

15. Marsh/Ronner Infertility Survey; Viguers, *With Child*, 27–28.

16. Helen McNamara, "Doctor, Am I Too Old to Have a Baby?" *Good Housekeeping* 184 (January 1977): 77; Bachu, "Fertility of American Women," xi. In a related development, secondary infertility also began to receive more attention. See Sherwin A. Kaufman, M.D., "The Mystery of Second-Child Sterility," *Parents* 47 (February 1972): 48–49. On the cultural dimensions of amniocentesis and genetic screening, see Rayna Rapp, "Communicating about the New Technologies," in Judith Rodin and Aila Collins, eds., *Women and New Reproductive Technologies: Medical, Psychosocial, Legal, and Ethical Dilemmas* (Hillsdale, N.J.: Erlbaum, 1991), 135–52.

17. The feminist critique of reproductive technology was in an embryonic stage in the 1970s but has become far more visible since. Two representative works include Renate D. Klein, ed., *Infertility: Women Speak Out about Their Experiences of Reproductive Medicine* (London: Pandora Press, 1989); and Janice Raymond, *Women as Wombs: Reproductive Technology and the Battle over Women's Freedom* (San Francisco: HarperSanFrancisco, 1993).

18. Albert Rosenfeld, "Science, Sex, and Tomorrow's Morality," *Life* 66 (June 13, 1969): 39, 50.

19. Ibid., 52.

20. Shulamith Firestone, *The Dialectic of Sex* (New York: Morrow, 1970), 198–99, 11.

21. Paul Starr, *The Social Transformation of American Medicine* (New York: Basic Books), 391–92.

22. Arthur Herbst, Howard Ulelfelder, and David Poskanzer, "Adenocarcinoma of the Vagina," *NEJM* 284 (April 22, 1971): 878–81; FDA Drug Bulletin, *Diethylstilbestrol Contraindicated in Pregnancy* (November 1971); "FDA Warns Ingestion of DES During Pregnancy May Cause Vaginal Cancer in Offspring Years Later," *BioMedical News* (December 1971): 12; "DES Link to Vaginal Cancer Questioned by California Ob," *Ob.Gyn. News* (August 15, 1972): 1, 29; Edito-

rial, *Journal of the American Medical Association* 218 (December 6, 1971): 1564. By the late 1970s, data indicated that the cancer occurred in from 1 in 1,000 to 1 in 10,000 of the exposed daughters. Adenosis is a proliferation of the glandular tissue of the cervix, extending into the vagina. See Cynthia Cooke, M.D., and Susan Dworkin, *The Ms. Guide to a Woman's Health* (New York: Berkeley Books, 1981), 399–402.

23. Walter W. Williams, "Evaluation of Clomiphene Therapy for Anovulation," *OB/GYN Digest* (December 1970): 31.

24. Dr. Amir Ansari, head of the Department of Reproductive Physiology at New York's St. Luke's Hospital, mentioned the low conception and high miscarriage rates of clomiphene-treated patients, although he suspected that the problem was dosage. "Hormone Inequality Key to Dysmaturity," *Ob/Gyn Observer* (November 1971): 7. For a description of how Clomid works, see Cooke and Dworkin, *Ms. Guide to Health*, 115.

25. *New York Times*, February 25, 1970, 1.

26. *New York Times*, February 26, 1970, 41, 50; see also "Flurry over Fertility," *Medical World News* (March 13, 1970): 130.

27. Robert W. Kistner, *Gynecology: Principles and Practice*, 3d ed. (Chicago: Year Book Medical, 1979): 496–500.

28. John Rock to Juan Z. Zanartu, M.D., September 23, 1969, John Rock Papers, Rare Books and Manuscripts Division, Countway Library of Medicine, Harvard University; Edward Tyler quoted in the *Boston Globe*, June 24, 1971, clipping in Rock Papers.

29. See *Ob.Gyn. News* 3 (August 15, 1968), clipping in Rock Papers.

30. Edward Tyler, a pioneer in sperm freezing, told a reporter for the *Boston Globe* that in most of his recent cases, this was the way he had utilized the frozen sperm. Tyler, *Boston Globe*, June 24, 1971, clipping in Rock Papers. See also "Insemination Success Rate Is 70% with Frozen Semen," *Ob.Gyn. News* 3 (August 15, 1971): 1.

31. *Life* poll in Rosenfeld, cited in n. 18, above; "Poll Yourself: What Do You Think about Test Tube Babies?" *Parents Magazine* 53 (November 1978): 148ff.

32. For physicians' points of view, see editorial (Herbert Horne), "Artificial Insemination, Donor: An Issue of Ethical and Moral Values," *NEJM* 293 (October 23, 1975): 873–74; letters in response, *NEJM* 294 (January 29, 1975): 280–81; editorial (S. J. Behrman), "Artificial Insemination and Public Policy," *NEJM* 300 (March 15, 1979): 619–20; and Martin Curie-Cohen et al., "Current Practice of Artificial Insemination by Donor in the United States," *NEJM* 300 (March 15, 1979): 585–90.

33. James Hefley and Marti Hefley, "Babies in Question," *Today's Health* 48 (August 1970): 56.

34. Emily Patt, "A Pathfinder on Artificial Insemination," *Legal Reference Services Quarterly* 8, 1/2 (1988): 122–30; Behrman, "Artificial Insemination," 620; Curie-Cohen et al., "Current Practice of Artificial Insemination," 588. See also

"Life without Father," *Newsweek* 86 (September 22, 1975): 87; "The Artificial Insemination Option," *McCall's* 102 (August 1975): 36; and "Medical Mailbox," *Saturday Evening Post* 250 (December 1978): 131.

35. Hefley and Hefley, "Babies in Question," 56; Horne, "Artificial Insemination," 874; letter to *NEJM* from Ronald Strickler, David Keller, and James C. Warren, 294 (January 29, 1976): 281.

36. Hefley and Hefley, "Babies in Question," 18.

37. Loretta McLaughlin, *The Pill, John Rock, and the Church* (Boston: Little, Brown, 1982), is the only full-scale biography of John Rock.

38. Quotations from "In Vitro Fertilization," May 12, 1963, typescript, Rock Papers.

39. R. G. Edwards, B. D. Bavister, and P. C. Steptoe, "Early Stages of Fertilization in Vitro of Human Oocytes Matured in Vitro," *Nature* 221 (February 15, 1969): 632–35. See "In Vitro Fertilization of Human Ova and Blastocyst Transfer: An Invitational Symposium," *Journal of Reproductive Medicine* 11 (November 1973): 192–204, esp. 201–2.

40. Leon Kass is quoted in Department of Health, Education and Welfare, Ethics Advisory Board, *Report and Conclusions: HEW Support of Research Involving Human in Vitro Fertilization and Embryo Transfer* (May 4, 1979), report reprinted in Clifford Grobstein, *From Chance to Purpose: An Appraisal of External Human Fertilization* (Reading, Mass.: Addison-Wesley, 1981), quote on 182. See also Leon Kass, "Babies by Means of in Vitro Fertilization: Unethical Experiments on the Unborn?" *NEJM* 285 (November 18, 1971): 1174–79; and Firestone, *Dialectic of Sex,* 11, 198–99.

41. Georgeanna Jones expressed strong feminist views. See her presidential address, "Women—The Impact of Advances in Fertility Control on Their Future—A Presidential Address," *Fertil. Steril.* 22 (June 1971), esp. 347, 349. We do not wish to argue that reproductive technology is in itself either feminist or antifeminist, but it is unfair to target all practitioners of reproductive medicine as people who desire to control women's bodies. On a range of issues—abortion rights and birth control, for example—a number of the gynecologists and specialists in reproductive medicine did not hold the conservative views toward women that had been the hallmark of their gynecological forefathers. It is certainly true that many male gynecologists deserved to be targeted by feminists in the 1970s, as they were repeatedly, for their attitudes toward women; however, there was another gynecological community, represented by men like John Rock and women like Sophia Kleegman, people with progressive views on a spectrum of issues.

42. "Symposium" cited in n. 37 above, 192–94.

43. Jones, "Presidential Address," 348.

44. Firestone, *Dialectic of Sex,* 197.

45. "Test Tube Babies Stir Medical, Moral Issues," *Boston Pilot,* February 6, 1971, clipping in Rock Papers.

46. Nicholas Panagakos, "Life in a Test Tube: Nearer Than You Think," *Boston Herald Traveler,* October 11, 1970, 8.

47. See "Invit: The View from the Glass Oviduct," *Saturday Review* 65 (September 9, 1972): 68; David M. Rorvik, "The Test-Tube Baby Is Coming," *Look* 35 (May 18, 1971): 83–88; and David R. Zimmerman, "Test-Tube Babies: How Soon?" *Ladies Home Journal* 87 (September 1970): 32.

48. See "Test Tube Bereavement," *Newsweek* 92 (July 31, 1978): 70.

49. Grobstein, *From Chance to Purpose,* discusses the ethics board in considerable detail and reprints its entire report.

50. Naomi Pfeffer, *The Stork and the Syringe: A Political History of Reproductive Medicine* (Cambridge, England: Polity Press, 1993), 165. See Ira M. Golditch, "Laparoscopy: Advances and Advantages," *Fertil. Steril.* 22 (May 1971): 306–10.

51. See "Fertilization outside Womb," *Science Digest* 69 (January 1971): 90.

52. See Pfeffer, *Stork and Syringe,* 165; and Robert Edwards, *Life before Birth* (New York: Basic Books, 1989), esp. 1–11.

53. Edwards, *Life before Birth,* 7–8. The popular news sources that we used for this account of Louise Brown's birth are "The Test-Tube Baby," *Newsweek* 92 (July 24, 1978): 76; "The First Test-Tube Baby," *Time* 112 (july 31, 1978): 58; "Louise: Birth of a New Technology," *Science News* 114 (August 5, 1978): 84; "Test-Tube Baby: It's a Girl," *Time* 112 (August 7, 1978): 68; and "All about That Baby," *Newsweek* 92 (August 7, 1978): 66.

54. Indeed, Bevis said shortly after making this explosive comment that he planned to stop doing such research and would have no further comments on the matter. If Bevis was indeed the first, there is no evidence other than his announcement. See "Test-Tube Babies: Now a Reality?" *Science News* (July 20, 1974): 106; "The Baby Maker," *Time* 104 (July 30, 1974): 58; "Test Tube Babies: Reaction Sets In," *Science News* 106 (July 27, 1974): 53; and "Test-Tube Babies?" *Newsweek* 84 (July 29, 1974): 70.

55. See "Test-tube Bereavement," 70; Doris Del Zio as told to Suzanne Wilding, "I Was Cheated of My Test-Tube Baby," *Good Housekeeping* 188 (March 1979): 202; and "Detour on the Road to Brave New World," *Science* 210 (August 4, 1978): 424–25.

56. See *Newsweek,* "Test-tube Baby," 76.

57. See "It's a Girl," 68.

58. See *People* 10 (August 1, 1978): 30.

59. See "A Young Couple Await Their Test-Tube Baby," *Ebony* 34 (November 1978): 33–39.

60. Grobstein, *From Chance to Purpose,* 114.

61. See "Hearings Asked on Va. Clinic for Test-Tube Babies," *Washington Post,* January 15, 1980, B2; see also February 2, 1980, A3, and May 17, 1980, A2; Richard Cohen, "Test-Tube Babies: Why Add to a Surplus?" *Washington*

Post, February 3, 1980, B1; Ellen Goodman, "The Baby Louise Clinic," *Washington Post,* January 15, 1980, A15; and editorial, *Washington Post,* January 19, 1980, A14.

62. "Nation's First 'Test-Tube' Baby Due within Days in Program at Norfolk," *Washington Post,* December 25, 1981, A6-A7; *New York Times,* December 29, 1981, 1, C1.

63. See, for example, "Government Urged to Actively Support Test Tube Baby Research," *Washington Post,* January 4, 1982, A3; "U.S. Scientist Barred from Speaking at Workshop," *Washington Post,* September 14, 1982, C3; and "Norfolk Team in Forefront of Test-Tube Baby Boom," *Washington Post,* September 13. 1982, A2. We discuss acceptance of IVF in the Epilogue.

Epilogue. The Past in the Present

1. See "Woman, 59, Gives Birth to Twins," *Washington Post,* December 28, 1993, A8; Andrea Kott, "Dr. Mark V. Sauer Helps 55–Year-Old Have Babies," *Medical Tribune* (February 24, 1994), 15; Nancy Wartik, "Making Babies," *Los Angeles Times Magazine* (March 6, 1994): 18–21ff.; Gina Kolata, "Young Women Offer to Sell Their Eggs to Infertile Couples," *New York Times,* November 10, 1991, 1, 30; and Ellen Hopkins, "Tales from the Baby Factory," *New York Times Magazine* (March 15, 1992): 40–41ff.

2. Surrogate motherhood is not an infertility treatment but a means by which a man can have a biological child, either if his female partner is infertile, or, in some cases, if he does not have a female partner. Because it is a recent phenomenon without the same kinds of historical precedent as the other issues discussed in this book, we believe that it would be impossible for us to do justice to this complex subject. Two of the many works that do deal with issues of surrogacy are Audrey Wolfson Latourette, "The Surrogate Mother Contract: In the Best Interests of Society?" *University of Richmond Law Review* 25 (fall 1990): 53–92; and Martha A. Field, *Surrogate Motherhood: The Legal and Human Issues,* expanded ed. (Cambridge: Harvard University Press, 1990).

3. Susan Lang, *Women without Children: The Reasons, the Rewards, the Regrets* (New York: Pharos Books, 1991), 125; Deborah Valentine, ed., *Infertility and Adoption: A Guide for Social Work Practice* (New York: Haworth Press, 1988), 2. Soon after we began working on this book, the historian of us took a course for general obstetrician/gynecologists called "Managing the Infertile Couple," given under the auspices of the American College of Obstetricians and Gynecologists. The lecturers were several of this country's leading infertility experts, who were convinced that infertility was increasing at a significant rate.

4. Primary infertility is the term used for those couples who have never been able to conceive. Until the last thirty years, figures on secondary infertility, or what used to be known as "one-child sterility," were even more elusive.

5. It is probably the higher number of women reporting primary infertility—

500,000 in the mid-1960s versus 1,000,000 in the 1980s—that has caused so much alarm. But we must also keep in mind that this later generation is more than 22 million larger than the earlier one. Data from Office of Technology Assessment, U.S. Congress, *Infertility: Medical and Social Choices* (Washington, D.C.: Government Printing Office, 1988), 50–52.

6. William D. Mosher and William F. Pratt, "Fertility and Infertility in the United States," *Advance Data* (December 4, 1990): 3–5. For a very good discussion of infertility statistics, see Arthur L. Griel, *Not Yet Pregnant: Infertile Couples in Contemporary America* (New Brunswick: Rutgers University Press, 1991), 27–28; also John A. Robertson, *Children of Choice* (Princeton: Princeton University Press, 1994), 225–27.

7. Lang, *Women without Children*, 43; see also Griel, *Not Yet Pregnant*, 33. Margarete Sandelowski has written the most detailed analysis of the way in which infertility is seen as a result of certain kinds of behavior. Although we agree with her in terms of the present attitude toward infertility, we do not agree, as will become clear below, that such an attitude has consistently informed views of the causes of infertility. Margarete J. Sandelowski, "Failures of Volition: Female Agency and Infertility in Historical Perspective," *Signs* 15 (spring 1990): 475–99.

8. Federation CECOS, D. Schwartz, and M. J. Mayaux, "Female Fecundity as a Function of Age: Results of Artificial Insemination in 2193 Nulliparous Women with Azoospermic Husbands," *NEJM* 306 (February 18, 1982): 404–6. The earlier study had been conducted in the 1950s by Allen Guttmacher. Women under twenty-five had a median "conception time" of two months to their first pregnancy; women between the ages of thirty-five and forty-four had a median time to conception of 3.8 months.

9. Alan H. DeCherney and Gertrud Berkowitz, "Female Fecundity and Age," editorial, ibid., 424–26.

10. *Infertility: Medical and Social Choices,* 50–52; Sandelowski, "Failures of Volition," 475–77.

11. See Chapter 6. Most gynecologists who specialized in infertility in the postwar period did, however, believe that stress could affect ovulation, but that is an entirely different matter.

12. Anne Taylor Fleming, *Motherhood Deferred* (New York: Putnam, 1994) held herself responsible for an infertility problem that was brought on because she contracted a sexually transmitted disease from her husband. But because it never affected his sperm count, *she* was the one with the problem.

13. Edith Brickman and John Beckwith, Letter to the Editor, *NEJM* 307 (August 5, 1983): 373.

14. Donors, typically young women in their early twenties, earn between $1,500 and $2,000 each time they "donate." Although some advocates of this procedure have compared egg donation to sperm donation, the two processes are not equivalent. Egg donors take fertility drugs to increase the number of eggs they produce, and the process of removing the ova requires an invasive procedure.

Wartik, "Making Babies," 18–21ff., quotation on 21; Kolata, "Young Women Offer," 30.

15. Wartik, "Making Babies," 21; "Result of New Fertilization Method Due in October," *Washington Post*, August 23, 1993.

16. We remind the nonmedical reader that in some ways these figures are misleading, since some conditions that cause infertility are much more easily remedied than others. Microsurgical techniques have vastly increased the rates of pregnancy among women with certain kinds of tubal problems. New treatments for endometriosis have emerged that have arrested the disease at an earlier stage. And drugs such as Clomid and Pergonal are very effective. However, such conditions as premature ovarian failure, azoospermia, or severe tubal blockages cannot be treated (although they can sometimes be circumvented by donor eggs, donor insemination, and in vitro fertilization). In short, how successful one's treatment can be depends on the diagnosis.

17. There are some centers that include in their pregnancy rates what is called a "chemical pregnancy," which simply means that the hormone levels are elevated for a few days. Wartik, "Making Babies," 21; Hopkins, "Tales from the Baby Factory," 41.

18. Susan Lang has described the "baby boomlet" of the 1980s, as births had climbed by 1990 to an average of 2 births per woman of childbearing age, up from 1.7 in 1976. Lang, *Women without Children*, 48.

19. There is an enormous literature on the experience of infertility. One of the best of the memoirs is Susan T. Viguers, *With Child: One Couple's Journey to Their Adopted Children* (New York: Harcourt Brace Jovanovich, 1986). For representative examples of scholarly studies, see Aline P. Zoldbrod, *Men, Women, and Infertility* (New York: Lexington Books, 1993); Griel, *Not Yet Pregnant;* and Margarete Sandelowski, *With Child in Mind* (Philadelphia: University of Pennsylvania Press, 1993). Several British studies confirm the American experience; see, e.g., James Monach, *Childless, No Choice: The Experience of Involuntary Childlessness* (New York: Routledge, 1993); also Robert Snowden et al., *Artificial Reproduction: A Social Investigation* (London: Allen and Unwin, 1983).

20. Nancy Felipe Russo, "Overview: Sex Roles, Fertility, and the Motherhood Mandate," *Psychology of Women Quarterly* 4 (fall 1979): 7–9; Sandelowski, *With Child in Mind*, 75; Griel, *Not Yet Pregnant*, 56–57.

21. Zoldbrod, *Men, Women, and Infertility*, 12, 111. She suggests that women's greater emotional investment may be, at least in part, because men are expected to be less expressive, but in fact most of her evidence supports the fact that they are truly less affected. Griel, *Not Yet Pregnant*, 77; Monach, *Childlessness, No Choice*, 117.

22. Renate D. Klein, ed., *Infertility: Women Speak Out about Their Experiences of Reproductive Medicine* (Cambridge, England: Pandora Press, 1989), cover quote; Janice Raymond, *Women as Wombs: Reproductive Technology and*

the Battle over Women's Freedom (San Francisco: HarperSanFrancisco, 1993), viii.

23. One of the clearest summaries of this point of view is Raymond, *Women as Wombs,* esp. vii–xxxiii.

24. See Hopkins, "Tales from the Baby Factory," 80.

25. Griel, *Not Yet Pregnant,* 76–77; Zoldbrod, *Men, Women, and Infertility,* 111; Fleming, *Motherhood Deferred.*

26. Sandelowski, *With Child in Mind,* esp. chap. 4; quotation on 39.

27. We were surprised to discover the extent to which infertility services were available in northeastern urban voluntary hospitals for much of the twentieth century, and from Planned Parenthood in the post–World War II era. While we are not arguing that the poor everywhere had access to such services—the rural and segregated South comes immediately to mind—nevertheless, in urban America infertility services were more widely available to the poor forty years ago than they are now.

28. Hopkins, "Tales from the Baby Factory."

29. Wartik, "Making Babies," 42.

Index

Abell, Mrs. L. H. G., 32
Aberle, Sophie, 139–40
abortion: and infertility, 45, 80, 153;
  medical opposition to, 84; in nineteenth century, 45, 80; opposition to,
  231; struggle over rights to, 218
Adams, Clover (Marian Hooper),
  99–100
Adams, Henry, 99–100
Addison's disease, 134
adoption: "black market" and, 127, 169;
  in colonial era, 17–20; laws governing,
  106, 108; and pregnancy, 168–69,
  204–6; "putting out," 19; rates of,
  169, 204; reluctance toward, 107–8; as
  response to childlessness, 35–37, 38,
  105–7, 110–11, 168–69, 204–5, 210,
  229; "sentimental," 110, 125–27; in
  twentieth century, 125–27, 168–69,
  204–6, 210
adrenal glands, 134

African Americans: adoption and, 107;
  childlessness among, 92–93, 117, 143;
  donor insemination and, 203; fertility
  of, 77, 92, 185–86; infertility and,
  92–93, 103–4, 187–88; in vitro fertilization and, 238–39; medical experimentation and, 50–51
age, and infertility, 208, 243–44, 246–48
Alcott, William, 31
Allen, Edgar, 140
Allen, Gracie, 168, 170
amenorrhea, 16. *See also* menstruation:
  retention of, suppression of; anovulation
American Association of Obstetricians
  and Gynecologists, 80–81
American Fertility Society, 227, 231,
  239. *See also* American Society for Reproductive Medicine; American Society
  for the Study of Sterility
American Gynecological Society, 80, 81;
  woman members, 88

Library of Congress Cataloging-in-Publication Data

Marsh, Margaret.
  The empty cradle : infertility in America from Colonial times to the present / Margaret Marsh and Wanda Ronner.
       p.   cm. — (The Henry E. Sigerist series in the history of medicine)
  Includes bibliographical references and index.
  ISBN 0-8018-5228-5 (hc : alk. paper)
    1. Infertility—United States—History.   I. Ronner, Wanda.   II. Title.   III. Series.
[DNLM: 1. Infertility—therapy.   2. Reproduction Techniques—trends.   3. History of Medicine, 18th Cents.   WP 570 M363e 1996]
RC889.M368   1996
616.6'92'00973—dc20
DNLM/DLC
for Library of Congress   95-35525
                                                                                                        CIP